LANGE REVIEW™

COMPUTED TOMOGRAPHY EXAMINATION

Sharlene M. Snowdon, MSEd, RT(R)(CT)(M)
(Former) Director of the Computed Tomography Internship Program
Radiology Technology Education
Penn Medicine at the Hospital of the University of Pennsylvania
Philadelphia, Pennsylvania

Mc
Graw
Hill
Education

New York   Chicago   San Francisco   Athens   London   Madrid
Mexico City   Milan   New Delhi   Singapore   Sydney   Toronto

Lange Review™: Computed Tomography Examination

1 2 3 4 5 6 7 8 9   ROV   21 20 19 18 17 16

ISBN 978-0-07-184386-7
MHID 0-07-184386-8

Notice

Medicine is an ever-changing science. As new research and clinical experience broaden our knowledge, changes in treatment and drug therapy are required. The author and the publisher of this work have checked with sources believed to be reliable in their efforts to provide information that is complete and generally in accord with the standards accepted at the time of publication. However, in view of the possibility of human error or changes in medical sciences, neither the author nor the publisher nor any other party who has been involved in the preparation or publication of this work warrants that the information contained herein is in every respect accurate or complete, and they disclaim all responsibility for any errors or omissions or for the results obtained from use of the information contained in this work. Readers are encouraged to confirm the information contained herein with other sources. For example and in particular, readers are advised to check the product information sheet included in the package of each drug they plan to administer to be certain that the information contained in this work is accurate and that changes have not been made in the recommended dose or in the contraindications for administration. This recommendation is of particular importance in connection with new or infrequently used drugs.

This book was set in Minion Pro by Aptara®, Inc.
The editors were Catherine A. Johnson and Peter J. Boyle.
The production supervisor was Richard Ruzycka.
Project management was provided by Amit Kashyap, Aptara, Inc.

Library of Congress Cataloging-in-Publication Data

Names: Snowdon, Sharlene M., author.
Title: Lange review : computed tomography examination / Sharlene M. Snowdon.
Other titles: Computed tomography examination
Description: New York : McGraw-Hill Education, [2016] | Includes
    bibliographical references and index.
Identifiers: LCCN 2016014064| ISBN 9780071843867 (pbk.) | ISBN 0071843868
    (pbk.)
Subjects: | MESH: Tomography, X-Ray Computed | Examination Questions
Classification: LCC RC78.7.T6 | NLM WN 18.2 | DDC 616.07/5722—dc23 LC record
available at http://lccn.loc.gov/2016014064

McGraw-Hill Education books are available at special quantity discounts to use as premiums and sales promotions, or for use in corporate training programs. To contact a representative, please visit the Contact Us pages at www.mhprofessional.com.

To my husband, Greg whose trust, love, and support helped me achieve my greatest dreams.
Without you my life would not be complete.
And to my grandchildren, Kayleigh and Zachary, your growth provides a constant source of joy and pride.

Contents

To access your complimentary online practice exams, visit www.MHEAlliedHealth.com.

Acknowledgments

The inspiration for this review book came to me from the many interns I had the pleasure of teaching. Their hunger for knowledge and to become certified CT technologists made teaching and researching most enjoyable.

The material in this book was gathered from numerous authors with expertise in patient care, cross-sectional anatomy and physiology, and medical physics. Without their intense research, this book could not be possible.

Many thanks to Elsevier, Lippincott Williams & Wilkins, and McGraw-Hill for granting permission to reproduce the medical images seen throughout this book.

I have confidence these images will provide a more in-depth explanation of the text and greater confidence when reviewing images.

A special thanks goes to my reviewers for taking time out of their busy personal life and work schedule to review this book's content for correctness and integrity.

I am especially grateful for the staff of McGraw-Hill for having the confidence in me to produce a review text that will help enhance the knowledge and skills of technologist preparing for their CT certification examination.

Introduction

ARRT CERTIFICATION AND ELIGIBILITY REQUIREMENTS

The structure of the computed tomography (CT) examination is to assess the knowledge and cognitive skills fundamental to the duties typically required of technologists who perform CT. Technologists who are about to take on the rewarding challenge of successfully completing the post-primary examination in CT are required to meet the professional requirements specified in the American Registry of Radiologic Technologists (ARRT) rules and regulations, along with documentation of structured education and clinical experiences. The ARRT strives to promote high standards of patient care and a high standard of ethics among its registered technologists and among candidates for certification and registration. All candidates must comply with the rules of ethics contained in the ARRT Standards of Ethics, found on the ARRT website: *The American Registry of Radiologic_Technologists Ethics Requirements for Computed Tomography (CT) Certification and Registration* (https://www.arrt.org/certification/computed-tomography).

Candidates for post-primary certification and registration in CT must be certified and registered by the ARRT in one of the following primary categories:

- Radiography
- Nuclear medicine
- Radiation therapy

It is imperative for you to uphold certification and registration in your primary discipline at all times to be eligible for certification and registration in the CT post-primary category. By dropping your certification and registration of your primary discipline between applying for and taking your examination, your eligibility is revoked. If this were to occur, your examination fees would be sacrificed, and your examination results would be canceled. This cancellation counts as one attempt and is not available for reporting. The maximum number of examination attempts is three and they must be completed within a 3-year period from the time of your initial examination window start date (e. g., if your first attempt was on January 01, 2016, your third attempt has to be completed by December 31, 2019). If you have not successfully passed on the third attempt, you will then be required to perform another set of clinical experiences starting after December 31, 2019 and these experiences must follow any new or updated requirements.

STRUCTURED EDUCATION

The CT technologist must document a total of 16 hours of structured education earned within the 24-month period immediately preceding submission of an application. The educational undertakings must be distributed among the current ARRT content specifications and at least 1 hour of structured education must be related to each of the following content areas:

- Patient care
- Safety
- Imaging procedures
- Physics and instrumentation

Your remaining 12 hours can be distributed among the above four categories in any manner as long as the educational curriculums meet the same standards as any CE activity, that is, the course or lecture must be approved by a Recognized Continuing Education Evaluation Mechanism (RCEEM or RCEEM+, (https://www.arrt.org/Registration/RCEEMs) or meet the definition of an approved academic course. An approved academic course is a formal course of study that is pertinent to the radiologic sciences and/or an associated patient care course, which is offered by a post-secondary educational accredited institution that is recognized by ARRT. Any activity that is only approved by a state licensing agency will not fulfil these requirements.

COMPUTED TOMOGRAPHY CONTENT SPECIFICATIONS

The following information describes the major content categories covered on the examination, and indicates the number of test questions in each category along with a detailed list of the specific topics addressed in each category. The CT examination consists of 165 scored questions and 20 embedded pilot unscored questions. The purpose of the pilot questions is to evaluate them for appropriateness for future examinations. These questions appear just like any other question on the test, but the ARRT allows you extra time for completion and these questions do not affect your score in a positive or negative manner. You will be asked approximately 36 questions covering Patient Care and Safety, 75 questions on Imaging Procedures (which consist of anatomical locations, pathology, and imaging protocols) and 54 questions on Physics and Instrumentation. For a detailed breakdown of each category, visit the ARRT website *The American Registry of Radiologic Technologists Content Specifications* (https://www.arrt.org/content-specifications).

CLINICAL EXPERIENCE REQUIREMENTS

Technologist applying to take the CT post-primary examination must document clinical performance of a minimum of 125 repetitions of procedures outlined by the ARRT. Your clinical experiences obligation is to be completed and documented within a 24-month timeframe prior to your application. The diagnostic quality studies must be documented, verified, and submitted when complete by way of the online tool accessed through your *My ARRT info* account at the *American Registry of Radiologic Technologist* website: www.arrt.org. The verification process must be performed by a registered technologist, supervisor, or physician. To view the specified clinical experience requirements, visit the ARRT website *American Registry of Radiologic Technologist Clinical Experience Requirements* (https://www.arrt.org/certification/computed-tomography).

STUDYING TIPS AND TEST-TAKING STRATEGIES

The first piece of advice I can give you is to start looking at the material at least 6 months or longer prior to taking the examination—in other words do not procrastinate.

Procrastination has many side effects, with the major one being stress, and the other being your inability to focus. You can avoid procrastination by organizing your time and spacing out your studying. Probably, most of you studying for this examination are full-time technologists; therefore, finding the perfect time to study may be your number one task. Study on a specific schedule to retain the material in your long-term memory. You should find a comfortable and quiet place, one with little distractions. It is best to eat something prior to studying to give your body energy. Stay away from too much sugar and caffeine (eliminates your highs and lows). If you are one that needs background noise in order to study, listen to relaxing music, such as classical or jazz and keep the volume low. Make sure all your study material is in front of you that way you are not interrupting your train of thought. It is best to review your lecture or course material as soon as possible so that those concepts stay fresh in your mind and if you have any questions, you can ask them at your next class or contact the lecturer for better clarification. Learn the general theories first and make sure you understand them before tackling the detailed material, do not try to memorize the material. Memorization limits your critical thinking skills, which are so important when it comes to analyzing the board questions. Take a 5-minute break per hour, because you retain more at the beginning and end of a session then in the middle and it also allows your brain to relax. Most individuals have a particular subject they find difficult. Tie that subject with a subject you find easier or like better so you don't lose interest or become bored with that subject. My last piece of advice is to keep a positive attitude. It is better and easier to study when you are relaxed than when you are stressed out.

DAY OF THE EXAMINATION

It is best to choose your testing time wisely. If you are a morning person, arrange your examination time during the mid-morning hours. On the other hand, if the morning hours are not your cup of tea, elect to take your test mid-afternoon. No matter what time you selected, make sure you eat something even if it is a light meal, to give your body and brain energy. I always advised my students not to study the day before the examination, try to do something fun and relaxing, but avoid late-night parties. Make sure you get a good night sleep, at least 7 hours, so you don't feel groggy or fall asleep during the examination. If you are unsure of the location of the testing center, take a dry run and estimate how long it will take to get there, adding extra time for morning or afternoon traffic. Arrive at the testing center at least 20 to 30 minutes prior to your examination time. This will give you time to relax, increase your confidence, and narrow your focus. You will be given a short introduction, which includes an ethics disclaimer, and test instructions. Listen to these instructions carefully in order to decrease your test-taking anxiety. Decide how you are going to use your allocated testing time, pacing yourself accordingly, and don't overthink a particular question. Complete the questions you are familiar with first and flag the questions you may need more time on and go back to them later. This will increase your confidence and make completing the examination easier.

MULTIPLE CHOICE AND MULTIPLE RESPONSE APPROACHES

All students, from elementary school through college, feel these standardized examination tests are meant to trick you, but in reality, they are an intended tool to utilize your critical thinking skills. Approach the questions with a positive attitude and use deductive reasoning. Read each question in its entirety making sure you understand what the question is asking before glancing at the options given. Answer the question in your head and then read the question again inserting your answer to determine if your thought process is the correct choice. If your answer is there choose that option and move on. This strategy will avert you from talking yourself out of the correct answer. If you are not sure of the answer, or your answer was not one of the choices, eliminate choices you know are absolutely incorrect before selecting the answer you believe is correct. If you find two answers to be correct, choose the **best** answer, determining this by inserting the answer in a true/false statement. Convert the question into a statement with each of the possible answers, and select one that is true. When a word like not, never, or none is in the stem of the question, the correct answer must be a fact or absolute. When the question states **"which of the following is false,"** make sure you look for the negative answer. In many cases the correct answer contains more information than the other possibilities. For multiple response questions, look for answer options that are similar and don't be sucked in to that since it states multiple response; more than one option should be chosen. Review all four options, pick what makes sense; contradictory choices are usually incorrect. If you have a good reason to change your answer, change it, otherwise leave it alone.

You probably have noticed I used the word confidence several times. Confidence is the key to a successful result. Remember you have attended hours of classes or lectures; you have studied the material presented and have incorporated your learning material into your clinical experience; so have faith in yourself that you are ready to undertake this challenging post-primary board examination.

Good Luck!!!!

Master Bibliography

ACR Committee on Drug and Contrast Media. *ACR Manual on Contrast Media, Version 9.* http://www.acr.org/quality-safety/resources/contrast-manual. Published 2013.

ACR. *ACR Practice Parameter for Performing and Interpreting Diagnostic Computed Tomography (CT).* http://www.acr.org/quality-safety/resources/contrast-manual. Res. 35–2011, Amended 2014 (Res. 39). Published 2014.

Adler AM, Carlton RR. *Introduction to Radiologic Sciences and Patient Care.* 5th ed. St. Louis, MO: Saunders Elsevier; 2012.

BD Medical. *BD Angiocath™ Autoguard™ Shielded IV Catheters. Shielded IV catheters.* http://bd.com/infusion/pdfs/D13779.pdf. Published 2004–2015. Updated 2015. Retrieved July 2015.

Boas EF, Fleischmann D. CT artifacts: causes and reduction techniques. *Imaging Med.* 2012;4(2):229–240. doi:10.2217/iim.12.13.

CDC. *Center for Disease Control and Prevention Saving Lives, Protecting People.* Page maintained by: Office of the Associate Director for Communication, Digital Media Branch, Division of Public Affairs. http://www.cdc.gov/Features/HandWashing/. Updated December 2013. Retrieved August 2015.

Davis M, Elizabeth RE, Matthew M. *The Relaxation & Stress Reduction Workbook.* 5th ed. Oakland, CA: Publishers Group West; 2000.

Ehrlich RA, Coakes DM. *Patient Care in Radiology: With an Introduction to Medical Imaging.* 8th ed. St. Louis, MO: Mosby Elsevier; 2013.

Fadem SZ, Rosenthal B; National Kidney Foundation. *GFR Calculators: Serum Creatinine and Cystatin C.* http://nephron.org/cgi-bin/MDRD_GFR/cgi. Published 2009. Updated 2013. Retrieved July 2015.

Fadem SZ, Rosenthal B; National Kidney Foundation. *Pediatric Calculators: CKiD Schwartz and Bedside Schwartz.* http://www.kidney.org/professionals/kdoqi/gfr_calculatorPed. Published 2000–2015. Updated February 2015. Retrieved July 2015.

Fishman E. *CTisus. John Hopkins University, Department of Radiology.* http://www.ctisus.com/. Updated 2015. Retrieved April 2015.

Foley TA, Mankad SV, Anavekar S, et al; European Cardiology. *Measuring Left Ventricle Ejection Fraction Techniques and Potential Pitfalls.* http://www.radcliffecardiology.com/articles/measuring-left-ventricular-ejection-fraction-techniques-and-potential-pitfalls. Summer 2012. Retrieved March 2015.

Gray ML, Ailinani JM. *CT and MRI Pathology: A Pocket Atlas.* 3rd ed. New York, NY: McGraw-Hill; 2012.

Gurley LT, Callaway WJ. *Introduction to Radiologic Technology.* 6th ed. ST. Louis, MO: Mosby Elsevier; 2011

Hale SE; Integrated Science Support, Inc. *Dose Reduction and Artifacts in CT.* http://issphysics.com/. Published 2013. Retrieved April 2015.

Honours LL. Model-based iterative reconstruction: a promising algorithm for today's computed tomography imaging. *J Med Imaging Radiat Sci.* 2014;45(2):131–136.

Indrajit IK, Sivasankar R, D'Souza J, et al. Pressure injectors for radiologists: a review and what is new. *Indian J Radiol Imaging.* 2015;25(1):1–10.

Kalendar WA. *Computed Tomography: Fundamentals System Technology, Image Quality, and Applications.* 3rd ed. Erlangen, Germany: Publicis; 2011.

Keller DM; Medscape. *Iodinated Contrast Media Raises Risk for Thyroid Dysfunction.* http://www.medscape.com/viewarticle/757345. Published January 2012. Retrieved July 2015.

Kelley LL, Petersen CM. *Sectional Anatomy for Imaging Professionals.* 3rd ed. ST. Louis, MO: Mosby Elsevier; 2013.

Madden ME. *Introduction to Sectional Anatomy.* 3rd ed. Philadelphia, PA: Wolters Kluwer, Lippincott Williams & Wilkins; 2013.

Madden ME. *Introduction to Sectional Anatomy: Workbook and Board Review Guide*. 3rd ed. Philadelphia, PA: Wolters Kluwer, Lippincott Williams & Wilkins; 2013.

Mayo Clinic Staff; Mayo Clinic. *Mayo Foundation for Medical Education and Research Blood Urea Nitrogen (BUN) Test*. http://www.mayoclinic.org/tests-procedures/blood-urea-nitrogen/basics/definition/prc-20020239. Published 1998. Updated 2014. Retrieved July 2015.

Mayo-Smith WW, Hara AK, Mahesh M, et al. How I do it: managing radiation dose in CT. *Radiology*. 2014;273(3): 657–672.

MedRad; Stellant D. *Description Guide*. 2014.

Musculoskeletal Imaging and Intervention Section; University of Wisconsin Imaging Protocols. *Imaging Protocols & Scanning Parameters*. https://www.radiology. wisc.edu/sections/msk/protocols.php. Updated May 2011. Retrieved March 2015.

National Institute of Health (NIH). National Heart, Lung, and Blood Institute. *What Does a Coronary Calcium Scan Show?* http://www.nhlbi.nih.gov/health/health-topics/topics/cscan/show. Published 2012. Retrieved March 2015.

Nayab N; Bright Hub Project Management. *How Are You Communicating to Your Team?* http://www.brighthubpm. com/methods-strategies/. Published October 2014. Retrieved July 2015.

Pozgar GD. *Legal Aspects of Health Care Administration*. 11th ed. Sudbury, MA: Jones and Bartlett; 2011.

Prokop M, Galanski M. *Computed Tomography of the Body: Spiral and Multislice*. Stuttgart, NY; Thieme; 2003.

Righini M, Van ES, Den Exter PL. Age-adjusted D-dimer cutoff levels to rule out pulmonary embolism. *JAMA*. 2014;311(11):1117–1124.

Romans LE. *Computed Tomography for Technologists: A Comprehensive Text*. Baltimore, MD: Wolters Kluwer, Lippincott Williams & Wilkins; 2011

Saia DA. *Radiology PREP*. 9th ed. New York, NY: McGraw-Hill; 2012.

Seeram E. *Computed Tomography: Physical Principles, Clinical Applications, and Quality Control*. 3rd ed. St. Louis, MO: Saunders Elsevier; 2009.

Sprawls P; Sprawls Global Collaborative Teaching Network. *The Sprawls Resources for Study, Review, Reference and Teaching*. http://www.sprawls.org/resources/. Published 2014. Retrieved March 2015.

The American Registry of Radiologic Technologists. *Clinical Experience Requirements*. https://www.arrt. org/certification/computed-tomography. Published 2015.

The American Registry of Radiologic Technologists. *Content Specifications*. https://www.arrt.org/content-specifications. Published 2015.

The American Registry of Radiologic Technologists. *Ethics Requirements for Computed Tomography (CT) Certification and Registration*. https://www.arrt.org/certification/computed-tomography. Published 2015.

The American Registry of Radiologic Technologists. *Recognized Continuing Education Evaluation Mechanism (RCEEM or RCEEM+)*. https://www.arrt.org/Registration/RCEEMs. Published 2015.

Webb WR, Brant WE, Major NM. *Fundamentals of Body CT*. 3rd ed. St. Louis, MO: Saunders Elsevier; 2006.

Weir J, Abrahams PH, Spratt JD, et al. *Imaging Atlas of Human Anatomy*. 4th ed. ST. Louis, MO: Mosby Elsevier; 2011.

Woolfolk A. *Educational Psychology*. 10th ed. Boston, MA: Pearson; 2007.

CHAPTER 1

Patient Care and Safety

Patient care is fundamental to all medical procedures. A patient's uneasiness may be overlooked due to the complexity of the imaging technology and the pressure to increase the number of studies performed. We must remember the patient is our primary concern and we as technologists must concentrate on that individual patient and give them the best care possible. Care is identified as services rendered by members of the health professions for the benefit of a patient. It is imperative to establish an initial rapport with the patients in order to put them at ease and make the computed tomography (CT) procedure less imitating. It is the technologists' responsibility to ensure patients leave the institution feeling respected and cared for as individuals. Our first step in developing this specific care is in communication.

COMMUNICATION

Communication is defined by the National Joint Committee for the Communicative Needs of Persons with Severe Disabilities as "any act by which one person gives to or receives from a person information about that person's needs, desires, perceptions, knowledge, or affective states". Communication may be intentional or unintentional, may involve conventional or unconventional signals, may take linguistic or nonlinguistic forms, and may occur through spoken or other modes." As stated in the definition there are two forms of communication, verbal and nonverbal.

Verbal Communication

Verbal communication is the most effective way of explaining intangible concepts, as problem areas can be readily addressed and explained. Clear well-defined speech habits are always essential, regardless of the communication circumstance. It is important to speak face to face with your patients, so that they can see your eyes and expressions.

Take notice of your listeners' response and modify your approach if they seem confused or anxious. The key to good verbal communication is to have your patients believe they have your full attention and concern.

Nonverbal Communication

Nonverbal communication is any kind of communication not involving words. Approximately 90% of our communication comes from nonverbal cues. A person's verbal communication may convey one meaning while their vocal intonation and body language communicates something totally different. This mixed communication causes the listener to choose between the verbal and nonverbal message and most often they choose the latter creating tension and distrust. Nonverbal communication can be in the form of facial expressions, eye contact, posture, and gestures, but while these are important elements of nonverbal communication, they are not the only ones. Nonverbal communication can be incorporated in a person's dress. A patient will give more respect to a technologist whose appearance is simple and neat. The setting where communication takes place also lends a meaning to words apart from their literal definition. When asking patients' confidential questions, it should be performed in a private area out of earshot of other individuals. The use of touching as an element of communication is called haptic communication, and its meanings are very culture-dependent. A positive touch can be reassuring giving the individual a sense of trust and caring, but must be used cautiously. In some societies, this might be a perplexing act or an embarrassing invasion of personal space. A technologist must be fully aware of the use of the eyes as an element of nonverbal communication. Direct eye contact is usually looked upon as an expression of interest and/or concern, but the intention may not be understood in all cultures. Nonverbal communication is by far the largest form of communication transferred by individuals, so it is critical for technologists to think before communicating with patients and put aside any mental distress they are experiencing. Remember that a patient is our main concern and should be treated as if he/she were a family member.

PATIENT PREPARATION

Consent

Consent stems from the ethical and legal right of the patient and is a voluntary agreement by a person who possesses appropriate mental capacity to make an intelligent choice concerning his/her medical treatment. Medical personnel determine a patient's decision-making capacity by assessing the individual's ability to:

- understand the risks, benefits, and alternatives of a proposed test or procedure.
- evaluate the information provided by the physician.
- express his/her treatment options/plan.
- voluntarily make decisions regarding his/her treatment plan without undue influence by family, friends, or medical personnel.

Consent must be obtained from the patient or, in the case of a patient being deemed incompetent, from a person authorized to consent on the patient's behalf before any procedure can be performed. The three types of consent appropriate for most CT examinations include simple expressed, informed consent, and implied consent.

Simple Expressed Consent

Simple expressed consent is the process of obtaining a patient's permission to perform a procedure and is generally utilized for noninvasive procedures. It is as straightforward as explaining the procedure to the patients and then asking them whether they agree to have the examination. A technologist should never assume consent.

Informed Consent

Informed consent is required for CT examinations that have a more invasive nature such as biopsies, aspirations, drainages, radiofrequency ablations, and cryotherapy ablations. This is a written consent providing visible proof of a patient's wishes. This consent must be procured by the radiologist performing or involved in the procedure. The informed consent form must possess the following elements:

- The nature of the patient's illness or injury
- The procedure or treatment consented to

- The purpose of the proposed treatment
- The risk and probable consequences of the proposed treatment
- The probability that the proposed treatment will be successful
- Any alternative methods of treatment and their associated risks and benefits
- The risks and prognosis if no treatment is rendered
- An indication that the patient understands the nature of any proposed treatment, the alternatives, the risks involved, and the probable consequences of the proposed treatment
- The signature of the patient, physician, and witness
- The date the consent is signed

It is pertinent a patient has full understanding of that to which he/she has consented and at any time during the procedure, the patient may withdraw the consent.

Implied Consent

Implied consent is utilized when a patient's decision-making capabilities are compromised due to their medical condition and consent cannot be taken from an appropriate designee in a timely manner. In these situations a "reasonable person" can authorize consent and the required procedure may be performed without liability for failure to attain consent. A "reasonable person" is one who has full knowledge and understanding of the situation and would consent to the procedure under these circumstances.

SCHEDULING AND SCREENING

Patient screening begins the moment the patient calls for a CT appointment. Proper screening ensures a seamless examination. Reviewing the physician's request with the patient will define the correct CT protocol. For studies that require oral and intravenous contrast media, the patient should be questioned regarding their tolerance of both agents and a clear explanation of the purpose of each media. The proper instruction necessary will optimize the examination quality. All abdomen and pelvis examinations should be scheduled prior to any fluoroscopic GI examinations. The oral contrast media used for such studies contain 4% barium sulfate, which is too dense causing streaking artifacts on the CT examination if the media are not properly eliminated. CT examinations requiring IV contrast must be scheduled 8 weeks prior to a nuclear medicine thyroid scan, since the iodine from the contrast media will inhabit the uptake of the radiopharmaceuticals.

PATIENT EDUCATION

Patient education can be divided into three phases: pre-procedural phase, procedural phase, and postprocedural phase. The preprocedural phase began at the time of scheduling and continues when the technologist encounters the patient. This phase includes the following points:

Patient identification
- two unique identifiers confirm patient identification
  - patient's full name and date of birth
- purpose for establishing proper identification include:
  - assuring the correct patient receives the correct test
  - establishing initial rapport with the patient
  - assessment of the patient's comprehensive level

Patient screening/health history
- proper medical history is essential

Physical examination/laboratory studies
- patient's receiving IV contrast must have the appropriate laboratory studies prior to the examination

Giving the patient proper instructions on the procedure
- explain the procedure to the patient in a language he/she understands and try to avoid any technical details unless the patient shows interest
- material can be in an oral and/or written format
- review each step with the patient
- make sure the patient understands the process by having him/her repeat the steps back to you

Ensuring that proper consent has been obtained as required by legal and institutional policies
- this consent will be in the form of simple expressed or informed consent

The procedural phase commences when the patient enters the CT examination room. This important phase includes:

Patient's health history assessment
Patient's experience while the study is taking place
- both ensure the patient's risk and cooperation during the procedure

The postprocedural phase is just as important as the prior phases and includes the following:

Determine if the patient needs any other studies before letting him/her leave the facility
Instruct the patient to drink extra fluids
- preferably 64 oz of water over the next 24 hours

Explain the IV contrast will filter through their kidneys, but they will not notice anything different in their urine
They may notice something white in the stools
- if they were given barium sulfate as an oral contrast

Explain your institution's policy of when their physician will receive a report
Make sure the patient does not need to take the images
If the patient is diabetic
- determine the medication the patient is taking
- if on Metformin or derivative oral agent
  - drug should be discontinued 48 hours post IV injection

Immobilization

Immobilization is the process of limiting patient motion through the use of various devices. The purpose of utilizing restriction methods is to reduce radiation dose to the patient from repeated scans. The following are suitable devices that are not categorized as restraints and do not require a physician's orders:

Sponges
Velcro straps
Tape
- use a cloth or a tissue to protect the skin from the adhesive surface
- twist the tape so that the nonadhesive side is against the patient

PATIENT ASSESSMENT

Clinical History

A focused evaluation is necessary to assess the patient's degree of risk for adverse events during the CT procedure and confirms the proper procedure is being performed for the patient's specific signs and symptoms. When taking a medical history, questions should be open-ended to give the patient the opportunity to speak freely about his/her condition. This one-on-one attention establishes an initial rapport with the patient and also assesses the patient's comprehensive level. Most institutions provide a written health assessment questionnaire for the patient to complete, but it is vital the technologist reviews the questions with the patient. A medical history assessment form may incorporate the following questions:

Patient's name
Date of birth
Date
Height/weight
Medical record number
Do you know what kind of examination you are scheduled for?
What complaints prompted your doctor to send you for a CT scan?

Have you ever had surgery?

If so

- when and why?

Do you have any known allergies?

- if yes
  - they need to list them and what was their reaction

Are you being treated for:

- asthma
  - these patients have a higher chance of bronchial spasms
  - check to determine the extent of diseases
  - those on steroid inhalers on a daily basis should follow their institution's protocol

Have you ever had IV contrast before?

- when was your last injection?
  - maximum dose is 200 mL in 24 hours
  - patients should not receive another dose for 24 hours and a new GFR and/or creatinine MUST be drawn

DID YOU HAVE A REACTION?

- if yes what was the reaction?
  - how were you treated for the reaction?

Are you diabetic?

- determine the medication the patient is taking
  - if on Metformin oral agent or derivative
  - drug should be discontinued for 48 hours post IV injection
  - follow your institution's guidelines

Do you have heart disease?

- these patients have an increased incident of cardiovascular side effects
  - CHF
  - pulmonary edema, cardiac arrest

Is there any possibility of pregnancy?

- nonemergency cases should be scheduled while the patient is menstruating
  - if there is a doubt
    - administer a pregnancy test

Lactating mothers

- it is safe for the mother and baby to breast-feed following the administration of IV contrast according to the American College of Radiology (ACR)
- less than 1% of contrast is excreted into breast milk out of which only 1% is absorbed by the infant

Do you have hyperthyroidism?

- contrast media can increase the thyroid hormone
  - causing life-threatening conditions when a dangerous high level is reached

Remember the technologist is the liaison between the patient and the radiologist and this interaction leads to a good imaging interpretation.

Monitoring

Level of Consciousness

The technologist should understand a patient's level of consciousness to determine if the questions being asked are answered properly. Level of consciousness can be described as the state of wakefulness, awareness, or alertness in which most human beings function while not asleep. It is also a sudden change in mental activity, which may indicate a serious problem occurring and can be divided into the following five categories:

Clouding—mild form of mental status change

Confusional—disorientation, bewilderment, and difficulty following commands

Stupor—only vigorous and repeated stimuli will arouse the individual

Lethargy—severe drowsiness

Coma—state of unarousable unresponsiveness

Vital Signs

Vital signs are a measure of various physiological statistics, taken by health professionals, in order to assess the most basic body functions. The act of taking vital signs involves the following:

- Pulse
- Respiration
- Blood pressure
- Temperature
- Oxygen saturation

Pulse (Heart Rate)

It is defined as the rate at which the heart beats in 1 minute. The pulse can be palpable where an artery is near the surface of the body. The feeling of the pulse comes from the surge of blood against the arteries when the left ventricle contracts. The rhythm and strength of the heartbeat can also be noted, as well as whether the blood vessel feels hard or soft. Changes in a patient's heart rate or rhythm, a weak pulse, or a hard blood vessel may be caused by heart disease or an indication of an adverse reaction (Fig. 1.1).

Adult Ranges

Normal adult

- 60–100 BPM

Bradycardia—slow heart rate

- Below 60 BPM

Tachycardia—rapid heart rate

- Above 100 BPM

Well-trained athlete

- 40–60 BPM

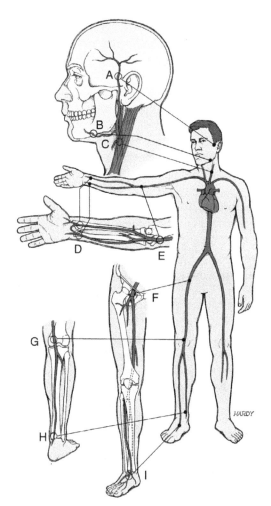

Figure 1.1. Illustration of anatomical pulse points. **(A)** Temporal, **(B)** facial, **(C)** carotid, **(D)** radial, **(E)** brachial, **(F)** femoral, **(G)** popliteal, **(H)** posterior pedal, **(I)** dorsal pedal. (Reproduced, with permission, from Romans LE. *Computed Tomography for Technologists: A Comprehensive Text.* Baltimore, MD: Wolters Kluwer Lippincott Williams & Wilkins; 2011.)

Pediatric Ranges

Age 1–8 years
- 80–100 BPM

Infants (1–12 months)
- 100–120 BPM

Neonates (1–28 days)
- 120–160 BPM

Respiration

Respiration is counted in breaths per minute and is often performed after the pulse is counted. If it is difficult to see the individual's chest rising and falling, place one hand on the diaphragm to get an accurate count. Respiration can be described as shallow, deep, labored, panting, and/or noisy.

Adult Ranges

Normal adult
- 12–20 BPM

Bradypnea—slow breathing that can produce cyanosis
- 12 or below

Tachypnea—rapid breathing that causes hyperventilation or syncope (fainting)
- 25 or above

Pediatric Ranges

Ages 1–8 years
- 15–30 BPM

Infants (1–12 months)
- 25–50 BPM

Neonates (1–28 days)
- 40–60 BPM

Blood Pressure

As the heart beats, it contracts and pushes blood through the arteries to the rest of your body. This force creates pressure on the arteries known as *systolic blood pressure*. *Diastolic blood pressure* indicates the pressure in the arteries when the heart rests between beats. Blood pressure is measured utilizing a sphygmomanometer. Baseline or average pressure is established by taking three readings over a period of time.

Adult Ranges

Normal adult range
- systolic 90–120 mm Hg
- diastolic 60–80 mm Hg

Prehypertension
- systolic 120–139
- diastolic 80—89

Hypertension
- stage 1
  - systolic 140–159
  - diastolic 90–99
- stage 2
  - systolic 160 or higher
  - diastolic 100 or higher

Hypotension
- below 90 systolic
- below 50 diastolic

Temperature

The body's ability to generate and get rid of heat is referred to as body temperature. The body is very good at keeping its temperature within a narrow, safe range in spite of large variations in temperatures outside the body. Your body temperature can be measured in many locations on your body. The mouth, rectum, and armpit are the most commonly used places, but temperature can also be measured in the ear and forehead. The device used to measure the temperature is a thermometer. They are calibrated in either degrees Fahrenheit (°F) or degrees Celsius (°C), depending on the custom of the region.

Normal
Oral
- 98.6°F
- 37°C

Rectal
- 0.5–1°F higher

Axillary
- 0.5–1°F lower

The conversion factor for Fahrenheit and Celsius are as follows:

- $°C = (°F - 32)/1.8$
- $°F = 1.8*(°C) + 32$

Pulse Oximetry

Pulse oximetry is a method used to determine the O_2 saturation—SaO_2 and desaturation of blood in a continuous noninvasive fashion through the use of a spectrophotoelectric instrument. The mechanism is applied to the finger, toe, or earlobe in which the small increase in absorption of light during the systolic pulse is used to calculate oxygen saturation of hemoglobin. A patient's pulse oximetry is measured on room air.

Normal range
- 95–100%

Mild hypoxia
- 91–94%

Moderate hypoxia
- 86–90%

Severe hypoxia
- 85% or below

Cardiac Cycle

The cardiac cycle is the sequence of events that occurs when the heart beats and consists of two phases, the diastolic and systolic. The *diastolic phase* is the point of relaxation while the *systolic phase* is when the ventricles contract. The cycle begins with the first diastolic phase; the right atrium receives deoxygenated blood from the SVC, IVC, coronary sinus, and cardiac veins that drain the myocardium. The tricuspid valve opens and the SA node triggers the atria to contract, allowing blood to empty into the right ventricle. The first systolic phase begins when the right ventricle receives impulses from the Purkinje fibers causing contraction of the right ventricle and the opening of the pulmonary semilunar valve forcing blood into the pulmonary arteries to be oxygenated. The second diastolic commences with oxygenated blood from the pulmonary vein entering the left atrium. The SA node triggers the mitral valve to open, emptying the oxygenated blood into the left ventricle. An impulse from the Purkinje fibers prompts the left ventricle to contract pumping blood into the aorta via the aortic semilunar valve completing the second systolic phase. The aorta carries oxygenated blood throughout the body. The events in the first and second diastolic and systolic phases occur simultaneously.

Laboratory Values

Laboratory values are an essential part of a patient's medical history. Renal function values determine if the individual is able to receive IV contrast safely. When undergoing an interventional procedure, there are particular tests that verify if the individual has a potential risk for excessive bleeding or hemorrhaging.

Renal Function Test

Blood Urea Nitrogen

Blood urea nitrogen (BUN) measures the amount of urea nitrogen in the blood, which reveals how well the liver and kidneys are working. The liver produces ammonia, which contains nitrogen. The nitrogen combines with other elements, such as carbon, hydrogen, and oxygen, to form urea, which is a chemical waste product of the body. Urea travels from your liver to your kidneys through your bloodstream. When the kidneys are healthy, they filter urea and remove other waste products from your blood. The filtered waste products leave your body through urine. Normal adult levels range from *7 to 20 mg/100 mL* and vary depending on the reference range used by the laboratory, and your age. BUN alone is not an accurate test for renal function, but used in conjunction with serum creatinine, it can provide information about the hydration status of a patient.

Creatinine

Creatinine is a chemical waste molecule that is generated from muscle metabolism. It is transported through the bloodstream to the kidneys. The kidneys filter out most of the creatinine and dispose of it in the urine. Normal levels are approximately 0.6–1.3 mg/dL depending on the laboratory reference values. Any value >1.3 mg/dL is an indication of renal impairment.

Glomerular Filtration Rate

Glomerular filtration rate (GFR) is the best test to measure kidney function and to determine stages of kidney disease. It is calculated from the results of the patient's blood creatinine test, age, race, and gender. Some useful GFR calculators are the MDRD (Modification of Diet in Renal Disease) calculator at: http://nephron.org/cgi-bin/MDRD_GFR/cgi and the Cockcroft-Gault at: http://www.mdcalc.com/creatinine-clearance-cockcroft-gault-equation. According to the National Kidney Foundation a normal GFR is approximately *90–100 mL/min/1.73 m²*. Patients with GFR results *<60 mL/min/1.79 m²* are at risk for kidney disease.

Interventional Test

Prothrombin Time

Prothrombin time (PT) measures the time required for prothrombin to be converted to thrombin for coagulation to occur. There are approximately 12 clotting factors present, with prothrombin being the second factor. Prothrombin is synthesized by the liver with the use of vitamin K.

Normal values and critical limits of PT are *10.7–15.0 seconds*. Twice the time should be considered normal for patients receiving anticoagulation therapy. A result >30 seconds is considered the "danger zone."

Partial Thromboplastin Time

Partial thromboplastin time (PTT) measures the time required for clot formation in normal plasma. The normal PTT range is *30–45 seconds*, whereas normal activated partial thromboplastin time (APTT) range *is 25–40 seconds*. Patients on blood thinner have a 1.5–2.5 times greater range. A result >100 seconds indicates spontaneous bleeding.

Platelet Count

A platelet count measures the amount of platelets in the body. Platelets also known as thrombocytes are blood cells whose function is to stop bleeding at the site of eruption. Normal test values range from *150,000 to 400,000 platelets per microliter (mcL)*. A patient whose platelet levels are below 100,000 platelets per microliter (*mcL*) is at a greater risk for bleeding.

International Normalized Ratio

International normalized ratio (INR) was established in an effort to standardize PT and PTT results, which varies greatly among laboratories. It's purpose is to measure the extrinsic pathways of coagulation. INR, PT and PTT are used to determine the clotting tendencies of blood, the regulation of warfarin dosage, the extent of liver damage, and a patient's vitamin K status. A result of *1–2 is normal*. A result >2 means the individual has a high chance of bleeding, while a range <1 indicates a high chance of clotting.

D-Dimer

A D-dimer test is of clinical use when there is a suspicion of deep venous thrombosis (DVT) or pulmonary embolism. When a tissue or blood vessel is injured and begins to bleed, a process called hemostasis is initiated by the body that creates a blood clot, in order to stop the bleeding. During this clotting process, thin protein threads called fibrin are formed, which together with the platelets eventually stop the bleeding by forming a blood clot. It is during the clotting process that D-dimer is formed as a fibrin degradation product. These protein fragments, though not usually present in blood, are otherwise detected in blood plasma when the coagulation system has been activated. The normal amounts for D-dimer in the blood should be around *0.5 mg/L of blood.*

Liver Function Tests (LFTs)

Albumin

Albumin (ALB) is a protein made by the liver. Albumin helps move many small molecules through the blood, including bilirubin, calcium, progesterone, and medications. It plays an important role in keeping the fluid from the blood from leaking out into the tissues. A serum albumin test measures the amount of this protein in the clear liquid portion of the blood. An elevated result usually indicates dehydration, while a below normal result can indicate liver dysfunction or insufficient protein intake.

Normal values: 4–6 grams per deciliter (g/dL)

Alkaline Phosphatase

Alkaline phosphatase (ALK PHOS) is an enzyme primarily concentrated in the liver and bone. Increased levels may indicate damage or disease of the liver or bone disease such as osteomalacia or Paget's disease. A result below normal is usually not significant.

Normal values: 25–100 units per liter (IU/L)

Alanine Aminotransferase (ALT or SGPT)

Alanine aminotransferase is an enzyme found in the liver, with smaller amounts in the kidneys, heart, muscles, and pancreas. The alanine aminotransferase (ALT) test is performed to identify liver disease, especially cirrhosis and hepatitis caused by alcohol, drugs, or viruses. When the liver is damaged or diseased, it releases ALT into the bloodstream, which makes ALT levels increase.

Normal values: 10–40 units per liter (IU/L)

Total Bilirubin (TBIL)

Bilirubin is a waste product from the breakdown of red blood cells. It is processed through the liver and is excreted in stool. Bilirubin flows through the liver's bile ducts and is dissolved in bile. An increased result indicates an impaired bile flow, which occurs in severe liver or gallbladder disease, or other bile conditions. This increase of bilirubin in the bloodstream may cause the skin and whites of the eyes to appear yellow. The yellowish appearance is known as jaundice and may be caused by liver disease (hepatitis), blood disorders (hemolytic anemia), or blockage of the tubes (bile ducts) that allow bile to pass from the liver to the small intestine.

Normal values: 0.3–1.9 mg/dL

Medication and Dosage

The technologist must review the patient's current medications for any contraindications to administering contrast media. Warfarin or any other anticoagulant therapies are blood-thinning agents given to patients that have had a heart attack or blood clots with the known side effects of causing excessive bleeding. Special attention should be taken with these patients when removing their IV access. Make sure to apply ample pressure at the IV site to avoid excessive bleeding or bruising. Another medication to be concerned with is Metformin. Individuals taking this medication or its derivative must abstain from its use for 2 days following the enhanced CT examination. There is a slight risk for renal impairment due to the retention of these medications in the body.

Medication Administration

The first important step in administering medication, whether it is oral contrast or IV contrast, is to implement the "six rights": the right patient, the right drug, the right dose, the right route, the right time, and with the right documentation. Documentation is imperative whenever IV contrast is administered and should include the following reconciliations:

Reason for venipuncture
Date and time of insertion
Site and gauge
Type of contrast media injected
- amount and flow rate
Number of attempts

Site assessment findings
Patient tolerance

Medication Container

Ampule—small glass vial that is sealed after filling and used chiefly as a container for a hypodermic injection solution
Bolus—single, relatively large quantity of a substance administered intravenously
Vial—small container holding several doses of medication
Infusion of medication—quantity of medication over time

Medication Routes

Enteral
- topical
- oral
- rectal

Parenteral—taken into the body in a manner other than through the digestive canal
- intradermal
- subcutaneous
- intramuscular
- intravenous
- intra-arterial
- intrathecal

Preprocedure Medication

Premedication is given to patients who are at risk for an adverse event. Several premedication regimens have been proposed to reduce the frequency and/or severity of reactions to contrast media. ACR utilizes the following as elective premedication:

Methylprednisolone (Medrol): 32 mg by mouth 12 hours and 2 hours before contrast media injection
Diphenhydramine (Benadryl): 50 mg intravenously, intramuscularly, or by mouth 1–2 hours before contrast media
- Benadryl is an optional drug

In emergency situations the following is used:

Hydrocortisone sodium succinate (Solu-Cortef)
- 200 mg intravenously starting 6 hours prior to injection every 4 hours (q4h) until contrast study
Diphenhydramine
- 50 mg IV 1 hour prior to contrast injection

Postprocedure Instructions

The patient must be educated on how the oral and IV contrast will be eliminated. All patients who received an enhanced CT examination must be informed that the contrast media will be filtered through their kidneys and eliminated with their urine. They will not see or feel anything different during elimination and must be instructed to drink at least 64 oz of water throughout the next 24 hours. The oral contrast is eliminated in their stools and there is a slight possibility that they may see some white stools if they were given barium sulfate. The patients should be instructed to contact their physician if they develop diarrhea, constipation, or scanty urine output. Tell the patients the hospital policy of when their referring physician will receive a report. And finally ask the patients if their physician requires a copy of their images.

CONTRAST ADMINISTRATION

Contrast Media

The purpose of contrast media is to increase the difference in attenuation between the adjacent structures. Since x-ray attenuation is directly related to the atomic number of the material in the path of the beam, we are able to assign an HU to the organ of interest making it possible for the radiologist to identify the biological nature of the variance or abnormality of the structure. Contrast aids in distinguishing between vessels, lymph nodes, and other organs of the body. All iodinated contrast media consist of three atoms of iodine per molecule.

Ionic Contrast Media

Ionic contrast is considered a high-osmolality contrast media (HOCM), which separates in water yielding two particles. The negatively charged anion consists of a benzene ring with a negatively charged amino acid group, while the positively charged cation consists of a sodium or methylglucamine complex. Ratio of iodine atoms to active particles is 3:2. Body must maintain a constant number of particles within the blood serum; by injecting an ionic contrast media there is an increase in the osmolality in the blood serum resulting in the total number of particles to increase. Due to this increase in atomic particles, water will be drawn into the blood stream from the tissues to compensate for the increased concentration of particles. This increase in water increases the total blood volume forcing the heart to work harder in order to pump the larger load. This phenomenon is referred as increased osmotic pressure. The results of this pressure include:

- Hypervolemia—increases blood volume
- Blood vessel dilation
- Shock—can occur in severely dehydrated patients

Renal effects are especially significant with HOCM resulting in constriction of the renal arteries due to release of vasoconstrictors. This constriction diminishes the blood supply to the kidneys, thereby decreasing renal function.

Nonionic Contrast Media

Nonionic contrast is considered a low-osmolality contrast media (LOCM) that does not separate in water. The iodine concentration is maintained without increasing the number of particles in solution; therefore, it does not increase the osmolality of the blood serum and does not change the osmotic pressure in the bloodstream. Ratio of iodine atoms to active particles is 3:1. It is safer for patients with compromised cardiac status.

Its advantages include:

- hemodynamic effect is less
- more water soluble
- hydrophilic (tendency to dissolve in water)
- less likely to be reactive with the cells to trigger allergic effects

Iso-Osmolar Contrast Media

Iso-osmolar contrast is the most recent class of agents. They are dimers that consist of a molecule with two benzene rings each with three iodine atoms. They do not dissociate in water; consequently, they are considered nonionic agents. The toxicity of contrast agents decreases as osmolality approaches that of serum. This has been accomplished by developing nonionizing compounds and then combining two monomers to form a dimer. Ratio of iodine atoms to active particles is 6:1.

Osmolality

Osmolality is the measurement of the total number of particles in the contrast solution per kilogram of water. It is the direct measurement of the ionization of a solute in a solvent. The osmolality of human blood is approximately 300 mOsm/kg. The osmolality of water-soluble contrast ranges from 300 to 1,000 mOsm/kg. Utilization of a solution that exceeds the osmolality of blood serum (a term known as hyperosmolar) results in negative effects to the human body.

Viscosity

Viscosity is the amount of friction generated by the concentration and size of the contrast molecules. The higher the viscosity, the thicker the agent and the more difficult it is to inject. Rapid injection with a higher-viscosity agent can trigger the body's pressure sensors causing vessels to constrict and making injection painful. Heating the agent to body temperature reduces the viscosity of the agent. Heating can be achieved through:

- contrast warmer
- manually—using tepid water

It is important to remember nonionic media are more viscous than ionic media at similar iodine concentrations.

Dosing

It is important to avoid overdosing of iodine. Toxicity levels consist of 80–90 g of iodine.

Injection of these concentrations causes tremors, irritability, and tachycardia. If such symptoms occur, stop administration immediately and initiate emergency action. A 24-hour period between contrast injections is imperative to avoid not only contrast-induced nephropathy, but also toxicity.

Types of Oral Contrast Media

Positive agent
- barium sulfate
- water soluble (iodinated)

Negative agent
- air
  - administered orally in an effervescent solution of gas-generating granules mixed in water
  - administered rectally using an air bulb
- carbon dioxide
  - administered rectally via insufflation

Neutral
- water
  - administered when a positive agent would obstruct an area of interest

Barium Sulfate

Barium sulfate suspensions are utilized for the opacification of the gastrointestinal tract. They provide greater delineation of mucosal detail and are more resistant to dilution than iodinated agents. The suspensions used for CT examination consist of 2% barium sulfate suspended in water. The time for barium sulfate to travel throughout the GI tract is 45–90 minutes. Barium sulfate should not be used for patients suspected of:

- colon obstruction or gastrointestinal tract perforation
- tracheoesophageal fistula
- obstructing lesions of small intestine
- pyloric stenosis
- inflammation or neoplastic lesions of the rectum
- recent rectal biopsy

VoLumen

VoLumen is another oral contrast agent used when bowel distension is necessary (CT enterography). Its purpose is to outline loops of bowel. It contains 0.1% barium sulfate suspended in water. It contains sorbitol to reduce water absorption and gum to increase viscosity. These ingredients theoretically result in better bowel distention than water. Because it contains sorbitol (is a sugar alcohol, which the human body metabolizes slowly) some patients will experience diarrhea when used. Patients should be warned about this before leaving the radiology department. The usual dosage is 2 or 3 premixed volumes (450 mL each). For best opacification, the patient should drink the solution over a 30-minute period. Upon completion the CT study is done promptly using IV contrast material often as a CT enterography study with CT angiography.

Water-Soluble Contrast Media (Diatrizoate Meglumine/Diatrizoate Sodium)

Water-soluble contrast is ionic with high-osmolality properties. The agent is intended to be therapeutically and biologically inert when ingested/injected into the body for use in organ or tissue enhancement. It is particularly suited for times when a more viscous agent such as barium sulfate (not water soluble) is not feasible or is potentially dangerous.

SPECIAL CONTRAST CONSIDERATIONS

Contraindications to IV Contrast

Allergies
- patients with a known allergy to iodine have up to five-fold increased likelihood of experiencing a subsequent reaction
- shellfish allergies are no longer considered a risk for adverse reactions
  - The ACR handbook on IV contrast states: the predictive value of specific allergies, such as those to shellfish or dairy products, previously thought to be helpful, is now recognized to be unreliable. A significant number of healthcare providers continue to inquire specifically into a patient's history of "allergy" to seafood, especially shellfish. There is no evidence to support the continuation of this practice.
- patients with previous anaphylaxis reactions to one or more allergens are believed to be at high risk.

Atopic syndrome (predisposed toward developing certain allergic hypersensitivity reactions)

- have a two to three times more likelihood of contrast reaction compared with nonatopic patients
- risk is considered low, but should be considered in the context of risk versus benefits

Asthma
- indicates an increased likelihood of a contrast reaction

Renal sufficiency
- these patients may be forced into contrast-induced nephrotoxicity (CIN) and nephrogenic systemic fibrosis (NSF)

Cardiac status
- significant cardiac disease may prompt an increased risk for contrast reactions
- attention should be paid to limiting the volume and osmolality of the contrast media

Protocol Deviations for the Use of CM
Pheochromocytoma (adrenal tumor)
- HOCM produced an increase in serum catecholamine levels
- using LOCM shows no elevation of catecholamine levels
- direct injection into the adrenal or renal arteries
- can cause a hypertensive crisis

Sickle cell
- no evidence of any clinically significant risk, particularly after the injection of LOCM

Multiple myeloma
- known to predispose patients to irreversible renal failure after HOCM
- no data predicting risk with the use of low-osmolality or iso-osmolality agents

Pregnant patients
- contrast media have been shown to cross the human placenta and enter the fetus when given in usual clinical dose
- ACR recommends the patient be educated on the possible risks and benefits of the ionization radiation and the contrast media to the fetus
  - informed consent is recommended to document the patient understands the risk and benefits and alternative diagnostic method is applicable

Lactation
- available data suggest that it is safe for the mother to continue breast-feeding following the administration of IV contrast

If the mother remains concerned, she may abstain for 24 hours utilizing the pump and dump method

Always consult with a radiologist before making the decision not to administer IV contrast.

ADMINISTRATION ROUTES AND DOSE CALCULATIONS

IV

Intravenous administration is a medical term referring to the administration of fluids and medicine directly into a vein. Medical professionals agree that intravenous administration is the quickest way to deliver fluids and medicine to the body and many medications can only be given intravenously. The amount of iodine delivered to render attenuation properties depends on its concentration of iodine particles. For instance, a contrast media with strength of 370 possesses a higher concentration of iodine than strength of 300. Higher strengths are given to patients with above average body weight and when less amount of fluid is desired. The dosage of IV contrast media is 2 mL/kg of body weight. The conversion of kilograms to pounds is 1kg is equal to 2.2 lbs.

Oral

The purpose of oral contrast is to highlight the stomach, small and large bowels. The amount ingested totally depends on the clinical area of interest. CT examinations limited to the abdomen require 300 mL of contrast given 30-minutes prior to the commencement of the study with 150 mL given when the patient gets on the table to highlight the stomach. For a routine abdomen and pelvis it is recommended that the patient drinks 450 mL of contrast 60–90 minutes before the start of the examination with 150 mL as described above. When the area of interest is the distal large bowel or rectum a delay time of 4–6 hours is necessary. When this delay time is impossible to wait, rectal contrast may be employed.

Rectal

Rectal contrast is given in the form of an enema. A typical enema tip is used with the exception of recent rectal surgery, when a French catheter is employed. This type of catheter is used to prevent rectal perforation. A contrast dose of 150–500 mL will adequately fill the area. The rectal contrast helps to increase the sensitivity of the CT examination by outlining not only the large intestines but also the bladder, the uterus in female patients and other organs. In some circumstances, the radiologist may request the administration of small amount of air to fully distend the distal bowel.

Intrathecal

Intrathecal administration is the method used when contrast is injected with the use of a spinal needle directly into the subarachnoid space. Myelography is the most common imaging procedure that requires this type of injection. CT myelography is performed following the contrast injection for the evaluation of the spinal cord and nerve roots.

Catheters

Central venous catheters can be used for the administration of IV contrast media, when a peripheral venous line is not available, and only when it is of adequate type, material, and diameter. The most common types of catheters technologists should familiarize themselves with are:

Central venous line
- inserted into the subclavian vein

Port-a-Cath
- inserted into the subclavian vein
- mainly used for chemotherapy
- PSI 150 is imperative

Peripheral inserted central catheter (PICC)
- inserted in a peripheral vein, such as the cephalic vein, basilic vein, and brachial vein

The above catheter types will indicate, on the tubing extending outside the patient's body, the maximum allowable flow rates in cc/sec. These specification must be strictly adhered to, since devastating from the manufacturer's recommendations may cause a breakage of the internal catheter, resulting in possible venous obstruction or death.

Hickman (used for long-term intravenous access)
- inserted into the jugular vein
- **never to be used for bolus injections**

Intra-Articular

An intra-articular injection is a type of injection in which contrast and air are inserted into a joint. The patient is instructed to exercise the specific joint in order to mix the contrast and air into the surrounding area. The most common CT arthrography examinations are shoulder, hip, knee, and wrist.

Stoma

A stoma is a surgically formed opening in the body which connects the small or large bowel to the outside world. A colostomy or ileostomy patient may need oral contrast (barium sulfate or water-soluble iodinated) injected into the stoma for opacification of the bowel during a CT examination of the abdomen and/or pelvis.

VENIPUNCTURE

Venipuncture in CT is the process of puncturing a vein with a needle for the purpose of establishing an intravenous line for the administration of contrast media. Most CT venipuncture is done on the inner elbow area in the median cubital vein, since this vein is superficial and does not lie in close proximity to any large nerve groups. There are two types of venipuncture devices used for the administration of intravenous contrast media: angiocatheter and a butterfly needle. *Angiocatheter* is a two-part device consisting of a stylet that fits inside a flexible plastic catheter. These IV catheters feature a push-button shielding technology to safeguard healthcare workers from accidental needle stick injuries. Angiocatheters are effective in withstanding the pressure applied by a power injector. The needle lengths available are ¾–1¼ in with the optimal length for CT procedures being 1 in. The gauge ranges are from 14 to 24. The following are the recommended flow rates for each gauge:

- 24 gauge—utilizing injection flow rates <1
- 22 gauge—utilizing injection flow rates 1–2
- 20 gauge—utilizing injection flow rates 2.5–3.5
- 14–18 gauge—utilizing injection flow rates of >3.5

Butterfly needle is a bare, stainless steel, variable gauge needle with flat plastic projections on either side of the base, a flexible small-bore transparent tubing (often 20–35 cm long), and finally a connector. The plastic panels can be grasped and then anchored by tape to the patient's skin, which secures the needle at the puncture site, while the connector attaches to another device, such as a syringe. These types of needles are used for hand injections (pediatric patients) and should never be used with power injectors since the needle remains in the vein. The needle lengths available are ½–1¼ in with gauges ranging from 19 to 25.

Steps in Performing a Successful Venipuncture Stick

Step 1
Gather your supplies:

- Gloves
- Tourniquet
- Antiseptic or bacteriostatic solution such as alcohol or chlorhexidine prep pads
- Angiocatheter (choice of needle length and gauge depends on the CT examination and vein stability)
- Needle-free valve connector
- Normal saline flush
- Tape (preferably paper to eliminate pulling or tearing of the skin upon removal) or a transparent dressing such as Tegaderm
- Gauze
- Bandage

Step 2

Patient identification

- Two unique identifiers (name and date of birth) confirm patient identification
- Review requisition for type of CT study ordered to proper angiocatheter size and placement

Step 3

Handwashing and the use of universal precautions

Handwashing is easy to do and it is one of the most effective ways to prevent the spread of many types of infection and illness especially in a hospital setting. Listed below are the Center for Disease Control and Prevention's (CDC) recommendations on handwashing:

Wet your hands with clean, running water (warm or cold), turn off the tap, and apply soap

Lather your hands by rubbing them together with the soap

- be sure to lather the backs of your hands, between your fingers, and under your nails

Scrub your hands for at least 20 seconds

Need a timer

- hum the "Happy Birthday" song from beginning to end twice

Rinse your hands well under clean, running water

Dry your hands using a clean towel or air dry them

Universal precautions—in 1985 the CDC introduced this system in the acknowledgment that many patients with blood-borne infections were not recognized. Under this system all patients are treated as potential reservoirs of infection; therefore, the need to wear gloves and masks depends on the nature of the interaction instead of the specific diagnosis.

Step 4

Choosing the venipuncture site:

Determine appropriate site for venipuncture by looking at patients' arms and asking patients about their venipuncture history is helpful

Best choice:
- vein is palpable without tourniquet
- large veins well visualized through skin
- soft and elastic veins

Poor choice:
- veins that are barely palpable with tourniquet
- small veins
- corded, sclerotic, fragile veins

Some conditions warrant you to use one arm over the other:
- CVA
- dialysis patients with shunts

- mastectomy (use contralateral arm to prevent fluid retention)
- deep scarring

Step 5

Preparing the site of venipuncture

Apply tourniquet 3–4 in above the site of injection and select a vein
- have the patient open and close fist several times followed by a clenched fist to make veins more identifiable
- the tourniquet should never be applied for more than 1 minute

Appropriately position the arm
- eliminate awkward movements when inserting the needle

Prepare skin with antibacterial prep
- apply friction for a minimum of 30 seconds
- begin in the center and move peripherally in a circular motion, without repalpating or touching the skin
- the skin should be allowed to fully dry before the needle is inserted
  - wet alcohol can create an uncomfortable and unnecessary burning sensation for the patient

Grasp arm distally to point of entry, placing thumb about 1 in below expected point of entry, and pull skin downward so it is taut

Approach the vein slowly holding the angiocatheter so that the needle bevel is facing upward

Place needle in line with the vein at a 15–30-degree angle

Insert sterile angiocatheter into the patient's vein

Observe early flashback along the catheter (20, 22, and 24 gauge only)
- in larger gauge sizes, observe flash behind white button

Upon flashback visualization
- lower catheter almost parallel to the skin

Advance entire unit slightly before threading catheter

Thread catheter into vein while maintaining skin traction

Release tourniquet

Apply digital pressure beyond catheter tip

Gently stabilize catheter hub

Press the white button to remove needle

Secure catheter and apply sterile dressing

Attach saline flush to needle valve flushing slowly
- ensuring no extravasation of saline is present

Discard all needles and equipment in puncture-resistance, leak-proof sharps container

Documentation of venipuncture

Reason for venipuncture

Date and time of insertion

Site, gauge, and flow rate
Contrast media injected and amount
Patient tolerance
Site assessment findings

- presence–absence of redness, swelling, tenderness, and catheter patency

Aseptic Technique

Nosocomial infections are contracted by approximately 10% of patients admitted to hospitals and are the major source of patient mortality and increased cost related to lengthened hospital stays. The only way to prevent these events is the use of aseptic techniques. Aseptic techniques are employed to maximize and maintain asepsis (the absence of pathogenic organisms), in the clinical setting. The goals of aseptic techniques are to protect the patient from infection and to prevent the spread of pathogens. There are two types of aseptic techniques employed in the CT department, surgical and medical. Surgical asepsis or sterile technique is the process of eliminating microorganisms or spores from an area. This is accomplished through heat, gas, or other chemicals.

Medical asepsis or clean technique is the process of maintaining cleanliness to prevent the spread of pathogens and to ensure that the environment is as free from microbes as possible. It is accomplished through the use of soap, water, and many other types of disinfectant materials.

CT IV Contrast Administration Methods

Drip Infusion

Drip infusion is the use of an IV bag or a bottle containing iodinated contrast media. An infusion set is attached to the bag or bottle and then to the patient's IV line. The tubing's flow meter is left wide open to allow the contrast media to flow freely. Since this method depends on gravitational flow, it is too slow to reach arterial peak enhancement.

Hand Bolus

Hand bolus is the process of connecting a syringe filled with contrast media to the hub of the patient's IV line. The radiologist or designee injects the contrast media manually. This method produces inconsistencies and reproducibility is not attainable, due to the individual's pressure strength. The major disadvantage of this method is the risk of the operator receiving radiation exposure. This method has and is still in use for pediatric patients.

Power Injectors

Power injection is an important advance that when combined with state-of-the-art scanner technology has made risky and expensive exploratory surgery virtually a relic of the past. Power injectors have proven to be more beneficial than either the drip infusion or the manual technique. With the power injector the amount of contrast can be concentrated in the area of interest during the scan giving the technologist the ability to perform split injection studies with specific delay times. The timing of contrast delivery can be closely monitored, which is especially important when performing CT angiograms and cardiac studies. These injectors deliver consistent flow rates and volume from scan to scan making comparison studies easier to interpret.

Most modern models are constructed with a dual head component equipped with two 200-cc disposable syringes, a heating device, in order to maintain contrast at or near body temperature, and a programmable venous pressure limit mechanism, for the purpose of eliminating extravasations.

For technologists the advantage of a power injector is the ability to manipulate the flow rate, duration time, and the volume when the routine study is impossible to perform. For instance, there is a patient scheduled for a cancer screening CT abdomen, pelvis study, but the patient's veins are fragile and will not withstand the routine 2-cc/sec flow rate. Normal venous enhancement of the liver takes approximately 70 seconds utilizing 100cc of contrast media delivered at a rate of 2cc/sec. When lowering the flow rate to accommodate the patient's venous access, the contrast delay time also needs adjusting in order to produce a good venous phase in the liver, which is of utmost importance when screening for metastatic disease. Changes in flow rates or contrast volume and calculating the duration time of the injection will help determine the exact or/near exact injection delay. The following are the three power injection calculations:

$$volume = flow\ rate \times time$$
$$flow\ rate = volume \div time$$
$$delay\ time = volume \div flow\ rate$$

POSTPROCEDURE CARE

Contrast Extravasation

Contrast extravasation is the most common complication of intravenous injection. Extravasation of intravenous contrast media is an adverse event that can potentially cause serious injury and permanent harm to the patient. The causes of extravasation include leakage from the vein into the soft tissue (e.g., because of brittle veins in very elderly patients), previous venipuncture (such as from blood drawn for laboratory tests prior to therapy), and/or direct leakage from ill-positioned venous access device.

The patients at risk for contrast infiltrations are noncommunicative patients (children or elderly), severely debilitated patients, patients with multiple punctures in the same vein, and injections on the dorsum of the hand and foot. The possible complications include:

- bruising
- phlebitis
- air embolism
- pulmonary thromboembolism
- catheter fragment embolism
- infiltration/extravasation
- infection
- cellulitis
- nerve damage

Air Embolism

Air embolism principally is caused by the entry of air into the vascular system. The embolism is propelled into the heart, creating an intracardiac air lock at the pulmonary valve and preventing the ejection of blood from the right ventricle of the heart. The beating heart can then fragment the trapped air into smaller bubbles. These bubbles bear the risk of impairing blood circulation in smaller vessels, which is critical for the pulmonary circulation system. The possible symptoms or clinical signs of an air embolism involve:

- anxiety
- tachycardia
- dyspnea
- tachypnea
- chest pain
- altered level of consciousness
- agitation or disorientation
- severe hypotension/shock
- shortness of breath
- cardiac "mill wheel" murmur
- cyanotic appearance
- sudden loss of consciousness, circulatory shock, or sudden death

The symptoms and clinical signs of air embolism are related to the degree of air entry into the circulation system and usually develop immediately after embolization. Any amount of air that might enter the patient must be considered critical. The impact is directly correlated with the patient's condition, the volume of air, and the rate of accumulation. It has been reported that injecting more than 100 mL of air into the venous bloodstream can be fatal; therefore, prevention is the key.

When filling the power injector it is essential to place the injector in the upright position. Upon completing the filling process, advance the plungers to the top, to rid the syringes of all air, then bleed the connection tubing. Always use the "wet" of joining the tubing to the patient's IV line. When the examination is completed dispose the empty syringes immediately. This prevents the medical mistake of reusing a syringe completely filled with air.

Treatment for air embolism has three goals—to stop the source of the air embolism, to prevent it from damaging the body, and to resuscitate if necessary. In the case of air entering the patient's venous system, the first step is to contact the radiologist. Place the patient in the Trendelenburg or left lateral position, to help stop the embolism from traveling to the brain, heart, and/or lungs. It is recommended to give the patient 100% oxygen; this is intended to counteract ischemia and accelerate bubble size reduction. The administration of medications, such as adrenaline, will aid in keeping the heart pumping. As with all adverse reactions documentation is a must.

ADVERSE REACTIONS

Types

An adverse reaction can be described as an undesired effect including the many subjective side effects experience to some degree by most patients to whom contrast is administered. There are two types of adverse reactions associated with contrast media: chemotoxic and idiosyncratic. Chemotoxic reactions result from the physicochemical properties of the contrast media that can result in contrast-induced nephropathy or CIN. Idiosyncratic contrast reactions are unpredictable and do not occur in most patients. This type of reaction occurs when a patient is hypersensitive to the chemical composition of iodine and the way their body metabolizes or responds to the iodinated contrast. The ACR has divided adverse reactions to contrast agents into the following categories:

Mild
- occurs in 3% of patients

Moderate
- occurs in 0.2–0.4% of patients

Severe
- occurs in 0.04% of patients

Mild Reactions
- Limited nausea, vomiting
- Altered taste
- Warmth (heat)
- Dizziness
- Nasal stuffiness

- Headache
- Flushing
- Anxiety
- Sweats
- Cough
- Itching
- Rash
- Limited hives
- Pallor
- Swelling: eyes, face
- Chills
- Shaking

Treatment for Mild Reactions

Treatment for a mild reaction requires observation and reassurance. Usually no intervention or medication is required; however, these reactions may progress into a more severe category. Most reactions are classified as mild.

Moderate Reactions

- Pronounced cutaneous reactions
- Tachycardia
- Bradycardia
- Hypotension
- Bronchospasm
- Hypertension
- Dyspnea
- Laryngeal edema
- Pulmonary edema
- Wheezing

Treatment for Moderate Reactions

Treatment for moderate reactions entails prompt treatment with close observation, since most reactions frequently result in bronchospasm and laryngeal edema. Patients must also be monitored carefully for changes in cardiac rate and blood pressure.

Severe Reactions

- Laryngeal edema (severe or progressive)
- Profound hypotension
- Unresponsiveness
- Convulsions
- Cardiopulmonary arrest
- Clinically manifest arrhythmias

Treatment for Severe Reactions

For severe reactions immediate treatment is necessary and usually requires hospitalization.

Severe reactions, while infrequent, can rapidly escalate to a life-threatening situation known as anaphylaxis.

Anaphylaxis is rapid in onset and is believed to be caused by the release of histamine from certain cells of the lungs, stomach, lining of the blood vessels. These reactions are so severe that death can occur.

Vasovagal Reaction

Vasovagal reaction is one of the most common causes of fainting and, according to the ACR, is not considered an adverse reaction. A vasovagal response occurs when your body overreacts to certain triggers, as in this case the anxiety of the examination itself or the flushing feeling due to the contrast injection. It is characterized by bradycardia and hypotension.

The initial resuscitation should include elevating the legs and/or placing the patient in a Trendelenburg position with the administration of oxygen at the rate of 6–10 L/min.

IV fluids are used to treat hypotension and should be administered rapidly. A medication such as Atropine (a parasympatholytic agent), which is used to treat bradycardia at a dose of 0.6–1.0 mg injected intravenously with a maximum dose of 2 mg.

Recognition and Assessment

It is most important to recognize an adverse reaction. Always notify a radiologist or nurse of any reaction, and always err on the safe side. It is better to call a reaction than to disregard the symptoms. Patient anxiety can turn a mild reaction into a more severe reaction; therefore, behavior and conduct become important factors in your ability to successfully manage the patient. Always be aware of any changes in the patient's mental and physical characteristics, since these changes are signs that an adverse reaction may occur. Maintain and display an unruffled, orderly, deliberate, capable, and effective demeanor, one that elicits confidence and promotes a sense of well-being in the patient. Always remember that documentation is important and must include the preprocedure patient assessment through conclusion of the treatment.

Adverse Reaction Medications

Albuterol inhaler—a beta-2 agonist that causes bronchodilation and relieves bronchospasm
- dose
  - 2 puffs to start
  - may need to be repeated

Diphenhydramine—an antihistamine which is an H-1 receptor site blocker. In this capacity, it blocks circulating histamine from binding to target cells.

- dose
  - 25–50 mg IV or IM
  - caution: causes drowsiness
  - patient should not drive or operate machinery for 4–6 hours
  - Clonidine—a drug used to treat a hypertensive crisis
- dose
  - 200 mcg (0.2 mg). Bite, chew, and swallow

Epinephrine—a drug which is a basic sympathetic agonist
- alpha—peripheral vasoconstriction
- beta-1—cardiac: increase contractility and heart rate
- beta-2—bronchodilation
- dose
  - subcutaneous: 1:1,000 (1 mg/mL) 0.1–0.3 mL (0.1–0.3 mg)
  - intravenous: 1:10,000 (0.1 mg/mL) 1 mL IV slowly every 3–5 minutes

Diazepam—a benzodiazepine used to treat seizures
- dose
  - 5–10 mg IV push
  - maximum dose: 30 mg

Nitroglycerin—a vasodilator used to treat acute angina
- dose
  - 0.4 mg sublingual
  - may be repeated q5 min for a total of 3 doses

RADIATION SAFETY AND DOSIMETRY

Technical Factors Affecting Patient Dose

With the expanding use of CT in medicine the major concern relates to the potential for high radiation dose. There are three essential questions we need to ask ourselves:

1. Why are doses so high?
2. How can we reduce radiation dose?
3. What are doses in your institution?

Dosimetry is a term used to describe the instrumentation and methods used to measure patient dose from the CT scanner. The factors affecting radiation dose in CT include:

- peak kilovoltage
- constant milliamperage-second (mAs)
- effective mAs
- Z—Overscanning
- filters
- collimation
- pitch
- patient centering
- number of detectors
- automatic tube current modulation

Kilovoltage

kVp is the qualitative measure of the x-ray beam. An increase in kVp produces an increase in photon energy resulting in an increase in patient dose when milliamperage remains the same. The increase is dependent on whether the automated tube current modulation or a manual technique is being used. In CT the usual kVp ranges are from 100 to 140. Physicists and radiologists are now becoming aware of CT dose for patients and are beginning to lower kVp in CT examinations. The principle behind the benefit of lower kV in some clinical applications is the attenuation coefficient of iodine increases as photon energy decreases. It has been noted that when lowering the kVp for contrast-enhanced studies, there is superior enhancement of iodine, which improves the characterization of hypervascular or hypovascular pathologies. The images obtained using lower tube potentials tend to be much noisier, mainly due to the higher absorption of low-energy photons by the patient. There is a tradeoff between image noise and contrast enhancement. For noncontrast CT examinations, the benefit of lower kV has not been established since soft-tissue contrast is not highly dependent on the tube potential.

Constant Milliamperage-Second

The term constant mAs is the selection of exposure time (gantry rotation) and the x-ray tube current prior to scanning. Images taken with a rotation time of 1 second and a tube current of 100 will produce the same results as a scan performed with a rotation time of 2 seconds and a tube current of 50 keeping all other technical factors constant. Milliamperage-second determines the quantity of photons reaching the detectors, and is directly proportional to the dose; therefore, if the mAs is doubled, the dose will be doubled. An increase in mAs improves image quality by reducing noise with the negative result of increasing patient dose.

Effective Milliamperage-Second

The term effective mAs is utilized with multi-slice CT and signifies the mAs per slice. The mathematical equation is as follows:

$$Effective\ mAs = True\ mAs \div pitch$$

In other words, to keep the effective mAs constant, when increasing the pitch, the true mAs must also be increased to keep the same image quality and SNR.

Exposure technique factors (mA and kVp) do not directly affect image density and contrast respectively, as they do in film-based radiology, so they never look over-exposed. CT scanner manufactures provide an average technique to use for all protocols; hence, it is not common for technologists to decrease the mAs for patients below the average size, which in turn results in excessive dose to the patient. To remedy this situation, it is important to use the automated tube current modulation technique whenever possible. In times that it is not feasible, be in conscience of the patient's size, muscle mass, and pathology when setting manual mAs settings.

Z—Overscanning

In spiral/helical scanning an additional rotation before and after the planned length is necessary to provide inter-polation data for the image reconstruction process. In a single-slice scanner, a half to one additional rotation is required; whereas, in a multi-slice scanner the number of rotations depends on interpolation method, the pitch, and the reconstructed image width. This overscanning process for multi-slice scanners leads to greater patient dose than for single-slice scanners because the total beam width col-limation is usually greater. This technique may also lead to significant but unseen exposure to radiosensitive organs.

Filters

CT filters are added materials that increase effective x-ray energy by absorbing low-energy photons and designed to reduce patient dose. The two types of filters incorporated into all CT scanners are the adaptive filter and the bow-tie filter. Both filters are automatically selected when the technologist chooses the body part of interest. It is impor-tant to review all the technical factors prior to scanner to determine that all factors chosen will produce the lowest dose to the patient without sacrificing image quality.

Collimation

When speaking of collimation for multi-slice CT scanners we need to consider the z-axis geometry efficiency. In multi-slice scanners the beam width includes the beam falling on the detectors and the penumbra. Since the penumbra is not used to produce an image, the beam width is increased to extend the penumbra past the active detectors; therefore, the z-axis geometry can be defined as the ratio of the z-axis dose profile falling on the active detectors to the total z-axis profile. The z-axis geometry efficiency is greater at wider beam width collimations and decreases significantly for tighter collimation. As the effi-ciency decreases, dose increases, for instance, wider colli-mators lead to a 10% increase in dose when compared to

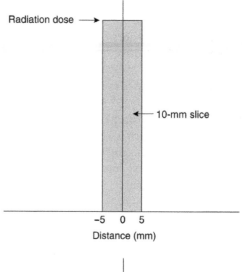

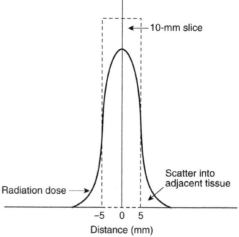

Figure 1.2. The implications of focal spot penumbra on dose. **(A)** Demonstrates the ideal dose profile of a single-slice scanner with a nominal collimation of 10 mm, taking into consideration no scatter radiation exists. **(B)** Demonstrates the actual dose profile including the scatter radiation, which is unavoidable and increases with the size of the object and the slice thickness. (Reproduced, with permission, from Romans LE. *Computed Tomography for Technologists: A Comprehensive Text.* Baltimore, MD: Wolters Kluwer Lippincott Williams & Wilkins; 2011.)

single-slice scanners; whereas, tighter collimations can result in a tripling or more in dose (Fig. 1.2).

Pitch

Pitch can be described as the ratio of the distance the table travels per one revolution of the x-ray tube to the total colli-mated beam width. If the mAs is kept constant as the table moves, the radiation dose is proportionally decreased as pitch is increased. A pitch of 1 means the table advances the same distance as the z-axis width of the total beam collima-tion, implying no gap of patient tissue exposure in the scan-ning region. When increasing the pitch by a factor of 2 and all other factors remaining the same the dose is decreased by one-half; therefore, pitch is inversely proportional to dose.

Patient Centering

Patient centering is sometimes overlooked as a factor affecting dose. When positioning the patient, they must be isocentered in the gantry for precise anatomical imaging. Incorrect centering degrades image quality and increases dose to the patient especially when utilizing the automated tube current modulation. If a patient is centered too close to the x-ray tube, there can be inappropriate magnification of the localizer image resulting in higher CT outputs and increased dose. It has been noted by Mayo-Smith et al. through a case study of a CT abdominal examination, when the patient was centered appropriately the overall $CTDI_{volume}$ was 15 mGy and the SSDE was 17.9 mGy. Another factor playing a part in centering is the bow-tie filter. Centering the patient outside the scan field of view underutilizes the bow-tie filter's performance. As stated earlier in the text, the purpose of this filter is to increase image quality while decreasing patient dose.

Number of Detectors

For multi-slice CT scanners, the number of detector rows dictates dose. As the detector rows increase from 4 to 64, the dose decreases. In other words, the number of detector rows is inversely proportional to the measured radiation dose.

Automated Tube Current Modulation

The purpose of automated tube current modulation is to regulate the pulse of current through different body tissues with the objective of reducing the overall radiation dose to the patient. It allows sufficient photons to pass through the widest parts of the patient without unnecessary dose to the narrower parts. ATCM aims to deliver a specified image quality across a range of patient sizes by varying the duration of the exposure. It tends to increase $CTDI_{volume}$ for large patients and decrease $CTDI_{volume}$ for small patients relative to a reference size. The reference mA chosen for a particular patient depends on the allowable noise in the final image reconstruction for image interpretation. This technique has been addressed as "the most important technique for maintaining constant image quality while optimizing radiation dose" (Seeram, 2009).

ATCM operates by adjusting the tube current (mA) in real time throughout the duration of the scan based on the differences in attenuation in the transverse or x–y axis and in the z-axis or longitudinal direction. The angular x–y axis modulation feature adjusts the tube current as the x-ray tube rotates around the patient to compensate for attenuation changes from the AP projection to the lateral projection. The angular tube current modulation guarantees there will be a constant uniform noise level throughout the entire scan.

Longitudinal (z-axis) tube current modulation feature adjusts the tube current as patient attenuation changes in the longitudinal direction (from head to toe) with the same principle of keeping a constant uniform noise level. The CT localizer radiograph is used to estimate patient attenuation along the scan length.

Angular–Longitudinal Tube Current Modulation

Angular–longitudinal tube current modulation feature incorporates the properties of both angular and longitudinal tube current modulation. It adjusts the tube current based on the patient's overall attenuation by modulating the tube current in the angular (x–y) and longitudinal (z) dimensions to adapt to the patient's shape. This technique is the "most comprehensive approach to CT dose reduction because the x-ray dose is adjusted according to the patient-specific attenuation in all three planes" (Seeram, 2009).

The common manufacturer names for angular modulation systems are:

- Smart Scan—GE Healthcare
- DOM-Dose Modulation—Phillips
- Care Dose—Siemens

The common manufacturer names for angular–longitudinal modulation systems are:

- Smart mA—GE Healthcare
- Z-DOM—Phillips
- Care Dose 4D—Siemens
- Sure Exposure—Toshiba

Gating

The most challenging CT examination is cardiac imaging. The coronary arteries are situated close to the heart muscle, because this muscle shows rapid movement during the cardiac cycle, it is imperative to freeze that motion for clear delineation of the individual arteries. Imaging of the heart is best attained when the heart is at rest or during the diastolic phase. During data acquisition, the patient's ECG is recorded, in order to synchronize the image reconstruction with the heart motion. There are two types of cardiac gating: prospective ECG triggering and retrospective ECG gating. Both techniques provide good image quality, but have different properties in regard to radiation dose.

Prospective ECG Triggering

The main advantage is its simplicity, since it is similar to conventional step-and-shoot CT imaging. The scan time is inversely proportional to the patient's heart rate, slice width, and number of detector rows. The radiation dose is

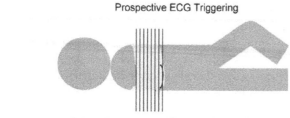

Prospective ECG Triggering

Conventional axial "partial scan" (step and shoot)

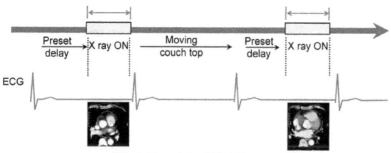

Preset delay → X ray ON   Moving couch top   Preset delay → X ray ON

ECG

Temporal resolution 200–250 msec
Radiation dose minimized
Limited data set

Figure 1.3. Diagram of prospective ECG triggering scan mode during a cardiac scoring protocol. Note images are acquired sequentially, lending to less radiation dose than for the retrospective gating mode. (Reproduced, with permission, from Seeram E. *Computed Tomography: Physical Principles, Clinical Applications, and Quality Control.* 3rd ed. St. Louis, MO: Saunders Elsevier; 2009.)

limited with this technique, since the x-ray source is only activated during image acquisition. With prospective triggering image quality may be degraded if irregular heart rhythms occur (Fig. 1.3).

Retrospective ECG Gating

During the retrospective gating method the scanner continuously acquires data in spiral mode, while the table travels at a constant speed with the data being acquired continuously by all detector rows. With this method pitch is of utmost importance. If pitch is too high and heart rate is too low, a gap in the table could exist in which no data are being recorded. If pitch is too low the scan is too long exposing the patient to too much radiation. Optimal pitch depends on heart rate and reconstruction algorithms (Fig. 1.4).

Retrospective ECG Gating

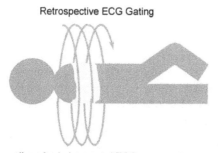

Continuous recording of spiral scan and ECG ⟶

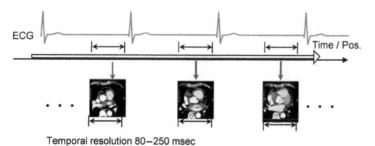

ECG

Time / Pos.

Temporal resolution 80–250 msec
Radiation dose higher than prospective triggering

Figure 1.4. Illustration of the retrospective ECG gating utilized for helical cardiac imaging. The retrospective data are reviewed with reconstruction occurring at the R-R interval, but the entire cycle can be reconstructed and used to determine ejection fraction. (Reproduced, with permission, from Seeram E. *Computed Tomography: Physical Principles, Clinical Applications, and Quality Control.* 3rd ed. St. Louis, MO: Saunders Elsevier; 2009.)

RADIATION PROTECTION AND SHIELDING

Gonadal shielding should be employed when the reproductive organs are within 4–5 cm of the x-ray beam, as long as it does not interfere with the area being examined, particularly important to shield children and adults of reproductive age. The types of shielding in CT include:

Flat contact (aprons)
- they are wrapped completely around the patient's gonadal region
- this method is known as above and below

Shaped contact
- designed to protect the male reproductive organs

Thyroid and breast shields
- constructed of bismuth germanium
- not actually considered a shield but a filter that eliminates low-energy photons from being absorbed into the patient
  - thus reducing dose
- to reduce artifacts
  - place a pad between body and shield

DOSE MEASUREMENT

Radiation Units

The milligray is a measure of the absorption of ionizing energy per unit mass of matter and is measured in joules per kilogram. This unit is used to measure the radiant ionizing energy from the scanner $CTDI_{volume}$ and absorbed radiation dose in the patient. Milligray is a measure of the absorption of ionizing energy per unit mass of matter and is measured in joules per kilogram. The milligray is used as a unit of measure for both the radiant ionizing energy from the scanner $CTDI_{volume}$ and absorbed radiation dose in the patient. The millisievert is the unit of effective radiation dose that is dependent on the amount of absorbed radiation (in milligrays) and the relative radiosensitivity of the exposed organs. It is derived from the absorbed dose to a generic reference for both sexes, all ages, standard-size patient, and is meant to normalize stochastic risk by a representative average whole-body dose.

CT Dose Index

CT dose index (CTDI) is used to quantitate patient exposure. It is measured by the manufacturer and checked by the on-site physicist utilizing an ionization chamber. It is the measurement of the radiation dose at the intended slice thickness as well as that from the penumbra. The values are estimated by software within the scanner and displayed in mGy along with the patient identification information in the DICOM header. The term CTDI was developed by the Food and Drug Administration (FDA); therefore, labeled $CTDI_{FDA}$. The $CTDI_{FDA}$ signifies the mean absorbed dose in the scanned plane object volume with the capability of measuring dose for the minimum slice thickness of 7 mm.

$CTDI_{100}$ was introduced to the community due to the shortcomings of the $CTDI_{FDA}$. This is a linear dose measurement allowed calculations of the index for 100 mm along the length of the entire pencil ionization chamber, regardless of the nominal slice width, permitting thinner slice thickness to be measured. $CTDI_{100}$ is not of clinical use because it does not account for the tissue variations of the human body.

To improve the accuracy of dose measurements, the weighted CTDI was introduced. This measurement accounts for the average dose in the x–y axis instead of the z-axis. $CTDI_w$ is calculated by using an ionization chamber positioned in the center and at the periphery of the phantom. It is simply calculated as:

$$CTDI_w = \left(\frac{2}{3}\right)(CTDI_{100})\, periphery + \left(\frac{1}{3}\right)(CTDI_{100})\, center$$

This equation demonstrates that $CTDI_w$ takes into account for the absorbed dose at skin level along with the absorbed dose in the center of the body.

When performing spiral examinations the $CTDI_w$ dose calculation is limited, since it does not report the dose measurement in the z-axis, so $CTDI_{volume}$ was devised to include the dose distribution in all three planes (x, y, and z). The formula for calculating dose distribution for modern CT scanners is as follows:

$$CTDI_{volume} = CTDI_w \div pitch$$

Volume CT dose index ($CTDI_{volume}$) is internationally recognized and perhaps the most important measure of the radiation output from the CT scanner. Its units are denoted in milligrays. $CTDI_{volume}$ is a measured quantity used only with CT. It is measured by using a pencil ionization chamber placed in a standard circular plastic (polymethyl methacrylate) phantom. $CTDI_{volume}$ reported by the scanner is an estimate of the average radiation dose within a volume of tissue when that tissue is the same size and attenuation as the plastic phantom. There are two sizes of phantoms used to measure $CTDI_{volume}$: a 16-cm phantom for adult head and pediatric head and torso calculations and a 32-cm phantom for adult torso measurements. Importantly, the method for calculating $CTDI_{volume}$ is standardized across all manufacturers and models using the two reference phantoms. Thus, $CTDI_{volume}$ is one of the key radiation descriptors in CT and is useful for comparing different scanner outputs from different imaging protocols and for comparing the same examination type on different CT machines. It is dependent on various machine settings, including x-ray tube current, voltage, z-axis collimation, and pitch. It is important to note that this measurement is independent of the patient size and length of body region scanned. With tube current modulation the $CTDI_{volume}$ displayed at the end of the scan is an average $CTDI_{volume}$ over the scanned length. Although the units (milligrays) are the same for both $CTDI_{volume}$ and patient absorbed dose, it is important to recognize that $CTDI_{volume}$ is not the true patient dose, it is only an approximation and guideline. It is mandatory that all CT scanners display $CTDI_{volume}$ on the CT operator's console before the scan begins. This allows the technologist to see what the radiation output will be before the scan actually starts and can modify the technique if needed. CT manufacturers are introducing a software technique called "dose check" to allow CT users to set a maximum $CTDI_{volume}$ value for each CT protocol and to alert the user when any change in scan parameters are chosen that can lead to values higher than the limit. Dose check was recently added as a requirement by the U.S. FDA to avoid radiation injuries.

Multiple-Slice Average Dose

Multiple-slice average dose (MSAD) was the first dose descriptor to be introduced into the CT world. This descriptor was based on the single-slice step-and-shoot scanners. To determine the dose, a series of scan are performed. As the scan proceeds, the patient is moved a particular distance, known as the bed index (BI), between each scan. Each slice delivers a characteristic bell-shaped dose. Regions where the bell curves overlap, dose is higher than from just on single scan. The dose from all scans is averaged to form the total patient dose.

Dose Length Product

The dose length product (DLP) is yet another dose descriptor that measures the total exposure the patient receives for the entire scan. If the $CTDI_{volume}$ and the scan length are known, the DLP can be easily calculated by the following equation:

$$DLP = CTDI_{volume} \times Scan\ Length$$

Radiation Quantities and Their Units

Absorbed Dose

Absorbed dose can be defined as the amount of energy absorbed per unit mass of the material. It measures the energy deposited in a unit mass at a certain position. The quantity of absorbed radiation within the body carries a certain amount or risks; therefore, it is the technologists' responsibility to monitor all patients' dose and utilize radiation protection methods at all times.

Effective Dose

Effective dose quantifies the risk from partial-body exposure to that from an equivalent whole-body dose. This dose accounts for the type of radiation and the radiosensitivity of different tissues. In other words, effective dose is related to the risk of carcinogenesis and with the possibilities of genetic effects. The effective dose from a CT examination is equivalent to natural background radiation.

Size-Specific Dose Estimate

Size-specific dose estimate (SSDE) is a newer CT measurement that incorporates patient size as a variable correction factor to better estimate patient dose. The SSDE is determined by multiplying $CTDI_{volume}$ by a conversion factor based on the patient's effective diameter. The effective diameter is defined as the square root of the product of the anterior–posterior and lateral patient diameter (Mayer-Smith). While not currently displayed with other CT parameters such as the $CTDI_{volume}$ or the DLP on the DICOM header of an individual patient's studies, SSDE could be calculated automatically by the scanner using patient localizer images.

PATIENT DOSE REDUCTION

Radiation Protection Principles

Radiation protection principles include:

Justification
- must be a benefit associated with every exposure

Optimization
- using the ALARA principle without degrading image quality

Dose limitation
- dose an individual receives annually or accumulates over a working lifetime
  - these doses were established by the ICRP and the NCRP

Pediatric

Children are at the highest risk from radiation damage, because their cells are still rapidly dividing as they are growing. Their cumulative effect over a lifetime of exposure may increase their lifetime risk of cancer; therefore, radiation protection is an integral part of the pediatric CT procedure. To minimize radiation dose to pediatric patients the following guidelines should be considered:

Have all CT request screened by the radiologist

Tailor the study to the diagnostic needs of the patient

Lead shielding should be employed using the "above and below" method

Immobilization provides patient safety and images free of motion artifacts

Utilize low-dose techniques when optimum spatial resolution can be spared

Gantry should be angled 20-degree cephalad when performing axial brain scans

- avoid exposure to the lens of the eyes

Adult

All radiology examinations cause an effective dose to the patient and should be considered as a potential risk. CT protocols should be tailored to specific patient size, anatomy imaged, and clinical indications for the examination. The goal is to customize each examination to its clinical implications for each patient. By doing so this would reduce variability in examination techniques. The following is a list of ways to modify CT protocols with the goal of dose reduction:

Taylor protocols to indications

Use tube current modulation

Consider varying tube voltage based on patient size and examination indication

Accurate patient centering

Only scan the region of interest on follow-up imaging

Limit the number of phases

- utilize the split injection protocols

Review protocols examining section collimation

Consider iterative reconstruction algorithm software

- to decrease image noise, allowing for lower-dose technique

Establish a dedicated CT protocol team

To continually monitor protocols and techniques to further reduce dose

(Mayer-Smith, 2014)

Radiation Dose Monitoring

With the increased awareness of CT dose in the communities, dose monitoring has become imperative. The ACR has developed a dose registry for individual institutions to review dose trends with a safety committee composed of radiologists, physicists, and technologists. Many institutions have their CT equipment connected to the ACR dose registry. This registry allows radiologists to compare their doses to other practices. With this program, you map your examination types to match the definitions of the ACR and the anonymized data are automatically sent electronically to the ACR from each scanner. The ACR then issues quarterly reports comparing parameters such as $CTDI_{volume}$, DLP, and SSDE by examination type and scanner for your institution and compares your practice's averages to national averages, to regional averages, and by type of practice. This dose-tracking software identifies outliers from your institution by scanner and examination type. The institution can then set alerts if the radiation dose for a particular examination's thresholds are exceeded and then quality metrics can be maintained in a retrospective fashion. When the outlier results are identified, then the examination can be reviewed by the site to determine if the protocol was followed and correct technique was used.

Review Questions

Multiple Choice: Select the one single best answer.

1. What dose descriptor is calculated with the following formula? $X = (2/3)(CTDI_{100})$ periphery $+ (1/3)(CTDI_{100})$ center

    (A) DLP
    (B) $CTDI_{volume}$
    (C) $CTDI_w$
    (D) MSAD

2. When evaluating a patient's laboratory results, an elevated creatinine level is an indication of what medical condition?

    (A) congestive heart failure
    (B) liver failure
    (C) impaired renal function
    (D) pregnancy

3. When performing an invasive CT examination, such as an RFA of the liver, a partial thromboplastin time (PTT) is drawn. What does a partial thromboplastin time test measure?

    (A) the time required to increase the platelet count by 10%
    (B) time required to manufacture prothrombin
    (C) time required to locate an decrease the platelet count by 10%
    (D) time for normal clot formation in plasma

4. What type of consent is obtained prior to a noninvasive CT procedure?

    (A) simple expressed
    (B) implied
    (C) written informed
    (D) informed

5. Which of the following methods must be utilized when placing an IV line in an antecubital vein?

    (A) the technologist must wash his/her hands prior to starting an IV line
    (B) the technologist should anesthetize the area using a topical agent
    (C) the technologist should release the tourniquet as the needle is being inserted
    (D) the technologist should make a minimum of four attempts in the arm before giving up

6. When administering IV contrast to a patient with a mastectomy, which vein should be chosen?

    (A) the vein on the same side as the removed breast
    (B) the vein on the contralateral side
    (C) the dorsal pedal veins
    (D) mastectomy patients should never receive intravenous contrast

7. What instrument is used to measure radiation exposure?

    (A) Geiger counter
    (B) ionization chamber
    (C) reference detector chamber
    (D) solid-state detector aperture

8. What method is used to lower the viscosity of contrast media before injecting?

   (A) heating the media to room temperature
   (B) heating the media to body temperature
   (C) mixing the media with a saline solution
   (D) viscosity of the media can never be altered

9. For radiation workers in the United States, what is their dose limitation per year?

   (A) 20 mSv
   (B) 50 mSv
   (C) 75 mSv
   (D) 100 mSv

10. A female patient arrives in the ER with severe right flank pain. The patient is 5′4″ weighing 100 lb. What technical factor would you change to reduce her radiation dose?

    (A) kVp
    (B) mAs
    (C) collimation
    (D) detector configuration

11. Which of the following is not part of the patient identification process?

    (A) establishing an initial rapport with the patient
    (B) obtaining informed consent
    (C) asking the patient to state his/her full name
    (D) asking the patient his/her date of birth

12. What is the premedication strategy for a patient with a prior allergic reaction to iodinated contrast media before a contrast-enhanced CT?

    (A) premedication with steroids and antihistamines
    (B) increase in fluids for 48 hours before the examination
    (C) having the patient stop his/her blood thinning medication
    (D) administration of a negative contrast agent

13. When a technologist examines a patient prior to placing an IV catheter for a contrast-enhanced CT study, which of the following veins would you most likely use?

    (A) vein of Galen
    (B) basilar vein
    (C) medial cubital vein
    (D) radial vein

14. Dose descriptors are used to identify approximate patient doses, which of the following is the dose descriptor utilized for modern multi-slice CT scanners?

    (A) multiple-scan average dose (MSAD)
    (B) dose profile
    (C) CTDI$_{volume}$
    (D) Roentgen

15. What type of needle is equipped with plastic projections on either side that aid in holding the needle during venipuncture?

    (A) butterfly needle
    (B) small gauge straight needle
    (C) angiocatheter
    (D) large gauge straight needle

16. What is the normal range of respiration for an adult?

    (A) 5–10 BPM
    (B) 12–20 BPM
    (C) 20–30 BPM
    (D) 35–50 BPM

17. What term refers to the number of ions formed when a substance dissociates in a solution?

    (A) solubility
    (B) osmolality
    (C) concentration
    (D) iodination

18. Which of the following is considered a severe reaction to an iodinated contrast reaction?

    (A) dyspnea
    (B) itching
    (C) nasal stuffiness
    (D) cardiopulmonary arrest

19. The dose to the central slice plus the dose from the scatter into nearby slices equals which of the following dose descriptors?

    (A) MSAD
    (B) SV
    (C) mAs setting
    (D) R

20. What is the dose descriptor that can be calculated if the length of the irradiated volume (scan length) and the $CTDI_{volume}$ are known?

    (A) $CTDI_{100}$
    (B) MSAD
    (C) DLP
    (D) Exposure

21. Of the following terms, which is a parenteral route of administering medication?

    (A) sublingual
    (B) intramuscular
    (C) oral
    (D) rectal

22. What is the measure of the total number of particles in contrast media per kilogram of water?

    (A) viscosity
    (B) osmolality
    (C) ionicity
    (D) iodination

23. Which of the following is a characteristic of ionic contrast media?

    (A) Higher osmolality
    (B) Does not increase the osmolality of the blood serum
    (C) Does not separate in water
    (D) Ratio of iodine atoms to active particles is 3:1

24. Of the following laboratory test listed below, which test can be utilized to evaluate the renal function of a patient?

    (A) D-dimer
    (B) INR
    (C) Glomerular filtration rate
    (D) PTT

25. The mAs for a particular procedure remains constant and the pitch changes from 2 to 1; what change does it have on dose?

    (A) decrease
    (B) increase
    (C) remains the same
    (D) there is no relationship between pitch and dose

26. Which of the following is deemed a moderate reaction to contrast media?

    (A) convulsions
    (B) seizures
    (C) dyspnea
    (D) nasal congestion

27. Which of the following is a property of nonionic contrast media?

    (A) it contains a negatively charged anion that consists of a benzene ring with a negatively charged amino acid group
    (B) iodine concentration is maintained without increasing the number of particles in solution; therefore, it does not increase the osmolality of the blood serum and does not change the osmotic pressure in the bloodstream
    (C) renal effects are especially significant
    (D) may result hypervolemia

28. What is the relationship between the dose and the number of detector rows?

    (A) as number of detector rows increase dose increases
    (B) as number of detector rows increases dose decreases
    (C) as number of detector rows increases dose triples
    (D) there is no relationship between dose and number of detector rows

29. Which of the following is a characteristic of a low-osmolality contrast media?

    (A) can decrease blood supply to the kidneys
    (B) can cause hypervolemia

(C) can cause shock in dehydrated patients

(D) less toxic

30. What is the principle behind the benefit of lower kV in some clinical applications?

   (A) superior enhancement of iodine

   (B) inferior enhancement of iodine

   (C) there is actually no benefit of reducing kVp

   (D) it increases patient dose

31. What radiation dose saving technique adjusts the tube current based on the patient's overall attenuation by modulating the tube current in the angular (x–y) and longitudinal (z) dimensions to adapt to the patient's shape?

   (A) angular–longitudinal tube current modulation

   (B) prospective ECG triggering

   (C) high-resolution CT

   (D) automated tube current modulation

32. What is the quantifying risk from partial-body exposure to that from the equivalent whole-body dose?

   (A) absorbed dose

   (B) effective dose

   (C) threshold effect

   (D) deterministic effect

33. Which of the following is a sign of an anaphylactic reaction?

   (A) diffuse urticarial

   (B) facial edema without dyspnea

(C) bronchospasm with significant hypoxia

(D) limited cutaneous edema

Multiple Response: Select one or more correct answers.

34. Which of the following statements are characteristics of power injectors?

   (A) they are only used for CT angiography studies

   (B) the maximum volume of each syringe is 200 cc

   (C) they cannot be used to inject ionic contrast

   (D) they have internal heating mechanisms to maintain the temperature of the contrast

35. Which of the following statements are part of the patient interaction process?

   (A) It is important to establish a feeling of trust with the patient

   (B) It is important to have the patient explain the procedure instructions back to you

   (C) Instructions should always be given orally, never using written material

   (D) It is important to access the patient's degree of anxiety

36. Which of the following are contraindications for the administration of IV contrast?

   (A) asthma

   (B) shellfish allergies

   (C) atopic syndrome

   (D) cardiac dysfunction

Answers and Explanations

1. **(C)** To improve the accuracy of dose measurements, the weighted CTDI was the introduction. This measurement accounts for the average dose in the x–y axis instead of the z-axis. $CTDI_w$ is calculated by using an ionization chamber positioned in the center and at the periphery of the phantom. *(Seeram, 3rd ed., p. 228)*

2. **(C)** Creatinine is a chemical waste molecule that is generated from muscle metabolism. It is transported through the bloodstream to the kidneys. The kidneys filter out most of the creatinine and dispose of it in the urine. Normal levels are approximately 0.6–1.3 mg/dL depending on the laboratory reference values. Any values >1.3 mg/dL is an indication of renal impairment. *(Ehrlich and Coakes, 8th ed., pp. 223–224)*

3. **(D)** Partial thromboplastin time measures the time required for clot formation in normal plasma. The normal PTT range is 30–45 seconds, whereas normal APTT range (activated partial thromboplastin time) is 25–40 seconds. Patients on blood thinner have a 1.5–2.5 time greater range. A result >100 seconds indicates spontaneous bleeding. *(Ehrlich and Coakes, 8th ed., p. 223)*

4. **(A)** Simple expressed consent is the process of obtaining a patient's permission to perform a procedure and is generally utilized for noninvasive procedures. It is as straightforward as explaining the procedure to the patient and then asking whether he/she agrees to have the examination. A technologist should never assume consent. *(Gurley, 7th ed., pp. 145–147)*

5. **(A)** Medically aseptic handwashing is an easy and effective method to control the transmission of disease. Handwashing with soap and water is still recommended by the CDC to physically remove spores from the surface of contaminated hands. Alcohol-based rubs should not replace handwashing with soap and water when hands are visibly soiled or contaminated with blood or body secretions. *(Ehrlich and Coakes, 8th ed., p. 171)*

6. **(B)** When a patient undergoes a mastectomy, many of the lymph nodes are removed. The removal of these nodes disrupts or damages the normal drainage pattern in the lymph nodes. Removing the axillary lymph nodes increases the risk for developing lymphedema; therefore, IV injections should be placed in the contralateral arm as not to cause an increase of fluid on the mastectomy side. *(National Breast Cancer Foundation)*

7. **(B)** An ionization chamber is used to measure dose. The chamber is positioned at the point of measurement. When radiation falls upon the chamber, it ionizes the air in the chamber to produce ion pairs. The measure of the amount of ionization produced in a specific mass of air by x-rays is exposure. This ionization indicates the amount of radiation to which a patient is exposed. *(Seeram, 3rd ed., pp. 219–220)*

8. **(B)** Solutions with high viscosity, as with nonionic contrast media, require greater injection pressures for administration. Viscosity may be reduced somewhat by warming the media to body temperature

before administering. *(Ehrlich and Coakes, 8th ed., p. 381)*

9. **(B)** Dose limitation addresses the dose that an individual receives annually or accumulates over a working lifetime. It ensures the dose is within the limits set by the International Council on Radiation Protection. The dose limitation for a radiation worker in the United States is 50 mSv/year. *(Seeram, 3rd ed., p. 220)*

10. **(B)** Of the technical factors listed, mAs is the most straightforward factor to change, since mAs is directly proportional to dose. *(Seeram, 3rd ed., p. 230)*

11. **(B)** The Joint Commission, which accredits healthcare organizations, recommends healthcare personal to utilize two forms of patient identification, the patient's full name and date of birth. This validates the right patient and the right study is being performed. *(Ehrlich and Coakes, 8th ed., pp. 111–113)*

12. **(A)** The American College of Radiology suggests the following two regimens: Prednisone—50 mg by mouth at 13 hours, 7 hours, and 1 hour before contrast media injection, plus diphenhydramine—50 mg intravenously, intramuscularly, or by mouth 1 hour before contrast media, or methylprednisolone—32 mg by mouth 12 hours and 2 hours before contrast media injection. An antihistamine (as in option A) can also be added to this regimen injection. *(The American College of Radiology Manual, p. 9)*

13. **(C)** The median cubital vein ascends in an oblique and medial course to create an anastomosis between the basilic and cephalic veins. The median cubital vein is a common site for venipuncture. *(Kelly, 3rd ed., p. 564)*

14. **(C)** To consider the dose in the z-axis, the $CTDI_{volume}$ was introduced. It is a standardized measure of the radiation output of a CT system, measured in a cylindrical acrylic phantom that enables users to gauge the amount of emitted radiation and compare the radiation output between different scan protocols or scanners. *(Mayer-Smith, 2014)*

15. **(A)** A butterfly needle is a bare, stainless steel, variable gauge needle with flat plastic projections on either side of the base, a flexible small-bore transparent tubing (often 20–35 cm long), and finally a connector. The plastic panels can be grasped and then anchored by tape to the patient's skin, which secures the needle at the puncture site, while the connector attaches to another device, such as a syringe. These types of needles are used for hand injections (pediatric patients) and should never be used with power injectors since the needle remains in the vein. *(Ehrlich and Coakes, 8th ed., p. 273)*

16. **(B)** The normal range of adult respiration is 12–20 breaths per minute. Slow breathing with fewer than 12 breaths is termed bradypnea, while rapid breathing with breaths exceeding 20 is called tachypnea. *(Ehrlich and Coakes, 8th ed., pp. 218–219)*

17. **(B)** Osmolality is the measurement of the total number of particles in the contrast solution per kilogram of water. It is the direct measurement of the ionization of a solute in a solvent. The osmolality of human blood is approximately 300 mOsm/kg. The osmolality of water-soluble contrast ranges from 300 to 1,000 mOsm/kg. When utilizing a solution that exceeds the osmolality of blood serum (a term known as hyperosmolar) results in negative effects to the human body. *(Ehrlich and Coakes, 8th ed., p. 474)*

18. **(D)** Cardiopulmonary arrest is a nonspecific end-stage result that can be caused by a variety of severe reactions, both allergic-like and physiologic. It is unclear what etiology caused the cardiopulmonary arrest. *(The American College of Radiology Manual, p. 102)*

19. **(A)** The value of MSAD is the average value of all profiles over one scan interval in the central portion of the profile. *(Seeram, 3rd ed., p. 226)*

20. **(C)** DLP replicates the radiation output and the potential biological effects attributed to the scan. The DLP can be calculated by the product of the $CTDI_{volume}$ and the scan length. *(Mayer-Smith, 2014)*

21. **(B)** Parenteral medication is taken into the body in a manner other than through the digestive canal. This form of medication route is classified as intradermal, subcutaneous, intramuscular, intravenous,

intra-arterial, and intrathecal. *(Ehrlich and Coakes, 8th ed., pp. 265–270)*

22. **(B)** Osmolality is the measurement of the total number of particles in the contrast solution per kilogram of water. It is the direct measurement of the ionization of a solute in a solvent. The osmolality of human blood is approximately 300 mOsm/kg. The osmolality of water-soluble contrast ranges from 300 to 1,000 mOsm/kg. When utilizing a solution that exceeds the osmolality of blood serum (a term known as hyperosmolar) results in negative effects to the human body. *(Ehrlich and Coakes, 8th ed., p. 273)*

23. **(A)** Ionic contrast is considered a high-osmolality contrast media (HOCM), which separates in water yielding two particles. The negatively charged anion consists of a benzene ring with a negatively charged amino acid group, while the positively charged cation contains a sodium or methylglucamine complex. Ratio of iodine atoms to active particles is 3:2. *(Ehrlich and Coakes, 8th ed., p. 381)*

24. **(C)** Glomerular filtration rate is the best test to measure kidney function and to determine stages of kidney disease. It is calculated from the results of the patient's blood creatinine test, age, race, and gender. *(National Kidney Foundation)*

25. **(B)** Pitch and dose are inversely proportional to each other. As pitch increases, the $CTDI_{volume}$ decreases and as pitch decreases, $CTDI_{volume}$ increases. *(Seeram, 3rd ed., p. 232)*

26. **(C)** Moderate reactions occur in approximately 0.2–0.4% of patients. Signs and symptoms are more pronounced and commonly require medical management. Some of these reactions have the potential to become severe if not treated. Moderate reactions include pronounced cutaneous reactions, tachycardia, bradycardia, hypotension, bronchospasm, hypertension, dyspnea, laryngeal edema, pulmonary edema, and/or wheezing. *(The American College of Radiology Manual, p. 101)*

27. **(B)** Nonionic contrast is considered a low-osmolality contrast media that does not separate in water. The iodine concentration is maintained without increasing the number of particles in solu-

tion; therefore, it does not increase the osmolality of the blood serum and does not change the osmotic pressure in the bloodstream. Ratio of iodine atoms to active particles is 3:1. It is safer for patients with compromised cardiac status. *(Ehrlich and Coakes, 8th ed., p. 381)*

28. **(B)** For multi-slice CT scanners, the number of detector rows dictates dose. As the detector rows increases from 4 to 64, the dose decreases. In other words, the number of detector rows is inversely proportional to the measured radiation dose. *(Seeram, 3rd ed., p. 233)*

29. **(D)** When a compound has lower osmolality, it contains fewer particles thus resulting in fewer or less severe adverse reactions. Low-osmolality agents have the tendency to be less toxic to the systemic system as compared to those containing a higher osmolality. *(Ehrlich and Coakes, 8th ed., p. 381)*

30. **(A)** The principle behind the benefit of lower kV in some clinical applications is that the attenuation coefficient of iodine increases as photon energy decreases. It has been noted that when lowering the kVp for contrast enhanced studies, there is superior enhancement of iodine, which improves the characterization of hypervascular or hypovascular pathologies. *(Mayer-Smith, 2014)*

31. **(A)** Angular–longitudinal tube current modulation feature incorporates the properties of both angular and longitudinal tube current modulation. This technique adjusts the dose according to the patient-specific attenuation in all three planes. *(Seeram, 3rd ed., pp. 237–238)*

32. **(B)** Effective dose is not actually a measurement of dose, but rather a model that predicts the stochastic risk, such as cancer, from a radiation exposure. The dose from a CT examination is comparable to natural background. *(Strategies for Reducing Radiation Dose in CT, Seeram, 3rd ed., p. 221)*

33. **(C)** Severe reactions, while infrequent can rapidly escalate to a life-threatening situation known as anaphylaxis. Anaphylaxis is rapid in onset and is believed to be caused by the release of histamine from certain cells of the lungs, stomach, lining of the blood vessels. These reactions are so severe that

death can occur. *(The American College of Radiology Manual, p. 102)*

34. **(B, D)** Most modern power injector models are constructed with a dual head component equipped with two 200-cc disposable syringes, a heating device, in order to maintain contrast at or near body temperature, and a programmable venous pressure limit mechanism, for the purpose of eliminating extravasations. *(MedRad Stellant D)*

35. **(A, B, D)** Patients scheduled for CT examinations are usually anxious, worried, and/or scarred due to the unknown results of their study. It is imperative the technologist speaks in an audible tone and uses language the patient can understand. This will promote a feeling of trust from the patients and will relieve some of their anxieties. Once the patient receives the instructions, the technologist should have the patient explain the procedure back to him/her to ensure the patient's comprehensive level and cooperation during the scan. *(Ehrlich and Coakes, 8th ed., pp. 208–211)*

36. **(A, C, D)** The predictive value of specific allergies, such as those to shellfish or dairy products, previously thought to be helpful, is now recognized to be unreliable. A significant number of healthcare providers continue to inquire specifically into a patient's history of "allergy" to seafood, especially shellfish. There is no evidence to support the continuation of this practice. *(The American College of Radiology Manual, p. 5)*

Subspecialty List

CHAPTER 2

Imaging Procedures

CROSS-SECTIONAL ANATOMY OF THE HEAD

The brain is one of the most complex and magnificent organs in the human body, but do not be afraid of its complexity. When studying the brain, just look at it like any other organ of the body, take each section at a time and since your brain's neurons record the memory of every event and thought in our lives, it will make this organ much easier to learn. Our brain gives us awareness, processing a constant stream of sensory data. It controls our muscle movements, the secretions of our glands, and even our breathing and internal temperature. Every idea, feeling, and plan is developed by our brain.

Cranial Nerves

The easiest way to study the cranial nerves is to remember this acronym, *On Old Olympus Towering Tops A Friendly Viking Grew Vines And Hops*

Olfactory (I)—sensory nerve for smell

Optic (II)—sensory nerve for vision

Oculomotor (III)—motor nerve for vision

Trochlear (IV)—motor nerve for vision

Trigeminal (V)—motor and sensory nerve of the face consisting of three major divisions
- Ophthalmic (V1)
- Maxillary (V2)
- Mandibular (V3)

Abducens (VI)—motor nerve of the eye

Facial (VII)—motor and sensory for the face

Vestibulocochlear (VIII)—sensory nerve for the ear

Glossopharyngeal (IX)—motor and sensory for swallowing

Vagus (X)—motor and sensory nerve for the neck, thorax, and abdomen

Accessory (IX)—motor nerve of the neck

Hypoglossal (XII)—motor nerve of the tongue

Internal Auditory Canal

Middle Ear

The middle ear is also known as the tympanic cavity. It communicates with both the mastoid antrum and the nasopharynx. Air is conveyed from the nasopharynx to the tympanic cavity through the eustachian tube. The auditory ossicles vibrate in response to sound waves received at the tympanic membrane and transmit these sound waves to the inner ear. The bones of the middle ear are the malleus, incus, and the stapes.

Inner Ear

The inner ear is also known as the bony labyrinth. It consists of the vestibule, semicircular canals, and the cochlea (Figs. 2.1 and 2.2).

Vestibule
- located between the semicircular canals and the cochlea
- two openings
  - oval window—footplate for the stapes
  - vestibular aqueduct—contains the endolymphatic duct

Semicircular canals
- continuous with the vestibule
- identified as three separate passages
  - superior, posterior, and lateral
    - located at right angles of each other
- control equilibrium and balance
- responsible for hearing

Cochlea
- conical structure lying on the internal auditory canal
- within the basilar turn
  - round window
    - allows fluid to move slightly
    - propagation of sound waves

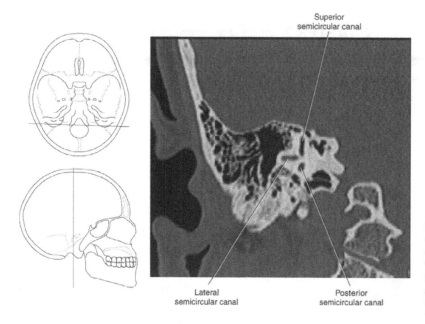

Superior
semicircular canal

Lateral
semicircular canal

Posterior
semicircular canal

Figure 2.1. Coronal image of the semicircular canal, notice the fine detail utilizing a bone/detail convolution kernel coupled with a bone window. (Reproduced, with permission, from Kelley LL, Petersen CM. *Sectional Anatomy for Imaging Professionals*. 3rd ed. St. Louis, MO: Mosby Elsevier; 2013.)

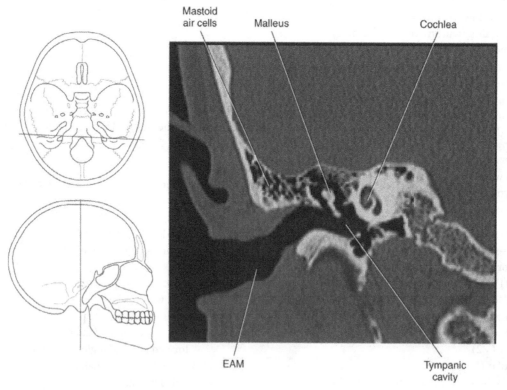

Mastoid
air cells   Malleus   Cochlea

EAM   Tympanic
cavity

Figure 2.2. CT image of the semicircular canal in the coronal position. Observe its position near the external auditory canal. (Reproduced, with permission, from Kelley LL, Petersen CM. *Sectional Anatomy for Imaging Professionals*. 3rd ed. St. Louis, MO: Mosby Elsevier; 2013.)

Pituitary Gland

The pituitary gland is an endocrine gland connected to the hypothalamus. It is nestled in the sella turcica at the base of the brain. It is known as the master gland, since it controls and regulates the functions of many other glands through the action of its six major types of hormones. Through production of its hormones, the pituitary gland controls metabolism, growth, sexual maturation, reproduction, blood pressure, and many other vital physical functions and processes.

Pineal Gland

The pineal gland is an endocrine structure that secretes the hormone Melatonin. This hormone aids in the regulation of the day–night cycles and is responsible for reproduction functions. It is not uncommon for the pineal gland to become calcified; therefore, it will be easily identified on cross sectional images.

Orbits

The bony orbits are cone-shaped recesses that contain the:
- globe, extraocular muscles, blood vessels, nerves, adipose, and connective tissue (Fig. 2.3)

- formed by the frontal, sphenoid, and ethmoid bones of the cranium and the lacrimal, maxillary, palatine, and zygomatic bones of the facial bones
- each orbit presents
  - roof, floor, medial and lateral wall, and an apex

Musculature of the Eye

There are six major muscles of the eye, which work together to control the eye's movement. The rectus muscle group comprises of four muscles, the superior, inferior, medial, and lateral. There function is to adduct and abduct the globe. The oblique muscle group consists of the superior and inferior. This muscle group functions to abduct and rotate the eyeball.

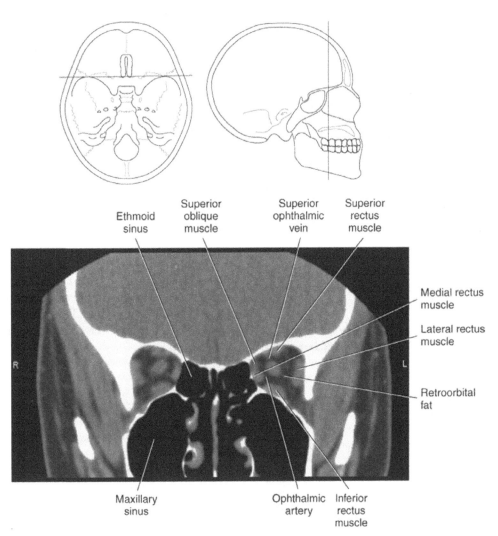

Figure 2.3. Coronal image of the right and the left orbital muscle group. This image scanned in the standard convolution kernel demonstrates good subject contrast between the soft tissue and the muscular tissue. (Reproduced, with permission, from Kelley LL, Petersen CM. *Sectional Anatomy for Imaging Professionals*. 3rd ed. St. Louis, MO: Mosby Elsevier; 2013.)

Muscles of Mastication

Temporalis Muscle

The temporalis is a thin fan-shaped muscle originating on the temporal fossa and inserts on the coronoid process of the mandible. Its role is to lower the mandible and close the mouth.

Masseter Muscle

The masseter muscle is the strongest muscle of the jaw. It arises from the zygomatic arch and inserts on the ramus at the angle of the mandible. It is the major muscle of mastication and serves primarily to elevate the mandible, while the deep tissues help to protract it forward.

Pterygoid Muscles

The pterygoid muscles consist of two muscles, one medial and one lateral. They originate at pterygoid process of the sphenoid bone and insert on the angle of the mandible. The purpose of the medial pterygoid muscle is to close the jaw, while the lateral pterygoid muscle opens the jaw, allowing the mandible to move forward and side to side.

Optic Nerve

The optic nerve commences at the posterior aspect of the globe and courses posteromedially to exit the orbit through the optic canal. The nerve is entirely surrounded by dura mater which is continuous with the meninges of the brain.

Paranasal Sinuses

The paranasal sinuses are air-filled cavities located within the facial bones and skull that communicate with the nasal cavity. Each set of sinuses is named after the bones in which they are located.

Ethmoid
- located within the labyrinths of the ethmoid bone

Maxillary
- located well within the body of the maxilla, beneath the orbit and lateral to the nose
- largest of the paranasal sinuses

Sphenoid
- this group is present at birth and continue to grow until the age of 12
- this paired group occupies the body of the sphenoid bone directly below the sella turcica
- on cross-sectional images they are the most posterior

Frontal
- paired group located inside the frontal bone
- separated along the sagittal plane by the septum

Maxillofacial Bones

The facial bones consist of:

- 2 maxilla
- 2 zygoma
- 2 lacrimal
- 2 nasal
- 2 palatine
- 2 inferior nasal conchea
- 1 vomer
- 1 mandible

Cranium (Fig. 2.4)
- 1 frontal
- 2 temporal
- 2 parietal
- 1 occipital

Cerebellum

The cerebellum is the second largest part of the brain, located in the posterior cranial fossa. It is seen behind the face and brain stem. Its purpose is to coordinates movement and maintains posture and balance. The cerebellum consists of two hemispheres. The falx cerebelli separates the right and left hemispheres consisting of intersecting folds of gray matter. This intertwining of the dura mater gives the cerebellum the appearance of cauliflower. The structure that connects these folds is termed the vermis.

Cerebrum

The cerebrum is the largest part of the brain consisting of two hemispheres. Similar to the cerebellum, the cerebrum contains two hemispheres that are joined by the corpus callosum, which is a large bundle of transverse fiber consisting of white matter. The corpus callosum is divided into three sections.

Genu
- anterior part
- transmits fibers between the frontal lobes

Body
- transmits fibers from the parietal and temporal lobes

Splenium
- posterior part transmitting fibers from the posterior parietal and the occipital lobe

The falx cerebri is the parting of the two hemispheres made up of dura mater that extends caudally from the upper calvarium and ends above the corpus callosum. Most regions of the cerebrum function as association areas

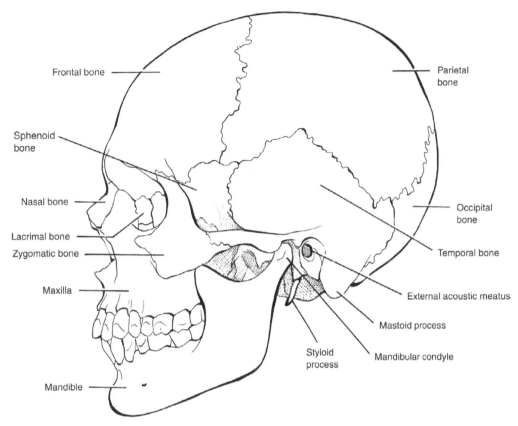

Figure 2.4. Illustration of the cranium in the sagittal projection demonstrating the frontal, parietal, temporal, and occipital bones. (Reproduced, with permission, from Madden ME. *Introduction to Sectional Anatomy.* 3rd ed. Philadelphia, PA: Wolters Kluwer; Lippincott Williams & Wilkins; 2013.)

related to memory, reasoning, judgment, intelligence, and personality. The cerebrum is divided into four lobes (Fig. 2.5):

Frontal
- located anterior to the central sulcus and above the Sylvian fissure

Parietal
- located between the central sulcus and the parieto-occipital fissure and found above the Sylvain fissure

Temporal lobe
- located inferior to the Sylvian fissure and anterior to an extension of the parieto-occipital fissure
- upper part contains the primary auditory area
- rest is part of the association areas

Occipital lobe
- posterior part of the cerebral hemisphere
- located behind the parieto-occipital fissure
- primary visual area

The area known as the tentorium cerebelli spreads out like a tent to form the partition between the cerebrum and the cerebellum.

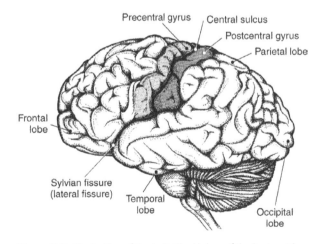

Figure 2.5. Illustration of the individual lobes of the brain with their associated fissures. (Reproduced, with permission, from Kelley LL, Petersen CM. *Sectional Anatomy for Imaging Professionals.* 3rd ed. St. Louis, MO: Mosby Elsevier; 2013.)

Meninges of Brain and Spinal Cord (Fig. 2.6)

Dura mater

- strongest double layered membrane
- continuous with the periosteum of the cranium
- located between the dura mater and the cranium
  - meningeal vessels
    - supply blood to the cranium and meninges
- epidural space
  - potential space between the dura and the cranium

Arachnoid mater

- middle layer between the pia and dura mater
- most delicate meningeal membrane
- the mater is made up of thin fibrous threads
  - resembling a spider web
- follows the contour of the dura mater
- subdural space
  - space between the dura mater and the arachnoid mater

Pia mater

- inner membrane and difficult to separate it from the nervous system structures
  - tightly adhered to the surface of the brain and spinal cord
- highly vascular
- subarachnoid space
  - space between the arachnoid mater and the pia mater
  - contains cerebral spinal fluid
    - circulates around the brain and spinal cord
    - provides further protection to the central nervous system

Cerebral Fissures

Cerebral fissure are natural division or groove in the brain, the longitudinal fissure divides the cerebrum almost completely in two hemispheres. The fissure of Rolando or central sulcus separates the frontal and parietal lobes of cerebrum, while the sylvian fissure or lateral sulcus runs between frontal and temporal lobes of cerebrum. The

Insula commonly called the inner lobe is located deep within the sylvian or lateral fissure. It may also be referred to as the island of Reil.

Gray and White Matter

The cerebrum is composed of both gray and white matter. The gray matter consists of unmyelinated nerve fibers, nerve cell bodies, and supportive tissues. The cortex receives sensory impulses and then transmits instructions to the necessary body structures and systems to initiate and control movement. White matter is mainly myelinated nerve fibers. These fibers serve as information highways for the impulses sent to and from the cortex. White matter is located within the interior of the cerebrum.

Brain Stem

The brain stem is the posterior part of the brain, adjoining and structurally continuous with the spinal cord (Fig. 2.7). It provides the main motor and sensory innervations to the face and neck and plays an important role in the regulation of cardiac and respiratory function. It includes the:

Medulla oblongata (myelencephalon)

- located in the lower brain stem just below the pons
- it is the communication between the brain and the spinal cord
- controls the vital functions of the body, such as respirations, heart rate, and blood pressure
- motor nerve fiber crossover causing one side of the brain to control the motor functions on the opposite side of the body

Pons (part of mesencephalon)

- can be found in the anterior section of the cerebellum
- this portion of the brain stem's fibers join the cerebellum to those of the cerebrum and spinal cord

Midbrain (mesencephalon)

- smallest section of the brain stem

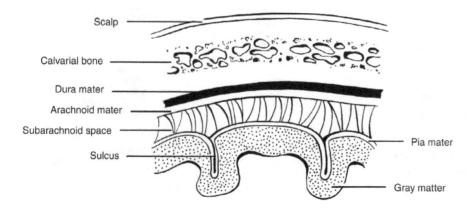

Figure 2.6. Illustration of the meninges of the brain and their internal relationship from the scalp to the gray matter. (Reproduced, with permission, from Madden ME. *Introduction to Sectional Anatomy.* 3rd ed. Philadelphia, PA: Wolters Kluwer; Lippincott Williams & Wilkins; 2013.)

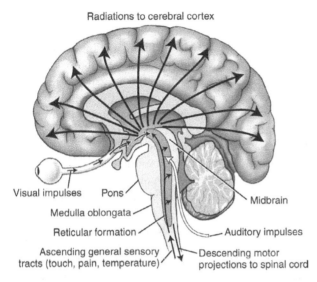

Radiations to cerebral cortex

Visual impulses — Pons — Midbrain
Medulla oblongata — Auditory impulses
Reticular formation —
Ascending general sensory — Descending motor
tracts (touch, pain, temperature) — projections to spinal cord

Figure 2.7. Sagittal illustration of the brain stem and its intricate reticular formation. (Reproduced, with permission, from Kelley LL, Petersen CM. *Sectional Anatomy for Imaging Professionals*. 3rd ed. St. Louis, MO: Mosby Elsevier; 2013.)

- located above the pons at the junction of the middle and posterior cranial fossa
- surrounds the cerebral aqueduct

Basal Ganglia

Basal ganglion is a collection of subcortical gray matter made up of the caudate nucleus, lentiform nucleus, and the claustrum (Fig. 2.8). The caudate nucleus is a C-shaped area of gray matter involved in muscle control found in the curve of the lateral ventricles. On cross-sectional images the head of the caudate nucleus can be found indenting into the floor of the anterior horns of the lateral ventricles. The tail is the tapered part of the nucleus and is seen at the roof of the inferior horn of the lateral ventricle. The lentiform nucleus is an area of gray matter located between the insula, caudate nucleus, and the thalamus. It is divided into the globus pallidus and the putamen. The internal capsule carries the sensory and motor nerve fibers connecting the cerebral cortex to the brain stem and spinal cord. These fiber tracks separate the thalamus from the caudate nucleus and the basal ganglia. The globus pallidus is in the medial section of the lentiform nucleus and can be seen on cross-sectional images between the thalamus and the putamen. The putamen is in the outermost area of the lentiform nucleus located next to the globus pallidus and medial to the external capsule. The external capsule is a thin layer of white matter between the claustrum and the putamen. The fibers originate from the insula. The sheet of gray matter bounded by laminae of white matter on either side of the external capsule is the claustrum. The thalamus is in the diencephalon and is a pair of large oval gray masses. It makes up a large portion of the walls of the third ventricle and is the relay station to and from the cerebral cortex for all sensory stimuli, except the olfactory nerves.

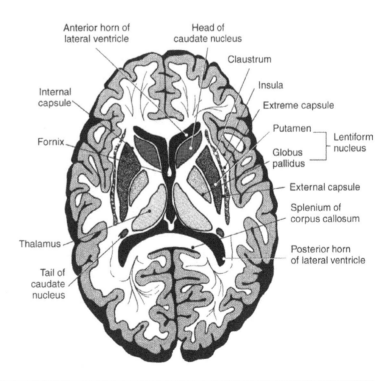

Anterior horn of lateral ventricle — Head of caudate nucleus
Claustrum
Insula
Internal capsule — Extreme capsule
Putamen — Lentiform nucleus
Fornix — Globus pallidus
External capsule
Splenium of corpus callosum
Thalamus — Posterior horn of lateral ventricle
Tail of caudate nucleus

Figure 2.8. Axial illustration of the basal ganglia. (Reproduced, with permission, from Kelley LL, Petersen CM. *Sectional Anatomy for Imaging Professionals*. 3rd ed. St. Louis, MO: Mosby Elsevier; 2013.)

Enhancement Patterns of the Brain: Blood–Brain Barrier

The brain has a unique triple layered blood–brain barrier (BBB) with tight endothelial junctions in order to maintain a consistent internal environment. Contrast will not leak into the brain unless this barrier is damaged. Many brain tumors can break down this BBB and will enhance. Extra-axial tumors such as meningiomas and schwannomas are not brain tumors, because they do not develop in brain tissue, therefore, they do not have a BBB, so they will also enhance. There is also no BBB in the pituitary, pineal, and choroid plexus region; therefore, they will enhance. Some noticeable lesions enhance because they can also break down the BBB and may simulate a brain tumor. These lesions include infections, demyelinating diseases (MS) and infarctions.

Ventricular System

The ventricular system provides a channel for the circulation of cerebral spinal fluid through the central nervous system (Fig. 2.9). The system consists of two lateral, a third, and a fourth ventricle. The choroid plexus produces CSF from the blood to fill the ventricles. Lateral ventricle is a C-shaped cavity that lies within each cerebral hemisphere. It is composed of the anterior horn, which is found within the frontal lobe. The roof of the ventricle is formed by the corpus callosum and the floor and lateral walls are formed by the head of the caudate nucleus. The medial wall is formed by the septum pellucidum. The Interventricular foramen also called the Foramen of Monro joins the lateral ventricle with the third ventricle. The third ventricle is a narrow opening found near the medium sagittal plane. The cerebral aqueduct located within the posterior part of the midbrain transmits CSF from the lateral and third ventricles to the fourth ventricle. The fourth ventricle is pyramid-shaped structure that rest on the pons and medulla oblongata. It receives CSF from the cerebral aqueduct and travels down to the spinal cord to communicate with the two foramina, the foramina of Luschka and the foramen of Magendie.

Vascular System of the Brain

The arterial system of the brain commences with the basilar artery. It is found at the midline on the anterior surface of the pons. It originates from the junction of the right and left vertebral arteries. It extends to the upper portion of the pons dividing and gives rise to the right and left posterior cerebral arteries. The cerebral arteries consist of a ring of vessels located within the subarachnoid space below the hypothalamus and the midbrain known as the circle of Willis. These arteries supply arterial blood to the cerebrum. The posterior cerebral artery originates from

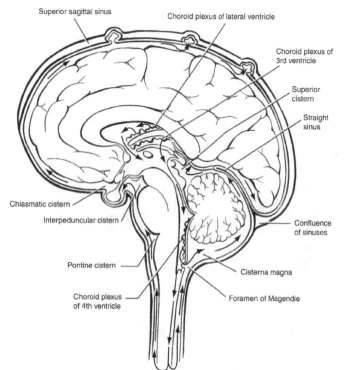

Figure 2.9. Sagittal view of the cerebral spinal fluid flow. (Reproduced, with permission, from Madden ME. *Introduction to Sectional Anatomy*. 3rd ed. Philadelphia, PA: Wolters Kluwer; Lippincott Williams & Wilkins; 2013.)

the basilar artery. It is located along the upper border of the pons and extends above the tentorium cerebelli supplying blood to the occipital lobe. As the posterior cerebral leaves the basilar artery, the posterior communicating artery connects to the internal carotid artery (ICA). The ICA bifurcates at the C3 level from the common carotid artery and enters the skull at the carotid canals. It passes the sella turcica and extends through the dura layers of the cavernous to enter the subarachnoid space. It branches to form anterior communicating and the middle cerebral artery. The middle cerebral artery is the major branch of the ICA extending laterally through the Sylvain fissure. Its purpose is to supply blood to the temporal and parietal lobes. The anterior communicating arteries are small vessels that provide blood flow to the right and left side of the anterior cerebral artery. The anterior cerebral artery is smaller in size than the middle cerebral and travels anteriorly into the interhemispheric fissure. It can be seen on cross-sectional images on either side of the falx cerebri, distributing blood to the frontal lobe and the medial part of the parietal lobe.

Dural Sinuses and Vein

The dural sinuses are large venous channels which drain the blood from the brain. The sequence of drainage flow is as follows:

- Superior sagittal sinus
- Inferior sagittal sinus
- Vein of Galen
- Straight sinus
- Confluence of sinuses
- Transverse sinus
- Sigmoid sinus

All venous output will drain into a venous sinus and then flow into the internal jugular vein.

The vein of Galen is an important landmark on cross-sectional imaging. It can be seen in the posterior region of a middle CT axial slice, since it runs between the corpus callosum and the pineal gland. When performing CT brain profusions, this vein is used as the reference vein for the washout process.

IMAGING PROCEDURES OF THE HEAD

CT procedures of the brain have been used since Hounsfield's first diagnostic procedure performed at Atkinson-Morley's Hospital, in London, England. It is a fast, noninvasive procedure for assessing intracranial pathological conditions, particularly in the acute stage.

Temporal Bones

The common indications for a CT procedure of the temporal bones include:

- Conductive hearing loss
- Pulsatile tinnitus
- Trauma
- Congenital malfunction
- Acoustic neuroma

There is basically no preparation required, with the only exception being pituitary gland procedures brain procedures for the diagnosis of primary tumor and metastatic disease. Patient's undergoing this procedure requires scans performed without IV contrast and then a post enhanced study. As with all IV contrast procedures special care is taken to ensure the patient does not have any contraindications for the use of IV contrast media.

Temporal Bone Acquisition Parameters

Anatomical coverage
- mastoid air cells through the petrous ridges

Slice thickness
- ≥1 mm

Interval
- overlap

DFOV
- 230 to 250 mm

Kernel
- standard/soft tissue
- bone/detail

Retrospective imaging
- right and left sides are reconstructed separately
- slice thickness/interval
  - same parameters as for the axial imaging
- DFOV
  - 100 mm
    - include all mastoid air cells
    - smaller DFOV increases spatial resolution
- kernel
  - standard/soft tissue
  - bone/detail

Reformats
- sagittal
- coronal

Pituitary Gland

Unenhanced Scan

Anatomical coverage
- anterior clinoid to posterior clinoid process

Slice thickness
- 1 to 2 mm

Interval
- overlap

DFOV
- 150 to 180 mm

Kernel
- standard/soft tissue

Retrospective imaging
- slice thickness/interval
- same parameters as for the axial imaging
- DFOV
- 150 to 180 mm
- kernel
  - bone/detail

Reformats
- sagittal
- coronal
  - display pituitary adenoma's best

Enhanced Scan

Same technical parameters as for the unenhanced

IV contrast
- 100 cc

Flow rate
- 2 to 3 cc/s

Delay time
- 3 to 5 minutes
  - radiologist preference

Orbits, Sinuses, and Maxillofacial Procedures

The orbits, sinuses, and maxillofacial bones utilize the same technical parameters; their only difference is positioning and anatomical coverage.

Indications for Nonenhanced Study

Trauma

Congenital abnormalities

Sinus disease
- fluid
- polyps

Evaluation for preoperative planning

Indications for Enhanced Study

Infection
- radiologist preference

Tumors

Vascular lesions

Anatomical Coverage

Orbits
- 2 cm below the orbital floor to 2 cm above the orbital roof

- eye position
  - looking upward to straighten out the
- optic nerve

Sinus
- alveolar process to above the frontal sinus

Maxillofacial
- 2 cm below the mandible to above the frontal sinus

Technical Factors

Head positioning
- neutral

Slice thickness
- ≤3 mm

Interval
- overlap

DFOV
- 140 to 160 mm or larger

Kernel
- bone/detail

Retrospective reconstructions
- slice thickness, intervals, and DFOV
  - same as the prospective imaging
- kernel
  - standard/soft tissue

Reformats
- sagittal
- coronal

Enhanced Scan

Same technical factors as for unenhanced imaging

IV contrast
- 100 cc

Flow rate
- 2 to 3 cc/s

Delay time
- 3 to 5 minutes
  - radiologist preference

Temporal Mandibular Joints

Indications
- Pain, includes headaches
- Inflammation
- Displaced meniscus
- Osteophyte

The temporal mandibular joints (TMJs) regulate both hinge movement and grinding movement. With the mouth in the closed position, the condyle of the mandible is located in a centric position in the mandibular fossa. In this position the joint is most stable. With the mouth in the open position, the condyle of the mandible is displaced anterior to the mandibular fossa, demonstrating the meniscus. Therefore, when scanning TMJs one scan is performed with the mouth in the open position and a second scan is done with the mouth closed. It is important to instruct the patient not to clench down in the closed position.

Technical Factors

Anatomical coverage
- 2 cm below the mandible to 2 cm above the zygomatic arch

Head positioning
- chin tucked

Slice thickness
- ≤1 mm

Interval
- overlap

DFOV
- 200 to 240 mm to encompass bilateral joints

Kernel
- standard/soft tissue

Retrospective reconstructions
- right and left sides are reconstructed separately
- slice thickness, intervals, and DFOV
  - same as for the prospective scanning

Reformats
- sagittal
- coronal
- 3D
  - volume rendered

Brain

Indications for Nonenhanced Study
- Trauma
- Subdural hemorrhage
- Epidural hemorrhage
- Fracture
- LOC
- Mental status change
- Vertigo
- Ventricular shunt placement or check
- Atrophy
- Dizziness

Indications for Enhanced Study
- Neoplasm
- Metastasis disease
- Abscess

Technical Factors

Anatomical coverage
- 1 cm below the occipital bone to the vertex

Head position
- chin tucked so the supraorbital meatal line is perpendicular to tablet top
  - eliminates bean hardening artifact
  - eliminates radiation to the eyes

Gantry angle
- 15- to 20-degree angulation from superior orbit to the skull base

Slice thickness/intervals
- 5 mm

DFOV
- 230 to 250 mm

Kernel
- standard/soft tissue

IV contrast—primary tumors or metastatic lesions
- 100 cc

Flow rate
- 2 to 3 cc/s

Delay time
- 5 to 10 minutes
  - radiologist preference

Retrospective reconstructions
- trauma and metastatic disease
- slice thickness
  - ≤3 mm
- interval
  - overlap
- kernel
  - bone/detail

Reformats
- sagittal
- coronal
- 3D
  - volume rendered
  - identify skull fractures

Brain Angiography

Indications
- Subarachnoid hemorrhage
- Vascular abnormality
- Aneurysm
- AVM

Technical Factors

Anatomical coverage
- C3 through skull vertex

Slice thickness
- ≤1 mm

Slice interval
- Overlap

DFOV
- 230 to 250 mm

Kernel
- standard/soft tissue

IV contrast
- 100 cc
- flow rate
  - 4 to 5 cc/s
- delay time
  - tracking or timing bolus
  - ROI on the ICA

Injection site
- ideally—right antecubital
- dumps directly into the SVC
- eliminates streak artifact

Retrospective reconstructions
- slice thickness
  - <1 mm
- interval
  - overlap
- DFOV
  - 120 to 150 mm (targeted at centered of Circle of Willis)
- kernel
  - standard/soft tissue

Reformats
- 3D
  - volume rendered

CT Perfusion

In cases of acute cerebral infarct, perfusion series may be performed first. The area to be scanned is from the inferior thalamus through top of lateral ventricles.

Flow rate
- 4 to 5 cc/s with 40 cc of contrast

Delay
- 3 to 5 seconds

Slice thickness
- 5 mm

Interval
- 0 mm

The purpose of perfusion studies is to obtain functional information about cerebral blood flow (CBF). A short IV contrast bolus is given, with 20 mm/40 mm of tissue irradiated for a total of 40 cycles.

Images are transferred to a workstation for analysis. The analyses parameters include: cerebral blood flow (CBF), cerebral blood volume (CBV), and the mean transit time (MTT). The CBF is the most important parameter. It indicates how much blood is flowing through the brain tissue in a specific period. The measurement is assessed on mL/blood/100 g of brain tissue/minute. The normal range is 50 to 80 mL/blood/100 g of brain tissue per minute. The CBV is the percentage of blood vessels in a specific volume of tissue. The functional parameter alters if vessel size changes in the context of vascular autoregulation system, thereby identifying infarcted tissue. The parameter for describing delayed (retarded) perfusion is MTT. This parameter is the time required for blood to pass through tissue in seconds. The CBF is calculated by CBV/MTT.

Perfusion Calculations

Reference artery
- anterior cerebral artery

Reference vein
- superior sagittal sinus

ROI placed on the reference artery and vein

Contrast enhancement curves can be generated

PATHOLOGY OF THE HEAD

Cholesteatoma

Cholesteatoma is a benign neoplasm of the external auditory canal or middle ear. Patients who acquire this disease range in age from 45 to 75. The tumors are generally unilateral, characterized by a soft tissue homogeneous mass with focal bone destruction. Surgery intervention is required.

Acoustic Neuroma

Acoustic neuroma is a benign tumor of Schwann cells covering vestibule portion of the eighth cranial nerve. These tumors are well encapsulated, but do not invade the nerve. It is often because of a genetic disorder called neurofibromatosis. This condition appears as a well-rounded hypodense or isodense mass on unenhanced images, when IV contrast media is injected the lesion becomes hyperdense. As with cholesteatoma, surgery is required.

Pituitary Adenoma

Pituitary adenomas are benign lesions that do not spread to other parts of the body. They are graded as nonfunctioning or functioning. Pituitary adenomas can lead to nerve damage, growth disturbances, and changes in hormonal balance depending on their ability to secrete hormones. They appear as central regions of hypodensity on unenhanced images, but will become isodense when IV contrast media is administered (Fig. 2.10).

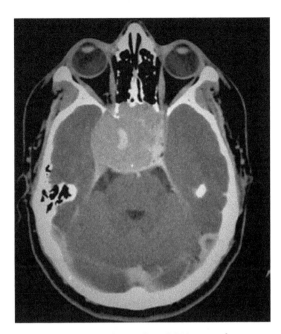

Figure 2.10. Contrast-enhanced axial CT image of an extremely large pituitary adenoma located within the sphenoid sinus. (Reproduced, with permission, from Seeram E. *Computed Tomography: Physical Principles, Clinical Applications, and Quality Control*. 3rd ed. St. Louis, MO: Saunders Elsevier; 2009.)

Orbital Hemangioma

Cavernous hemangiomas of the orbit are the most common benign orbital tumor. They occur more frequently in females of middle age. Visual disability results from an optic-nerve compression in most cases. Treatment for these tumors even though benign requires surgical intervention. Orbital imaging should be performed in both the axial and coronal planes due to the pyramidal shape of the bony orbit (Fig. 2.11).

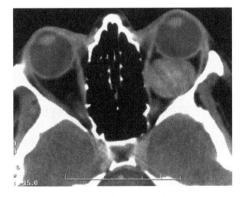

Figure 2.11. Axial CT image of the orbits demonstrating a hemangioma of the left orbit shifting the globe anteriorly. (Reproduced, with permission, from Grey ML, Ailinani JM. *CT and MRI Pathology: A Pocket Atlas*. 2nd ed. New York, NY: McGraw-Hill; 2012.)

Tripod Fracture

Tripod fractures can also be referred to as a Le Fort III fracture. These fractures have four visible components, not always all visible. The bones involved are the orbital floor, fracture of the lateral wall of the maxillary antrum, zygomatic arch fracture, and a widening of the zygomaticofrontal suture. High-resolution CT is the modality of choice, because of the complex anatomy and fractures of the facial bones, are shown extremely well by CT, and soft tissue complications can be evaluated to a far greater degree, due to CT's ability to perform multiplanar and 3D reformations.

Sinusitis

Sinusitis is a bacterial, viral, or fungal inflammation of the paranasal sinuses. A patient with acute sinusitis presents with thick green or yellow nasal discharge. CT imaging is one of the ways a physician diagnoses sinusitis. CT imaging (preferably in the coronal plane) may demonstrate mucosal thickening, opacification, or air-filled levels. Sinusitis can occur in one or more of the paranasal sinuses.

Epidural Hematoma

An epidural hematoma appears as a classic biconvex (lentiform or football), shaped lesion with the dura bulging inward. Blood collects between the dura mater and the skull that is mainly caused as a consequence of a blunt force trauma. These hematomas are caused by arterial tears. CT is an excellent modality for this pathology. In CT imaging during the acute stage, the hemorrhage appears hyperdense, but as it proceeds into the subacute and chronic stage, the hemorrhage becomes isodense to hypodense. CT retrospective reconstruction imaging utilizing high-resolution techniques usually demonstrates skull fractures in the area of the epidural hematoma.

Subdural Hematoma

Subdural hematoma is a form of "traumatic brain injury." Blood collects between the dura mater (the outer protective covering of the brain) and the arachnoid (the middle layer of the meninges). Subdural bleeding usually results from tears in veins that cross the subdural space. This type of hemorrhage results from the head striking an immovable object. Subdural hemorrhages can be caused by auto vehicle accidents, birth trauma, and child abuse. As with epidural hematomas, subdural hematomas appear on CT imaging as hyperdense lesions in the acute phase, isodense lesions in the subacute phase, and isodense lesions in the chronic stage.

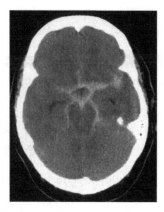

Figure 2.12. CT image in the axial projection of a subarachnoid hemorrhage, note the blood collection in the basal cisterns and Sylvian fissures. (Reproduced, with permission, from Grey ML, Ailinani JM. *CT and MRI Pathology: A Pocket Atlas.* 2nd ed. New York, NY: McGraw-Hill; 2012.)

Subarachnoid Hemorrhage

Subarachnoid hemorrhage is a collection of blood in the space between the arachnoid mater and pia mater. This hemorrhage is caused by trauma, a leak of a berry aneurysm in the circle of Willis, an AVM, or hypertension. On an unenhanced CT imaging study, this hemorrhage shows blood in the subarachnoid space, basilar cistern, and Sylvian fissure (Fig. 2.12).

Aneurysm

An aneurysm is a contained bulge of an artery resembling a balloon-like structure. This out pouching causes a weakness of the outer wall of the artery (tunica adventitia) resulting in the wall to rupture, allowing blood to flow into the subarachnoid space. On unenhanced CT images, the blood leakage shows as a hyperdensity within the brain parenchyma. A CT angiogram is one of the modalities to demonstrate the region in which the aneurysm occurred (Fig. 2.13).

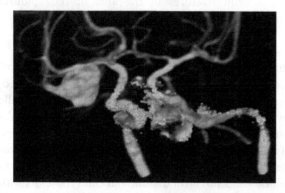

Figure 2.13. CT angiogram of the cerebral arteries with 3D volume-rendered reconstruction. This image demonstrates a large right middle cerebral artery aneurysm. (Reproduced, with permission, from Grey ML, Ailinani JM. *CT and MRI Pathology: A Pocket Atlas.* 2nd ed. New York, NY: McGraw-Hill; 2012.)

Stroke (Cerebrovascular Accident)

A CVA occurs when blood flow to a part of your brain is stopped either by a blockage or a rupture of a blood vessel. There are two main types of strokes. An ischemic stroke caused by a blockage, and a hemorrhagic stroke is caused by a breakage in a blood vessel. In both cases, part of the brain is deprived of blood and oxygen, causing the brain's cells to die. An ischemic stroke is caused by a clot preventing blood to flow freely. When a clot forms somewhere else in your body and gets lodged in a brain's blood vessel, it is called an embolic stroke. When the clot forms in a brain blood vessel, it is called a thrombotic stroke. A known common complication of cardiac surgery is thromboembolism and has been described in medical literature as a source of stroke.

CROSS-SECTIONAL ANATOMY OF THE NECK

Pharynx

The pharynx is a funnel-shaped fibromuscular tube 12 cm long that acts as an opening for both the respiratory and digestive systems. It extends from the base of the skull to the level of C6 and ends inferiorly as the continuation of the esophagus. The pharynx as it descends divides into three sections: the nasopharynx, the oropharynx, and the laryngopharynx (Fig. 2.14).

Nasopharynx

The nasopharynx is the most superior portion of the pharynx, located posterior to the nasal cavity allowing air to pass from the nasal cavity to the trachea; it extends from the base of the skull to the soft palate. The pharyngeal tonsils (aka adenoids) are seen in the roof of the nasopharynx.

Oropharynx

The oropharynx extends from the soft palate to the tip of the epiglottis. The palatine and lingual tonsils are found within the oropharynx and can be seen on the left and right sides at the back of the throat. The valleculae are spaces on either side of the glossoepiglottic fold. On cross-sectional images it can be seen posterior to the tongue and epiglottis. It is a common site for foreign bodies to lodge.

Laryngopharynx

The laryngopharynx continues from the oropharynx and lies between the hyoid bone and the entrance to the larynx, continuing as the esophagus at the level of the cricoid cartilage of the larynx. On both sides of the larynx are two cavities called the piriformis sinus (pear-shaped) that divert food away from the entrance of the larynx so that it can continue into the esophagus.

Larynx

The larynx is the bony skeleton that surrounds and protects the vocal cords (called the voice box) extending from the level of C3–C6. It begins at the laryngopharynx and continues to the trachea, marking the beginning of the respiratory passage. It consists of an outer skeleton made up of nine cartilages that extends approximately from the third to the sixth cervical vertebrae. These cartilages are connected to one another by ligaments and moved by various muscles.

Trachea

The trachea is the main airway in the body. It extends from the larynx which terminates into the main bronchi roughly at the C6–C7 vertebral level. On cross-sectional images it will be seen in the midline anterior to the esophagus and vertebral bodies.

Hyoid Bone

The hyoid bone is located at C2 and C3 vertebral level. Unlike other bones within the skeleton, the hyoid does not feature any major points of articulation and does not join with any other bone. It provides a place of attachment for many muscles associated with the mouth's floor, as well as the larynx, pharynx, and epiglottis. A hyoid fracture commonly is the result of strangulation.

Laryngeal Cartilages

There are three unpaired laryngeal cartilages, which include the thyroid, epiglottis, and cricoid cartilages. Thyroid cartilage is the largest and most superior made up of two plates, called laminae. They join together at the front of the neck and form a prominent structure commonly referred to as the Adam's apple. The epiglottis differs from the other cartilages in that it is elastic and allows movement. During swallowing it folds back over the larynx, preventing the entry of liquids and solid food from entering the respiratory passage. The cricoid forms a complete ring at the base of the larynx and marks the junction of the larynx and the trachea and the beginning of the esophagus.

They are also three paired cartilages including the arytenoid, corniculate, and the cuneiform. The arytenoids are shaped like pyramids and are situated on top of the cricoid cartilage. They are fundamental to the production of vocal sound. The muscular process, of this cartilage, attaches to the muscles of phonation which allow the movement of the arytenoid cartilage to adjust the tension

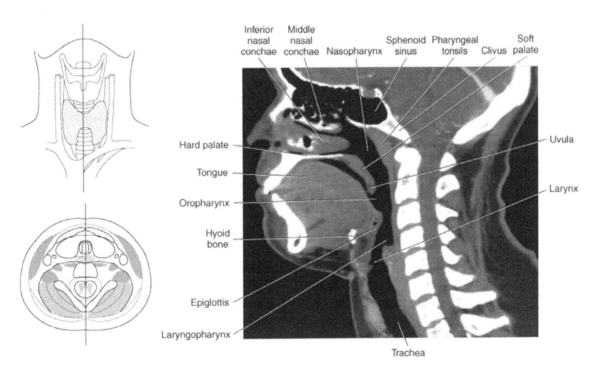

Figure 2.14. CT sagittal view utilizing the standard algorithm of the oropharynx, nasopharynx, and trachea. (Reproduced, with permission, from Kelley LL, Petersen CM. *Sectional Anatomy for Imaging Professionals*. 3rd ed. St. Louis, MO: Mosby Elsevier; 2013.)

of the vocal ligament and thus change sound pitch. The corniculate are small horn-shaped cartilages that articulate with the tops of the arytenoid cartilages involved in the opening and closing of the glottis for the production of sound. The cuneiform cartilages are small curved cartilages lying within the aryepiglottic folds and extend between the arytenoid cartilages and epiglottis.

Vocal Cords (True)

The vocal cords are two pairs of ligaments that extend from the arytenoid cartilages to the thyroid cartilage, which are separated by a space called the ventricle or glottic space. During phonation the cords extend toward the midline in a closed position, while in quiet respiration, they relax creating an opening between them called the glottis. The muscles on the cartilages move with respect to one another in order to change the tension of the ligaments controlling the sound emitted when air moves through the larynx.

Vestibular Folds (False Vocal Cords)

The false vocal cords are located superior to the glottis space. Dissimilar from the true vocal cords, they do not have ligament connections; therefore, they have little to do in the production of voice.

Esophagus

The esophagus is found at the terminal end of the pharynx at the approximate level of C6. It descends through the thoracic cavity ending at the stomach. On cross-sectional images, the esophagus is seen between the trachea and the vertebral bodies near the medial plane of the body.

Salivary Glands

The salivary glands collectively produce and empty saliva into the oral cavity by way of ducts to begin the process of digestion. They are three large paired glands: the parotid, the submandibular, and the sublingual.

The parotid gland is the largest of the salivary glands situated between the rami of the mandible and the sternocleidomastoid muscle. The gland extends inferiorly from the level of the EAM to the angle of the mandible. This gland differs from other gland because of the amount of fat they contain. The parotid duct also known as Stensen's duct passes lateral to the masseter muscle and enters the oral cavity through the buccal tissues adjacent to the mandibular first and second molars. The submandibular gland borders the posterior half of the mandible extending from the angle of the mandible to the hyoid bone. They can be palpitated as a spongy area below the latter half of the mandible. Saliva drains from this gland through a tube, known as Wharton's duct, which opens on the inside of the mouth under the tongue immediately behind the lower front teeth. This duct is a common site for stone development, which can be seen on CT images as small round, or oval hyperdense formations. Stones obstruct the food-related flow of salivary secretions. Calculi may cause stasis of saliva facilitating bacterial ascent into the gland and subsequent infection.

The sublingual glands are the smallest of the salivary glands lying anterior to the submandibular gland inferior to the tongue, as well as beneath the mucous membrane of the floor of the mouth. Each gland can be palpated on the floor of the mouth posterior to each mandibular canine. The Rivinus's duct is responsible for the flow of saliva within the mouth.

Thyroid Gland

The thyroid gland is an endocrine gland located at the level of the cricoid cartilage. In the axial plane they appear as a wedge-shaped structure hugging both sides of the trachea. The gland is located at the level of the cricoid cartilage containing two lobes connect by a narrowed area known as the isthmus on the anterior trachea. On CT cross-sectional images, they are seen as high-attenuation structures due to their iodine content.

Musculature of the Neck (Fig. 2.15)

Anterior Triangle Muscle

Sternocleidomastoid

The sternocleidomastoid muscle is a broad strap-like muscle that originates on the sternum and clavicle and inserts onto the mastoid tip. It function is to turn the head from side to side and turn the neck. Due it this muscles superficial position, it provides landmarks for identifying structures within the neck.

Posterior Triangle

Levator Scapulae

The levator scapulae muscle is located on the posterolateral portion of the neck arises from the transverse processes of the upper four cervical vertebra. This muscle inserts on the vertebral boarder of the scapula. Its action is to raise the scapula.

Trapezius

The trapezius muscle is a superficial muscle located on the posterior portion of the neck, originating from the occipital bone and spinous process of C7–T12. It inserts on the clavicle, acromion and spine of the scapula with the function of elevating the scapula.

Scalene Muscle Group

The scalene muscle group is located on the anterolateral portion of the neck. This group divides into the anterior, middle, and posterior scalene muscle. They originate from the transverse process of the cervical vertebra and insert on the 1st and 2nd ribs. The purpose of this muscle group is to elevate the upper two ribs and flex the neck.

Vascular System of the Neck

Carotid Arteries

The right common carotid artery arises from the brachiocephalic artery posterior to the sternoclavicular joint, while the left common carotid artery arises directly from the aortic arch. Both arteries lie medial to the internal jugular veins and bifurcate into the internal and external carotid arteries at the level of the thyroid cartilage (C3–C4). Their function is to supply blood to the head and neck.

Internal Carotid Arteries

The ICAs ascend the neck in an almost vertical plane, to enter the skull through the carotid canal of the temporal bone. The ICA supplies blood to the orbits and brain. The term siphon refers to the portion of the ICA as it enters the bony skull and bifurcates into the anterior and middle cerebral arteries.

External Carotid Arteries

The external carotid arteries (ECAs) ascend the neck, and pass through the parotid gland to the level of the temporal mandibular joint (Fig. 2.16). The ECA bifurcates into terminal branches to supply blood to the face and neck. Their location in relationship to the ICA changes through its course. The ECA is lateral to the ICA at the level of C1, whereas it is medial to ICA at the vertebral levels of C3–C2.

Jugular Veins

The jugular veins are the largest vascular structures of the neck. They drain blood from the face and neck. The IJV commence at the jugular foramen and descend the lateral portion of the neck to unite with the subclavian vein to form the brachiocephalic vein. The enlargement of the jugular foramen is the jugular fossa.

Retromandibular Vein

The retromandibular veins are two smaller veins on either side of the head, just posterior to the mandible. During their course, they pass through the parotid gland and terminate into the external jugular vein.

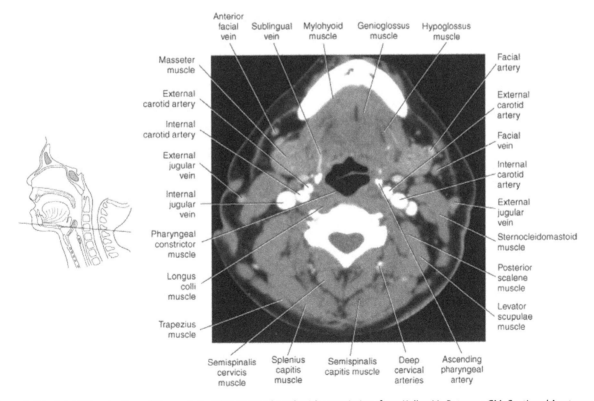

Figure 2.15. Axial CT projection of the neck muscles. (Reproduced, with permission, from Kelley LL, Petersen CM. *Sectional Anatomy for Imaging Professionals*. 3rd ed. St. Louis, MO: Mosby Elsevier; 2013.)

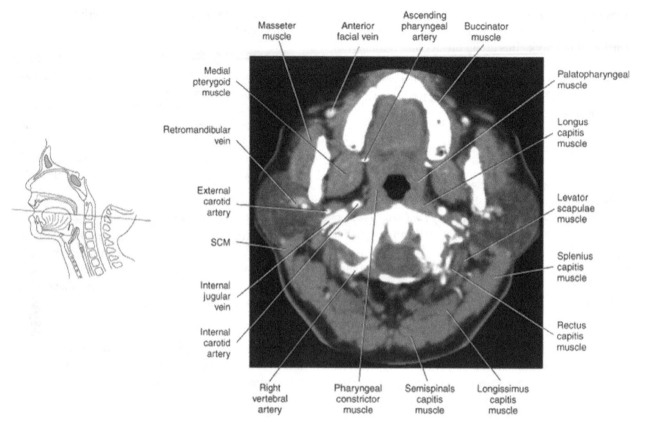

Masseter muscle • Anterior facial vein • Ascending pharyngeal artery • Buccinator muscle • Medial pterygoid muscle • Palatopharyngeal muscle • Retromandibular vein • Longus capitis muscle • External carotid artery • Levator scapulae muscle • SCM • Splenius capitis muscle • Internal jugular vein • Rectus capitis muscle • Internal carotid artery • Right vertebral artery • Pharyngeal constrictor muscle • Semispinals capitis muscle • Longissimus capitis muscle

Figure 2.16. Axial CT image of the external carotid artery at the level of C1. Note its lateral position to the internal carotid artery. (Reproduced, with permission, from Kelley LL, Petersen CM. *Sectional Anatomy for Imaging Professionals*. 3rd ed. St. Louis, MO: Mosby Elsevier; 2013.)

External Jugular Veins

The external jugular veins begin near the angle of the mandible and cross the SCM just beneath the skin to empty into the subclavian vein. A slow gentle pulse can be usually felt near the middle of the sternocleidomastoid muscle. These veins can be recognized after the parotid gland in the lateral portion of the neck.

Vertebral Arteries and Veins

The vertebral arteries begin as a branch of the subclavian artery and ascend the neck through the transverse foramina of C6–C1. At this point the arteries enter the foramen magnum to join together to form basilar artery. The basilar artery supplies blood to the posterior aspect of the brain.

Vertebral Veins

The vertebral veins descend within the transverse foramina in conjunction with the vertebral arteries. Their function is to drain blood from the spine emptying into the subclavian vein.

Imaging Procedures of the Neck

Patient Positioning and Preparation

Remove all jewelry
Removable teeth containing metal
Head first, supine
Mandible extended
- Ensure it is perpendicular to the table

Routine Neck

Indications for IV Contrast

- Parotid/submandibular gland lesion or infection
- Head and neck cancers
- Pharyngeal/retropharyngeal or tonsillar abscess
- Neck mass or abscess
- Tongue mass or lesion
- Tumors or infections involving the vocal cords

Nonenhanced Studies

- Stones
- Foreign body in the neck or upper airway

Technical Factors

- Anatomical coverage
  - trachea bifurcation through the frontal sinus
  - scan inferior to superior
  - direction of blood flow
- Slice thickness
  - ≤3 mm
- Interval
  - ≤3 mm
- DFOV
  - 180 to 250 mm
- Kernel
  - standard/soft tissue
- IV contrast
  - 100 cc
  - flow rate
    - 2 to 3 cc/s
  - delay time
    - 120 seconds (single injection)
      - radiologist preference
- Retrospective reconstructions
  - slice thickness
    - ≤1 mm
- interval
  - overlap
- kernel
  - standard/soft tissue
  - bone/detail
- Reformats
  - MPR
    - sagittal
    - coronal
  - 3D
    - volume rendered

Split Injection

First Injection

Volume/rate
- 40 cc at 2 cc/s

Delay
- 60 to 90 seconds

Second Injection

Volume/Rate
- 60 cc at 4 cc/s

Delay
- 25 seconds

Purpose

- The ability to visualize both the arterial and venous phases, while reducing radiation dose

Larynx

Scan routine neck then rescan through vocal cords

Image order
- hyoid through cricoid

Scan type
- step and shoot

Gantry angle
- parallel to the axis of the mandible

Slice thickness
- 2 mm

Increments
- overlap

Kernel
- standard/soft tissue

Reformats
- MPR
  - sagittal
  - coronal

Phonation employed
- visualize vocal cord function

Neck Angiography

Indications

- Vascular abnormalities
- Vascular bypass surgery
- Stenosis
- Dissection
- Blunt or penetrating injury to the neck

Technical Factors

Anatomical coverage
- aortic arch to skull base

Slice thickness
- ≤1 mm

Increments
- ≤1 mm

DFOV
- 200 mm

Kernel
- standard/soft tissue

IV contrast
- 100 cc

Flow rate
- 4 cc/s

Scan delay
- tracking bolus or timing bolus
  - triggering at aorta arch

Reformats
- MPR

- sagittal
- coronal

3D

- volume rendering

PATHOLOGY OF THE NECK

Submandibular Salivary Gland Abscess

Submandibular salivary gland abscesses are mucous-filled cysts caused by trauma or obstruction. On unenhanced CT images, stones may be visualized along Wharton's duct, while the enhanced images show these abscesses as hypodense interior masses with hyperdensity in their peripheral (Fig. 2.17).

Laryngeal Mass

Laryngeal masses may develop along the chains of lymph nodes, nerves, or vessels in the neck (Fig. 2.18). These tumors often metastasize causing a change in the tumor grade, treatment protocol, and survival rate of the individual patient.

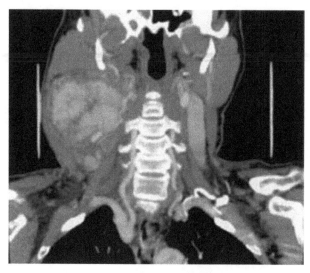

Figure 2.18. CT angiogram with coronal reformation demonstrating a large vascular carotid body laryngeal tumor. (Reproduced with permission from Seeram E. *Computed Tomography: Physical Principles, Clinical Applications, and Quality Control.* 3rd ed. St. Louis, MO: Saunders Elsevier; 2009.)

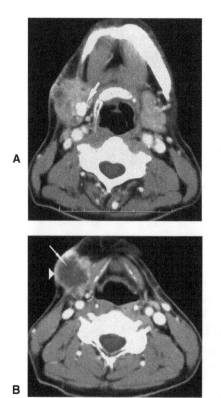

Figure 2.17. Contrast-enhanced axial CT projection of a large right submandibular abscess. The lesion consists of an enhanced peripheral and a low-density central region. (Reproduced, with permission, from Grey ML, Ailinani JM. *CT and MRI Pathology: A Pocket Atlas.* 2nd ed. New York, NY: McGraw-Hill; 2012.)

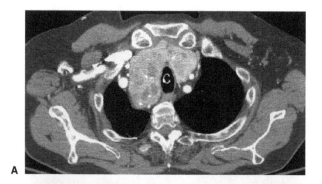
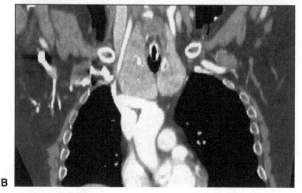

Figure 2.19. Contrast-enhanced axial CT image demonstrating an enlarged thyroid gland causing swelling in the anterior portion of the neck representing a thyroid goiter. (Reproduced, with permission, from Grey ML, Ailinani JM. *CT and MRI Pathology: A Pocket Atlas.* 2nd. ed. New York, NY: McGraw-Hill; 2012.)

Goiter

Goiters may be related to an increase in thyroid-stimulating hormone (TSH) due to a deficiency in normal hormone synthesis. On cross-sectional images they appear a multiple focal regions of low density (Fig. 2.19). An enlarged thyroid gland goiter can dip into the superior mediastinum and result in airway obstruction.

Carotid Artery Stenosis

Carotid artery stenosis is a narrowing of the carotid artery(s) caused by buildup of plaque inside the artery wall that reduces oxygen-rich blood flow to the brain. The process of plaque buildup is called atherosclerosis. Carotid stenosis is a major risk factor for stroke and can lead to brain damage.

CROSS-SECTIONAL ANATOMY OF THE CHEST

The thoracic apertures consist of the thoracic inlet and thoracic outlet. The inlet is superior and formed by the first thoracic vertebra, first pair of ribs and their costal cartilages and the manubrium. The thoracic outlet is inferior and formed by the twelfth vertebra, twelfth pair of ribs, and their costal cartilages and the xiphoid sternal junction.

Mediastinum

The mediastinum is a tissue compartment situated between the lungs containing the heart, great vessels, trachea, esophagus, thymus, considerable fat, and lymph nodes. These structures can be identified by their location, appearance, and attenuation. It is positioned on each side by the mediastinal pleura, anteriorly by the sternum and chest wall, and posteriorly by the spine and chest wall.

Lungs

The lungs are our air-filled organs of respiration. They are composed of sponge-like material called the parenchyma and enclosed by a layer of serous membrane. The right lung is divides into three lobes: upper, middle, and lower. The middle lobe does not completely separate the upper and lower lobes; therefore, in axial sections through the upper lung, both the upper and lower lobes are often demonstrated noting the lower lobe more posterior. The left lung contains two lobes: the upper and lower. In axial sections through the middle of the lung, both lobes will be seen due to the course of the oblique fissure.

Pleura

The pleura are the serous membranes covering the lungs and lining the walls of the chest cavity. It is divided into two layers: the visceral pleura which are the membrane surrounding the lung and the parietal pleura, the outer layer lining the chest wall. Between the visceral and parietal pleura there exists the pleural space that is the cavity between the layers that contains serous fluid. On cross-sectional images the pleural space is not distinguished unless there is an abnormality such as fluid or air.

Fissures of the Lungs

A lung fissure is a space separating lobes of the lungs. The right lung contains two fissures, the oblique fissure, is the space separating the upper and middle lobes from the lower lobe and the horizontal fissure, which is the detachment of the upper and middle lobes. Since the left lung only has two lobes an upper and lower, the fissure of the left lung is the oblique fissure.

Bronchi

The trachea bifurcates into left and right main stem (primary) bronchi posterior to the great vessels and anterior to the esophagus. This area is commonly termed the carina. The carina is seen near the level of the pulmonary arteries at the 5th thoracic vertebra. At the hilum the main stem bronchi enter the lungs and divide into secondary or lobar bronchi then further divide into tertiary or segmental bronchi. Each bronchial tree continues to divide into smaller bronchi termed bronchioles and each bronchiole divides further until it reaches the terminal end called the alveoli.

Musculature of the Chest

Pectoralis Muscles

The pectoralis muscles are two muscles found on the anterior surface of the chest with their primary function is to move of the upper limbs. The pectoralis major muscle is most anterior and aids in the flexion, abduction, and rotation of the arms. Its other function is to expand the thoracic cavity when during deep inspiration. The pectoralis minor muscle lies directly behind the pectoralis major on the anterior surface of the 3rd through 5th ribs. It acts to elevate and protract the scapula.

Intercostal Muscles

The intercostal muscles are situated in the intercostal space. They act to keep the intercostal spaces slightly rigid during respiration. These muscles also aid forced inspiration by elevating the ribs.

Vasculature of the Chest

Mediastinum Vascular Anatomy

The mediastinum vascular anatomy can be divided into three equal divisions. In adults each of these divisions is made up of about 15 contiguous 5-mm slices.

Supra-aortic
* thoracic inlet to the top of the aortic arch

Subaortic
* aortic arch to the superior aspect of the heart

Paracardiac
* heart to the diaphragm

Supra-Aortic Mediastinum

Great arterial branches of the aortic arch and the veins are the most important structures to recognize (Fig. 2.20). At the thoracic inlet the brachiocephalic veins are the most anterior and lateral branches visible lying immediately behind the clavicular heads. The left brachiocephalic vein crosses the mediastinum from left to right to join the right brachiocephalic vein thus forming the superior vena cava (SVC). These great arterial branches are posterior to the veins and lie adjacent to the anterior and lateral walls of the trachea. These vessels include left subclavian artery, the left common carotid artery and the brachiocephalic trunk (innominate). The left subclavian artery is most posterior and is situated adjacent to the left side of the trachea. The left common

carotid artery is anterior to the left subclavian artery and the brachiocephalic artery is usually anterior and somewhat to the right of the tracheal midline. The artery is usually oval, being somewhat larger than the other aortic branches.

Subaortic Mediastinum

The subaortic compartment contains many of the undivided mediastinal great vessels: the aorta, SVC, and pulmonary arteries. Along with the vessels it contains most of the important lymph nodes groups. These nodes may be abnormal in patients with lung cancer, infectious diseases, sarcoidosis, or lymphoma.

Aortic Arch Level

The anterior aspect of the arch passes to the left of the trachea and the posterior arch is usually lying anterior and lateral to the spine. The SVC is visible anterior and to the right of the trachea usually oval in shape, while the esophagus is somewhat to the left and posterior to the midline of the trachea. Anterior to the great vessels contains the thymus, lymph nodes, and fat.

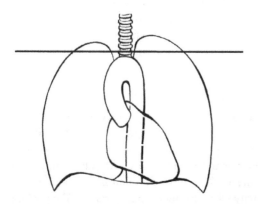

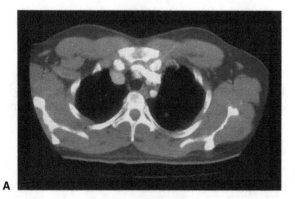

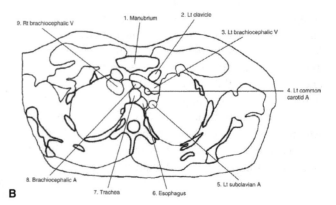

Figure 2.20. Axial CT image of the supra-aortic mediastinum. (Reproduced, with permission, from Madden ME. *Introduction to Sectional Anatomy.* 3rd ed. Philadelphia, PA: Wolters Kluwer; Lippincott Williams & Wilkins; 2013.)

Pulmonary Arteries (Fig. 2.21)

Main Pulmonary Artery

The main pulmonary artery also known as the pulmonary trunk arises from the left ventricle continuing posteriorly to form the right and left pulmonary artery. On cross-sectional images, as the trunk divides into the right and left arteries, it can be seen as a T-shaped structure. This structure is an important landmark when performing pulmonary embolism examinations. On the localizer image the pulmonary trunk is slightly lower than the bifurcation of the trachea on most patients. The pulmonary arteries carry deoxygenated blood to the lungs and are the only arteries in the body containing deoxygenated blood.

Right

The right pulmonary artery is posterior to the ascending aorta and SVC, and is anterior to the esophagus and right main stem bronchus to enter the hilum of the right lung. At the root of the right lung, it divides into two branches; the lower branch supplies the middle and inferior lobe, while the upper branch supplies the upper lobe

Left

The left pulmonary artery is shorter and smaller than the right artery. It arches over the left main stem bronchus entering the hilum of the left lung being the most superior of the pulmonary vessels and can be see superior to the left main stem bronchus. Similar to the right pulmonary artery, the left divides into lobar and segmental arteries.

Pulmonary Veins

The pulmonary veins commence in a capillary network where they are continuous with the capillaries of the pulmonary arteries and divide into four branches. There are two superior and two inferior extend from each lung to enter the left atrium. These veins are located inferior to the pulmonary arteries and on axial images; the pulmonary veins are anterior to the pulmonary arteries.

Azygos Venous System

The azygos venous system provides a collateral circulation between the SVC and the inferior vena cava and divides into the azygos and hemiazygos veins. These veins are a continuation of the right and left ascending lumbar veins. The azygos vein is located in the posterior thoracic cage ascending along the right side of the vertebral bodies. It drains blood from the posterior chest and superior abdomen into the SVC. The hemiazygos vein ascends along the left side of the vertebral bodies and crosses to the right behind the aorta to join the azygos vein at approximately the level of T7–T9. This vein drains blood from the inferior, posterior thoracic cage into the azygos vein.

CROSS-SECTIONAL ANATOMY OF THE HEART

The heart is a muscular hollow organ situated within the middle mediastinum approximately the size of a clenched fist containing four chambers:

- Right atrium
- Left atrium
- Right ventricle
- Left ventricle

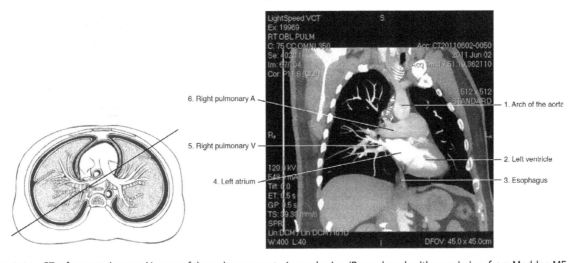

Figure 2.21. CT reformatted coronal image of the pulmonary arteries and veins. (Reproduced, with permission, from Madden ME. *Introduction to Sectional Anatomy*. 3rd ed. Philadelphia, PA: Wolters Kluwer; Lippincott Williams & Wilkins; 2013.)

The heart is not located centrally within the thoracic cavity, but obliquely having one-third of the heart lying to the right of the median plane and two-thirds lying to the left of the midline. In cross-sectional images, the chambers appear off-center with the right ventricle being the most anterior chamber and the left atrium the most posterior (Fig. 2.22). The base of the heart is superior formed by the two atria, while the apex is inferior portion projecting anteriorly and to the left.

Heart Wall

The heart is composed of three walls:

Epicardium
- thinner outer layer

Myocardium
- thick middle layer consisting of strong cardiac muscle

Endocardium
- thin layer lining the inner surface

The outer covering called the pericardium is a sac that surrounds the heart and the proximal portions of the great vessels entering and leaving the heart.

Chambers Atria

Right atrium
- forms the right border of the heart
- receives deoxygenated blood from the SVC, IVC, coronary sinus, and cardiac veins that drain the myocardium

Left atrium
- most posterior surface of the heart
- receives oxygenated blood directly from the lungs via the four pulmonary veins

Right and left atrium
- separated by interatrial septum

Chambers Ventricles

Right ventricle
- comprises the largest portion of the anterior surface
- receives deoxygenated blood from the right atrium and forces it into the pulmonary trunk for transportation to the lungs

Left ventricle
- forms the apex

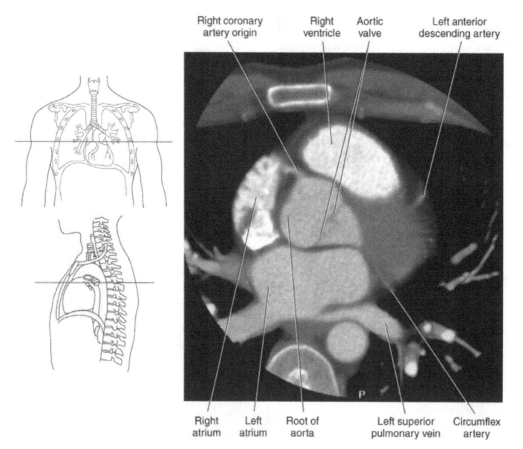

Figure 2.22. Axial CT image of the heart with the right coronary artery. (Reproduced, with permission, from Kelley LL, Petersen CM. *Sectional Anatomy for Imaging Professionals*. 3rd ed. St. Louis, MO: Mosby Elsevier; 2013.)

- receives oxygenated blood from the left atrium and pumps it into the aorta for distribution throughout the systemic circuit
- myocardium is three times thicker in the left ventricle than the right ventricle
  - reflecting the force necessary to pump blood throughout the systemic circuit

Heart Valves (Fig. 2.23)

Atrioventricular Valves

The atrioventricular valves function to maintain one-way directional blood flow throughout the heart. The tricuspid valve contains three leaflets and is located at the entrance of the right ventricle preventing blood to backflow into the right atrium. The valve located at the entrance of the left ventricle is the bicuspid or mitral valve. This valve contains two leaflets and stops blood from the left ventricle to enter the left atrium.

Semilunar Valves

The semilunar valves are the pulmonary and aortic. Pulmonary valve is located at the junction of the right ventricle and pulmonary artery. This valve prevents blood from the pulmonary trunk to drain back into the right ventricle. On cross-sectional axial images this valve is not well visualized. The aortic valve is located between the left ventricle and the aorta. Its function is to stop blood from the ascending aorta from entering the left ventricle.

Coronary Arteries (Fig. 2.24)

Right Coronary Artery

- Arises from the base or root of the aorta
- Passes anteriorly between the pulmonary trunk and right atrium to descend to the coronary groove
- At this point it communicates with the left anterior descending artery
- Supplies blood to the right atrium, right ventricle, interventricular septum, and the sinoatrial and atrioventricular nodes also supplying a portion of the left atrium and ventricle

Left Coronary Artery

Arises from the left aortic sinus

Passes to the left between the pulmonary trunk and left atrium to reach the coronary groove

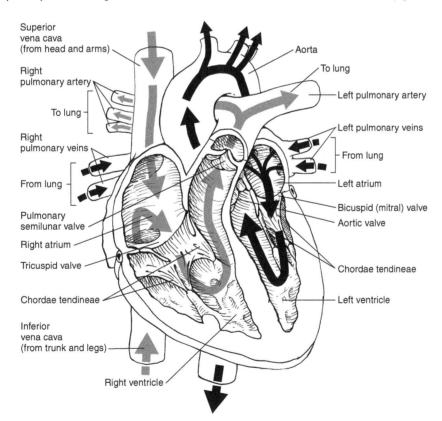

Figure 2.23. Illustration of the heart and heart valves. The *gray arrows* indicate blood flow from the SVC to the pulmonary arteries, while the *black arrow* demonstrates blood flow from the lungs (pulmonary veins) to the aorta. (Reproduced, with permission, from Saia, DA. *Radiology Prep*. 10th ed. New York, NY: McGraw-Hill; 2016.)

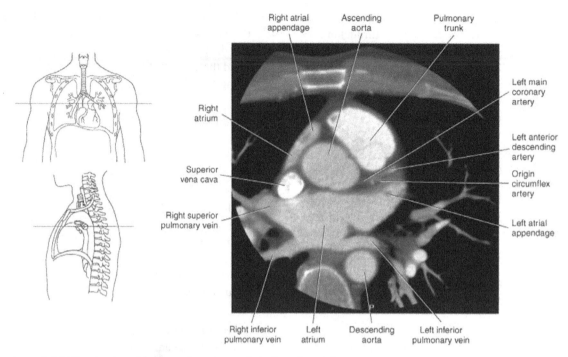

Figure 2.24. Axial CT projection of the ascending aorta with the branching left coronary vessels. (Reproduced, with permission, from Kelley LL, Petersen CM. *Sectional Anatomy for Imaging Professionals*. 3rd ed. St. Louis, MO: Mosby Elsevier; 2013.)

Divides into the circumflex and left anterior descending artery

- supplies the interventricular septum, the AV bundles, and most of the left ventricle and atrium

Coronary Veins

Coronary Sinus

Runs along the posterior section of the coronary sulcus and terminates in the right atrium (Fig. 2.25)

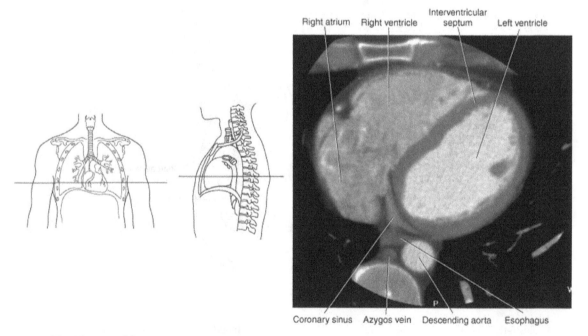

Figure 2.25. CT axial image of the coronary sinus. (Reproduced, with permission, from Kelley LL, Petersen CM. *Sectional Anatomy for Imaging Professionals*. 3rd ed. St. Louis, MO: Mosby Elsevier; 2013.)

Carries most of the venous return from the heart

Its tributaries include:

- great, small, and middle cardiac veins, left posterior ventricular vein, and the oblique vein of the left atrium

IMAGING PROCEDURES OF THE CHEST

Patient Preparation and Positioning

Remove all metallic objects

Including ECG leads and monitoring wires if possible

When IV contrast is utilized

- patient should be NPO for approximately 3 to 4 hours prior to injection
  - reduce the chance of aspiration if vomiting should occur

Arms should be raised above the head

- if both arms cannot be raised
  - attempt to raise at least one
  - preferably the arm being utilized for the iv contrast injection
  - optimize DFOV

If arms need to be included

- increase technical factors
  - compensate bone (beam hardening artifact)

Exclude the arms (best method)

Respiration

Significant importance for chest CT

Identifies air trapping in the lungs

- refers to the retention of excess gas in all or part of the lungs during any phase of expiration
- leads to hyperinflated lungs and lack of ability of the chest to expand and contract

Inspiration

- Air fills lungs and CT number is very low

Expiration

- Expel of air and CT number becomes higher
- Attenuation of the voxels is predominantly the result of interstitial tissue
- Patients with disease will fail to show an increase in attenuation

Indications for IV Contrast

- Mediastinal and hilar lesions
- Abscess or cyst
- Evaluation of trauma
- Survey for metastatic disease
- Evaluation of lung infiltrates
- Pleural disease

Use of IV Contrast Agent

- Allows precise definition of the aorta and its branches, SVC, IVC, and pulmonary veins
- Identifies mediastinum and hilar masses
- Critical in the evaluation of patients with lung CA
- Aids in the analysis of lung infiltrates
- Differentiates pneumonias from parenchyma lung CA
  - CA superficially look similar to pneumonias but will enhance

Routine Chest

Technical Factors

Anatomical coverage

- 2 cm above the clavicles through the adrenal glands

Slice thickness

- 5 mm
  - radiologist preference

Slice interval

- 5 mm
  - radiologist preference

DFOV

- 320 to 480 mm

Kernel

- standard/soft tissue

IV contrast

- 100 cc
  - flow rate
    - 2 to 3 cc/s
  - delay time
    - 40 seconds

Respiration

- full inspiration

Retrospective reconstructions

- slice thickness and intervals
  - 5 mm
  - 1 mm
- kernel
  - lung/detailed
  - if metastatic disease is of concern
    - bone/detail

Reformats

- MPR
  - sagittal
  - coronal
- 3D
  - volume rendered

High-Resolution Chest

High-resolution chest examinations provide remarkable resolution for visualizing the small pulmonary lobules and inflammation in the interlobular septa. They are able to asses diffuse disease at these sites.

Indications for Noncontrast High Resolution

- Asbestosis
- Suspected bronchiectasis
- Pulmonary fibrosis, sarcoidosis
- Diffuse pulmonary disease discovered on chest radiographs
- Quantification of the extent of air trapping
- Emphysema
- Asthma

Technical Factors

Routine nonenhanced CT followed by HRCT
Anatomical coverage
- just above the apices through the lung bases

Retrospective reconstruction
- from the routine chest scan
- slice thickness/slice increments
- 1 mm × 10 mm

Kernel
- lung/detailed

Expiration (low-dose technique)
- axial or helical acquisition

Retrospective reconstruction
- slice thickness/slice increments
  - 1 mm × 10 mm
- kernel
  - lung/detailed

If asbestosis is suspected a low-dose series is performed. The patient is scanned in the prone position utilizing inspiration and expiration respiration and the same technical factors as the high-resolution expiration scan.

Bolus Tracking/Triggering

Obtain localizer view
Obtain a single slice at the area of interest
Plan the diagnostic study parameters
Determine the target region
Obtain a single slice
Set the trigger threshold
- usually set at an HU of 100 to 130

Start the contrast injection
- when the area identified on the monitor scans reaches the threshold
- the scan will commence

May need to manually start the scan
- if the scan does not start within 30 seconds
  - due to patient pathology
  - patient moved and tracker ROI is not in correct place

Test Bolus

Obtain localizer scan
Obtain a single slice at the area of interest
Plan the diagnostic study parameters
Determine the target region
Obtain a single slice
Using the power injector
Inject 20 mL of contrast
Begin scanning at 8 to 15 seconds after start of the injection
Scans are taken every 2 seconds
- at the obtained slice
- slice interval is 0
  - AKA dynamic scanning

10 to 5 scans are taken
Bolus is evaluated by identifying the image that shows the maximum enhancement in the target region (ROI)
Determine the delay time
- trial scan delay + (2 × the image showing the maximum enhancement) + 4 seconds (breath hold delay—*varies per institution)

Example:
- trial scan delay was 10 seconds, image 4 shows maximum enhancement

Image 1 is at 10 seconds, then add 2 seconds to the remaining images, in this case 3 images
- 10 + (2 × 3) + 4
- 10 + 6 + 4 = 20
  - Scan starts 20 seconds following the start of the injection

Pulmonary Embolism

Technical Factors

Anatomical coverage
- 2 cm above the apices to 2 cm below the lung bases
- scan inferior to superior
  - follows blood flow
  - minimizes motion artifact

Slice thickness
- 1 mm

Slice interval
- 1 mm

DFOV
- 320 to 480 mm

Kernel
- standard/soft tissue

Respiration
- expiration
- if using high-speed MDCT
  - normal breathing will suffice

IV contrast
- 100 cc
- flow rate
  - 4 to 5 cc/s
- delay time
  - tracking bolus with ROI placement on the pulmonary trunk
  - HU threshold 100 to 150

Retrospective reconstruction
- slice thickness
  - 1 mm or less
- slice interval
  - overlap
- kernel
  - standard/soft tissue
  - bone/detail

Reformats
- MPR
  - sagittal
  - coronal
- 3D
  - MIP
    - coronal MIP's best method for demonstrating emboli
  - volume rendered

Deep Vein Thrombosis (DVT)

Additional scan of the lower extremities are performed to survey the legs for thrombi, scanning from the bifurcation of the IVC through the knees. A lower mAs is utilized to eliminate excessive radiation dose to the patient.

Slice-thickness intervals
- 5 mm

Slice intervals
- 5 mm

DFOV
- larger enough to encompass patient's width

Kernel
- standard/soft tissue

IV contrast
- 2.5 to 3 minutes following the initial injection

Scan delay
- 2.5 to 3 minutes from start of injection

Chest Dissection

Chest dissection protocols are performed using an unenhanced scan followed by biphasic series

Precontrast
- common anatomical structures

Postcontrast
- highlights arteries

Delayed postcontrast
- check for arterial leak

Technical Factors

Unenhanced

Anatomical coverage
- 2 cm above the aortic arch through the dissection

Slice thickness
- 5 mm

Slice interval
- 5 mm

DFOV
- 320 to 480 mm

Kernel
- standard/soft tissue

Respiration
- inspiration

Bolus/Arterial Phase

Anatomical coverage
- 2 cm above the aortic arch through the dissection

Slice thickness
- 1 mm

Slice intervals
- 1 mm

DFOV
- Same as for unenhanced scan

Kernel
- standard/soft tissue

IV contrast
- 100 cc
- flow rate
  - 4 to 5 cc/s
- delay time
  - Tracking bolus
  - trigger ROI on the aorta mid chest
    - HU threshold 100 to 150

Retrospective reconstruction
- slice thickness
  - 1 mm or less
- slice interval
  - overlap
- kernel
  - standard/soft tissue
  - lung/detail

Reformats

- MPR
  - sagittal
  - coronal
- 3D
  - MIP
  - volume rendered

Equilibrium/Delayed Phase

Anatomical coverage
- 2 cm above the aortic arch through the dissection

Slice thickness
- 5 mm

Slice intervals
- 5 mm

DFOV
- same as for unenhanced scan

Kernel
- standard/soft tissue

PATHOLOGY OF THE CHEST

Asbestosis

Asbestosis is the inhalation of asbestos fiber causing scarring of the lungs and can lead to lung CA (mesothelioma). The risk for this disease increases dramatically in smokers. High-resolution CT imaging will demonstrate pleural plaques, pleural thickening, and pleural calcifications.

Bronchogenic Carcinoma

Lung cancer is the leading cause of death in both men and women. Active cigarette smoking increases the risk for developing a lung neoplasm by a factor of 10, while passing smoking reduces the risk to a factor of 2. Bronchogenic carcinoma is characterized by early lymphogenous and hematogenous spread. On CT images the mass will appear irregular shaped with speculated margins (Fig. 2.26). There may also be central necrosis of the tumor as the tumor increases in size.

Lung Metastasis

The lungs are the most common site of metastatic disease from primary cancers outside the lungs. Primary cancers such as colon, breast, kidney, pancreas, and uterus are most likely to metastasize to the lungs. The disease spreads through blood circulation and lymphatic system. On CT images lung mets appear as multiple bilateral lung masses without calcification (Fig. 2.27). The patients may also have mediastinal lymphadenopathy. With the introduction of contrast media, the lesions will enhance.

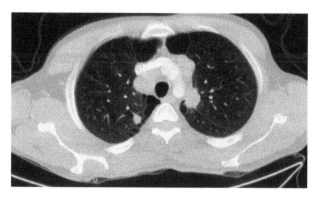

Figure 2.26. CT axial image of the chest scanned in a lung/detailed algorithm and lung windows demonstrating bilateral round lung nodules with irregular speculated margins typical of bronchogenic carcinoma. (Reproduced, with permission, from Grey ML, Ailinani JM . *CT and MRI Pathology: A Pocket Atlas.* 2nd ed. New York, NY: McGraw-Hill; 2012.)

Pleural Effusion

Pleural effusion is the accumulation of fluid between the pleural layers. Effusion can be seen on CT images when the volume of the fluid exceeds 15 mm (Fig. 2.28). The fluid is seen in the posteribasal region forming a crescent-shaped collection that borders the chest wall. CT aids in defining the etiology of the effusion.

Emphysema

Emphysema is considered a chronic obstructive pulmonary disease (COPD) that involves the destruction of the alveolar wall. This results in the surface area of the lung to reduce allowing the collection of free air on inhalation to collect in the lung tissue. On CT images the lungs are hyperinflated with lucent hypodense areas of the lung surrounded by normal lung parenchyma.

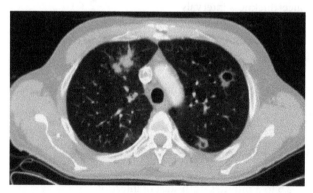

Figure 2.27. Axial CT projection of the chest with multiple enhanced solid lesions with smooth borders a characteristic of pulmonary metastatic disease. (Reproduced, with permission, from Grey ML, Ailinani JM. *CT and MRI Pathology: A Pocket Atlas.* 2nd ed. New York, NY: McGraw-Hill; 2012.)

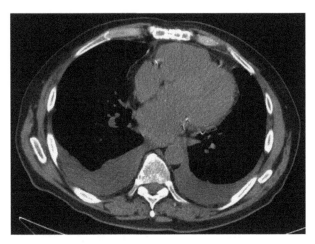

Figure 2.28. Unenhanced axial CT view showing bilateral pulmonary effusions. Fluid within the pleural space is easily noted due to the high subject contrast within the chest. (Reproduced, with permission, from Grey ML, Ailinani JM. *CT and MRI Pathology: A Pocket Atlas*. 2nd ed. New York, NY: McGraw-Hill; 2012.)

Pneumothorax

A pneumothorax is the separation of the pleural cavity by air. CT is highly sensitive in defining the visceral pleura from the air-filled pleural space. CT is an important tool in identifying pneumothorax for patients undergoing mechanical ventilation or anesthesia for surgery. It is also useful to search for instrumental subpleural bullae. These bullae may be congenital or have been formed in the setting of COPD or fibrotic lung disease.

Hodgkin Disease

Hodgkin disease is a primary malignancy of the lymphatic system. It presents itself with enlarged mediastinal lymph

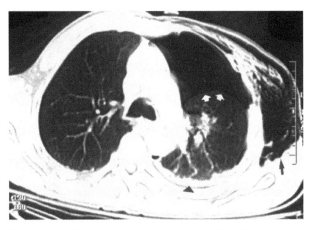

Figure 2.29. Contrast-enhanced axial projection of the chest demonstrating a left pneumothorax (*short arrows*), minimal hemothorax (*arrow heads*), and subcutaneous emphysema (*long arrows*). (Reproduced, with permission, from Grey ML, Ailinani JM. *CT and MRI Pathology: A Pocket Atlas*. 2nd ed. New York, NY: McGraw-Hill; 2012.)

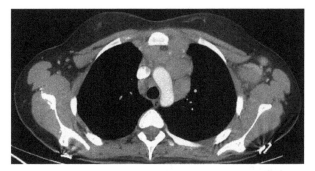

Figure 2.30. Contrast-enhanced axial CT image demonstrating enlarged mediastinal and left axillary lymph nodes typically present with patients with Hodgkin lymphoma. (Reproduced, with permission, from Grey ML, Ailinani JM. *CT and MRI Pathology: A Pocket Atlas*. 2nd ed. New York, NY: McGraw-Hill; 2012.)

nodes, spleen, and liver (Fig. 2.30). The symptoms of the disease are palpable lymph nodes, dry cough, and a greater than 10-lb weight loss. The exact cause of the disease is unknown.

Pulmonary Embolism

A pulmonary embolism is an obstruction in one or more of the main pulmonary artery or one of its branches. The general cause is from a thrombi developing in the leg veins. The risk factors include: long-termed hospitalized patients, COPD, CHF, recent surgery, advanced age, and/or patient immobility. A CT angiogram will demonstrate a hypodense filling defect cause by a clot within the artery (Fig. 2.31). The signs and symptoms are chest pain, SOB, hemoptysis and in some cases leg swelling, but more than 80% of patients with PE have no clinical signs.

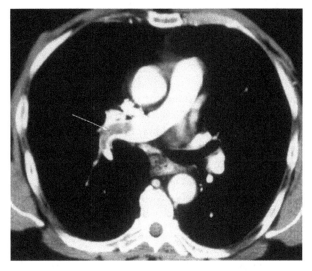

Figure 2.31. CT angiogram of the chest reveals a large pulmonary embolism located well within the right pulmonary artery. (Reproduced, with permission, from Grey ML, Ailinani JM. *CT and MRI Pathology: A Pocket Atlas*. 2nd ed. New York, NY: McGraw-Hill; 2012.)

Pulmonary Dissection

A pulmonary dissection is a tear in the wall of the aorta that causes blood to flow between the layers of the wall of the aorta and force the layers apart. Blood penetrates the intima and enters the media layer. The compositions of the arterial walls are as follows:

Tunica intima—direct contact with flow of blood
Tunica media—smooth muscle layer
Tunica adventitia—outermost layer
• made up of connective tissue

CROSS-SECTIONAL ANATOMY OF THE ABDOMEN

Abdominal Cavity

The abdominal cavity is the region located between the diaphragm and sacral promontory. Each section abdominal and pelvic cavities can be identified by the four surface landmark quadrants and nine Addison's planes regions (Fig. 2.32).

Four Quadrants

Right Upper Quadrant (RUQ)
• Right lobe of the liver, gallbladder, right kidney, portions of the stomach, small, and large intestine
Left Upper Quadrant (LUQ)
• Left lobe of the liver, stomach, tail of pancreas, left kidney, spleen, portions of the large intestine
Right Lower Quadrant (RLQ)
• Cecum, appendix, portions of small intestine, right ureter, right ovary, right spermatic cord
Left Lower Quadrant (LLQ)
• Most of small intestine, portions of large intestine, left ureter, left ovary, left spermatic cord

Addison's Planes

The four quadrants can then be subdivided by four planes into nine regions (Fig. 2.33). The horizontal planes are the transpyloric plane found midway between the xiphisternal joint and the umbilicus, passing midway through the L1 vertebrae and the transtubercular, which passes through the tubercles on the iliac crest at the L5 vertebral body. The sagittal planes are the midclavicular lines that run inferiorly from the midpoint of each clavicle to the midinguinal point.

Peritoneum

The peritoneum is the serous membrane that forms the lining of the abdominal cavity. It covers most of the intra-abdominal organs, and is composed of a layer of mesothelium supported by a thin layer of connective

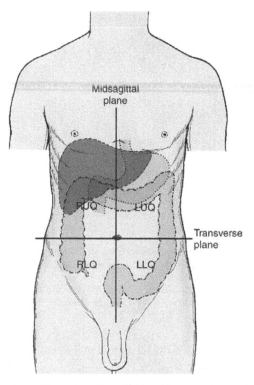

Figure 2.32. Illustration of the divisional four quadrants of the abdomen. (Reproduced, with permission, from Kelley LL, Petersen CM. *Sectional Anatomy for Imaging Professionals*. 3rd ed. St. Louis, MO: Mosby Elsevier; 2013.)

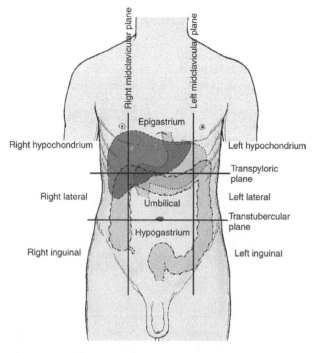

Figure 2.33. Illustration of the nine abdominal regions known as Addison's planes. (Reproduced, with permission, from Kelley LL, Petersen CM. *Sectional Anatomy for Imaging Professionals*. 3rd ed. St. Louis, MO: Mosby Elsevier; 2013.)

tissue. The peritoneum supports the abdominal organs and serves as a conduit for their blood vessels, lymph vessels, and nerves. The various recesses and spaces of the peritoneal cavity are easiest to recognize on CT images when ascites is present.

The peritoneal cavity encloses organs such as: liver (except the bare area), gallbladder, spleen, stomach, ovaries, and majority of intestines. In males the cavity is closed, but in females it communicates with the exterior through the uterine tubes, uterus, and vagina. It consists of two sacs: greater sac is located between the inner surface of the anterior abdominal wall and the outer surface of the abdominal viscera, while the lesser sac is located between the posterior surface of the stomach and posterior abdominal wall. Their communication is through the epiploic foramen or foramen of Winslow.

The mesentery is double layer of peritoneum that extends like a fan across the abdomen from the ligament of Treitz to the region of the right sacroiliac joint. The greater omentum is a double layer of mesentery that is attached to the stomach. The omentum encloses the nerves, blood vessels, lymph channels, and fatty connective tissue. It serves as fertile ground for implantation of peritoneal metastases.

Retroperitoneum

Retroperitoneum consists of structures posterior to the peritoneum. The retroperitoneal space is located between the diaphragm and the pelvic brim and is divided into the anterior pararenal, perirenal, and posterior pararenal compartments by the anterior and posterior renal fascia. It houses organs such as: the kidneys, ureters, adrenal glands, and pancreas, most of the duodenum, ascending and descending colon, aorta, inferior vena cava, and uterus.

Liver

The liver is divided into lobes according to surface anatomy or into segments according to vascular supply, right lobe, left lobe, caudate lobe, and the quadrate lobe. It is mostly located in RUQ, and extends partly into LUQ and can be seen between the 10th thoracic and 3rd lumbar vertebra. The liver is surrounded by a strong connective tissue capsule known as Glisson's capsule, which gives shape and stability to the soft hepatic tissue of the organ.

Liver Ligaments

Ligament Venosum

The ligament venosum is the remnant of the ductus venosus (umbilical cord) which carried blood directly from the umbilical vein to the inferior vena cava to bypass the liver in fetal circulation. It separates the caudate lobe from the left lobe and may be continuous with the round ligament of the liver.

Round Ligament (Ligamentum Teres)

The round ligament or ligamentum teres is the remnant of the fetal umbilical vein. It attaches the internal surface of the umbilicus within the free inferior margin of the falciform ligament. Prenatally and for a month or two after birth, the umbilical vein is patent, and subsequently degenerates to fibrous tissue. This ligament divides the left lobe into medial and lateral segments.

Falciform Ligament

The falciform ligament extends from the liver to the abdominal wall and diaphragm, divides the liver anatomically into right and left lobes. On the posteriorly surface of the liver, it is continuous with the coronary and triangular ligaments. Its free border, which extends from the umbilicus to the anterior border of the liver, contains the ligamentum teres between its two layers.

Coronary Ligament

The coronary ligament attaches the liver to the diaphragm forming the margins of the bare area of the liver. It consists of two layers which are separated from each other by a space equal to the breadth of the bare area of the posterior surface of the liver.

Bare Area of the Liver

The bare area of the liver is a large triangular surface of the liver devoid of peritoneal covering. This section of the liver is connected to the diaphragm by loose areolar tissue.

Blood Supply to the Liver

The liver consists of a dual supply system delivered by the hepatic artery and the portal vein. The hepatic artery is responsible for 15% to 25% of its blood supply, which accounts for the low attenuation values during the arterial phase of injection. The hepatic artery supplies oxygen to the liver allowing it to function. The portal vein then circulates the remainder 75% to 85% of the blood within the liver. As opposed to the arterial phase, the portal venous phase, with the proper delay time, shows a great amount of enhancement. Its function is to transport all material absorbed through the GI tract, whether it is nutrient or toxin.

Gallbladder and Biliary System

The gallbladder is located in RUQ, on the anterior aspect of abdomen under the inferior surface of the liver—associated with the main lobar fissure. It can be seen medial to the stomach between the 12th thoracic and 3rd lumbar vertebra. The biliary system is composed of the gallbladder and bile ducts, which serve to drain the liver of bile and then store it until it is transported to the duodenum. Its function is to aid digestion.

Bile Ducts (Fig. 2.34)

The bile ducts consist of:

Intrahepatic duct
- runs beside the hepatic arteries and portal veins through the liver eventually forming the right and left hepatic ducts

Right and left hepatic ducts
- unite at the portal hepatis to form the proximal portion of the common hepatic duct (CHD)

CHD
- marks the beginning the extrahepatic biliary system
- descends down joined from the right by the cystic duct to form the common bile duct (CBD)

CBD
- follows a grove on the posterior surface of the pancreatic head then pierces the medial wall of the duodenum along the main pancreatic duct (duct of Wirsung) through the ampulla of Vater
  - ends of both ducts are surrounded by circular muscle fibers of the sphincter of Oddi

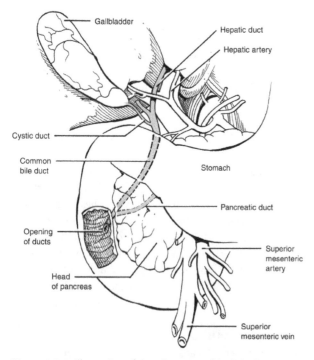

Figure 2.34. Illustration of the tributaries of the bile ducts. (Reproduced, with permission, from Madden ME. *Introduction to Sectional Anatomy.* 3rd ed. Philadelphia, PA: Wolters Kluwer; Lippincott Williams & Wilkins; 2013.)

Pancreas

The pancreas is a long narrow retroperitoneal organ lying posterior to the stomach and medial to the spleen. It is located in LUQ and RUQ between the 12th thoracic and 3rd lumbar vertebra. It is a collection of glandular tissue with little connective tissue having both exocrine and endocrine functions. The pancreas is divided into five distinct parts:

- Head
  - flat and inferior and to the right of the body and tail
  - nestles in the curve of the duodenum
- Uncinate process
  - medial and posterior extension of the head
  - it is sandwiched between the aorta, IVC, SMA, and SMV
    - the aorta and IVC are posterior while the SMA and SMV are anterior to the surface
- Body
  - largest and most anterior
  - extending transversely to the left
- Tail
  - superiorly and posteriorly portion of the body

Spleen

The spleen is the largest lymph node of the body located in LUQ. It is posterior to the stomach in posterior aspect of abdomen with a highly vascular and spongy parenchyma. The spleen produces white blood cells, filters abnormal blood cells, stores iron from red blood cells, and initiates the immune response. Due to its spongy structure, during the arterial phase of injection, its characteristic appearance is of a stripped tiger.

Stomach

The stomach is the dilated portion of the digestive system and acts as a food reservoir. It is responsible for the early stages of digestion. When the stomach is empty its inner surface creates prominent folds called rugae. This allows the stomach to expand with the ingestion of food. It is important when scanning the abdomen, the patient receive approximately 250 mL of oral contrast to fill these folds; otherwise, they appear as hypodensities within the stomach and can be interpreted as an abnormality. It can be seen on cross-sectional images anterior to the spleen under the left dome of the diaphragm. It resides mostly in LUQ, and partially in RUQ, between the 10th thoracic and 2nd lumbar vertebra. The stomach can be divided into three parts:

Fundus
- superior surface

Body
- largest portion
- between the two curvatures
  - lesser—medial
  - greater—lateral

Pylorus
- inferior portion
- consist of the pyloric antrum, angular notch, pyloric canal and pyloric sphincter
- empties into the duodenum through the pyloric sphincter

Small Intestines

The small intestines are located between the pylorus and ileocecal valve consisting of loops of bowel averaging 6 to 7 m in length. The small bowel is subdivided into three distinct portions:

Duodenum
- duodenal bulb

First 2 in

Superior portion
- descending portion

Next 4 in

Contains the ampulla of Vater
- horizontal

4 in long

Runs anterior to the SVC, aorta, IMA
- ascending
  - ascends to the left side of the aorta at the level of L2
  - meets the jejunum (duodenojejunal flexure)
  - fixed in place by the ligament of Treitz

Jejunum
- centrally located occupying all four quadrants (2.5 m)

Ileum
- centrally located except terminal ileum (RLQ) (3.5 m)
- ileocecal valve—junction of the ileum and the cecum
- sphincter that controls the flow of material from the ileum into the cecum
- receives blood from the branches of the SMA and are drained by the SMV

Large Intestines

The large intestines lye inferior to the stomach and liver and almost completely frames the small intestine. The longitudinal muscle of the large intestine forms three thickened bands called the taenia coli, which gathers the cecum and colon into pouch-like folds known as hastra. On the outer surface of the colon the epiploic appendages, which are fat-filled sacs of omentum attaching the intestine to the abdominal wall. The colon can be subdivided into four distinct portions:

Ascending
- located in both the RUQ and RLQ
- commences at the cecum and extends to the liver
  - hepatic flexure
  - vermiform appendix
  - attaches to the posteromedial surface of the cecum
  - a normal appendix may be difficult to visualize on cross-sectional imaging

Transverse colon
- located in both the RUQ and LUQ
- extends across the abdomen toward the spleen
  - Splenic flexure

Descending colon
- located in both the LUQ and LLQ
- extends inferiorly along the lateral abdominal wall to the iliac fossa

Sigmoid colon
- travels posteriorly and inferiorly in midline and LLQ, posterior and inferior to small intestines

Adrenal Glands

The adrenal glands are retroperitoneal organs located superior to each kidney. They are separated from the superior surface of the kidney by perirenal fat and enclosed along with the kidneys by Gerota's fascia. The right adrenal gland is lower and more medial then the left and commonly appears as an inverted V on cross-sectional images. The left adrenal gland is anteromedial to the upper pole of the left kidney with its appearance as a triangular or Y-shaped configuration. Both glands border the crus of the diaphragm. The outer cortex and inner medulla of the glands function independently.

Cortex
- produces more than two dozen steroids collectively
  - adrenocortical steroids or just corticosteroids

Medulla
- produces the hormones epinephrine and norepinephrine
  - accelerates metabolism and energy and are responsible for the body's "fight or flight" response

Urinary System

The structures include the kidneys, ureters, bladder, and urethra. The organs located within the abdominal cavity are the kidneys and ureters. The bladder and urethra are located in the pelvic cavity and will be discussed in the pelvic section.

Kidneys

Kidneys are retroperitoneal bean-shaped organs, located in RUQ and LUQ between the levels of the 12th thoracic and 4th lumbar vertebra. They are composed of an outer cortex and inner medulla.

Cortex

- comprises the outer one third of the renal tissue
- responsible for filtration of urine
- during the corticomedullary phase of injection only the renal cortex is enhanced

Medulla

- consists of segments called renal pyramids and function as the beginning of the collecting system
- during the nephrographic phase of injection IV contrast has to be filtered demonstrating the inner medulla to enhance

Collection System of the Kidneys (Fig. 2.35)

Minor calyces

- cup-shaped and arise from the apices of the pyramids
- 7 to 14 in each kidney
- merge into two or three major calyces

Renal pelvis

- joining of the major calyces–largest dilated portion and is continuous with the ureters

Ureters

- located medial to kidneys and lateral to IVC and aorta

The renal fascia (Gerota's fascia) is perirenal fat surrounding the kidneys. It functions to anchor the kidneys to surrounding structures in an attempt to prevent bumps and jolts to the body from injuring the kidneys.

Musculature of the Abdomen

Psoas

The psoas muscle extends along the lateral surface of the lumbar vertebrae to insert on the lesser trochanter of the femur. Its purpose is to flex the thigh and trunk. On axial images the large muscles are round and readily identified lying on either side of the vertebral column and aid in identification of the adjacent ureters and vessels.

Linea Alba

The linea alba is a longitudinal band of fiber that forms a central anterior attachment for the muscle layer of the abdomen. It is formed at the midline, extending from the xiphoid process to the pelvic symphysis, by interlacing of fibers from the rectus abdominis and oblique muscles.

Rectus Abdominis

The rectus abdominis muscle originates anteriorly at the pubic bone near symphysis and inserts into the costal

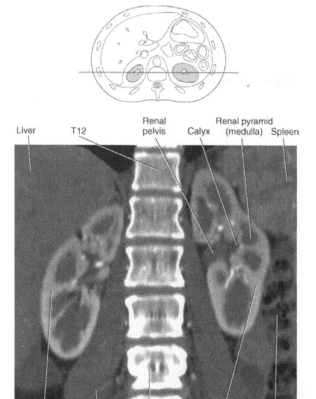

Liver   T12   Renal pelvis   Calyx   Renal pyramid (medulla)   Spleen

Cortex of right kidney   Psoas muscle   L4   Cortex of left kidney   Descending colon

Figure 2.35. Contrast-enhanced coronal reformatted image in the arterial phase demonstrating the renal collecting system. (Reproduced, with permission, from Kelley LL, Petersen CM. *Sectional Anatomy for Imaging Professionals.* 3rd ed. St. Louis, MO: Mosby Elsevier; 2013.)

cartilage of the 5th, 6th, and 7th rib, xiphoid process of sternum. The function of this muscle is to flex the lumbar vertebra and support the abdomen.

External and Internal Oblique Muscles

The oblique muscles are located on the outer lateral portion and extend from the cartilages of the lower ribs to the level of the iliac crest. They work together to flex and rotate the vertebral column. The external oblique is the most extensive of the abdominal muscles and contains a triangular opening, known as the inguinal ring, which allows for the passageway of the spermatic cord or the round ligament of the uterus.

Transverse Abdominis Muscle

The transverse abdominis lies deep in the internal oblique muscle. Its strong fibers provide maximum support for the abdomen viscera. When the trunk bends it compresses the abdominal viscera.

Quadratus Lumborum Muscle

The quadratus lumborum muscle forms the large portion of the abdominal wall. This muscle extends from the iliac crest to the inferior border of the 12th rib and transverse processes of the lumbar vertebrae. Its function is in aiding lateral flexion of the vertebral column.

Vascular System of the Abdomen

Aorta

The aorta is a retroperitoneal structure beginning as an extension of the thoracic aorta, at the aorta hiatus of the diaphragm. This artery passes posterior to the head of the pancreas delivering blood to the abdomen and pelvic organs and their structures. The aorta bifurcates into the right and left common iliac arteries at approximately the level of 4th lumbar vertebra.

Celiac Trunk (Fig. 2.36)

The celiac trunk is a very short vessel that leaves the anterior wall of the aorta just after the aorta passes through the diaphragm at approximately T12/L1. This vessel divides into three branches:

- Left gastric
- Common hepatic
  - Gives rise to the proper hepatic artery
  - Supplies the liver and gallbladder
- Splenic
  - Largest branch of the celiac trunk
  - Travels a tortuous path giving it a distinctive appearance
  - Spring or curly cue

Superior Mesenteric Artery

The superior mesenteric artery branches 1 cm below the celiac trunk at approximately the level of 1st lumbar vertebra and extends downward. It supplies the head of the pancreas and majority of the small and large intestines. Compared to the perpendicular origin of the celiac trunk, its oblique coursed can be a noticeable characteristic on axial images. Fat planes that surround the artery are preferential sites for the spread of pancreatic cancer.

Inferior Mesenteric Artery

The inferior mesenteric artery arises 3 to 4 cm above the bifurcation of the aorta at the L3/L4 level. It enters the

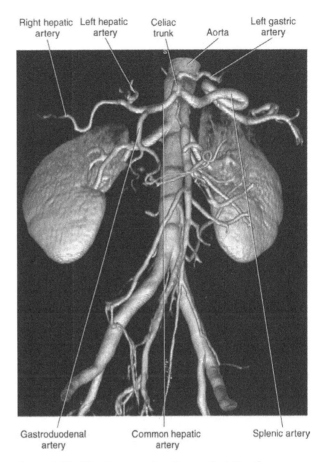

Figure 2.36. 3D volume-rendered image depicting the branches of the celiac trunk (common hepatic, splenic, and left gastric artery). (Reproduced, with permission, from Kelley LL, Petersen CM. *Sectional Anatomy for Imaging Professionals*. 3rd ed. St. Louis, MO: Mosby Elsevier; 2013.)

mesentery to supply blood to the distal half of the large intestine.

Renal Arteries

The renal arteries arise on the lateral aspect of the aorta just below the superior mesenteric artery and supply blood to the kidneys. Once the artery enters the hilum of the kidney it divides into each section of the kidney. The right renal artery is slightly longer than the left due to the fact it passes behind the IVC and the right renal vein. It is not uncommon to see more than one renal artery especially on the left.

Common Iliac Arteries

The common iliac arteries are bilateral arteries arising from the aorta. As they enter the pelvis, they diverge laterally. Each artery then bifurcates to give rise to the internal and external iliac arteries.

Venous System of the Abdomen (Fig. 2.37)

Inferior Vena Cava

The IVC is the largest vein of the body carrying blood to the heart from the lower limbs, pelvic organs, abdominal viscera, and abdominal wall. This vessel is formed by the union of the common iliac veins at approximately level of the 5th lumbar vertebra. The IVC is similar in arrangement of branches to aorta except ovarian and testicular vein arrangement. The right ovarian or testicular vein empties directly into IVC, while the left ovarian or testicular vein empties into the renal vein, then the renal vein, and then empties into IVC. As it ascends the abdominal cavity, it passes the posterior surface of the liver and pierces the diaphragm at the caval hiatus to enter the right atrium of the heart.

Portal Vein

The portal vein carries nutrient-rich blood to the middle of the visceral surface of the liver and lies adjacent to the hepatic bile ducts and the hepatic artery. Lying adjacent to the hepatic bile duct and the hepatic artery proper, it forms part of the porta hepatis. This vein is found in the Retroperitoneum by a joining of the splenic vein and superior mesenteric. Porta hepatis is a transverse fissure on the visceral surface of the liver, where the portal vein and hepatic artery enter and the hepatic ducts leave.

Splenic Vein

The splenic vein transverses the abdomen posterior to the stomach and the pancreas. Its function is to drains nutrient-rich blood from the spleen to the inferior mesenteric vein into the portal vein. As opposed to the splenic artery the course of the vein is linear.

Inferior Mesenteric Vein

The inferior mesenteric vein drains blood from the rectum, sigmoid colon, and the ascending colon to the splenic vein. During its course, the vein lays within the mesentery attaches the intestine to the posterior abdominal wall.

Superior Mesenteric Vein

The superior mesenteric vein drains blood from the stomach, duodenum, jejunum, ileum, cecum, appendix, ascending colon, transverse colon, and pancreas. This vessel lies within the mesentery and carries nutrient-filled venous blood from the intestines to the portal vein.

Renal Veins

The renal veins pass inferior to the renal arteries to empty into the IVC at about the level of the 2nd lumbar vertebra.

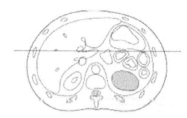

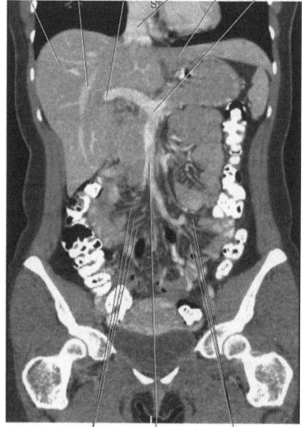

Figure 2.37. CT coronal reformatted image of the portal venous system. (Reproduced, with permission, from Kelley LL, Petersen CM. *Sectional Anatomy for Imaging Professionals.* 3rd ed. St. Louis, MO: Mosby Elsevier; 2013.)

The left renal vein sasses posterior to the superior mesenteric artery and anterior to the aorta on its route from the kidney to enter the left lateral wall of the IVC. It receives the left gonadal vein, left inferior phrenic vein, and generally the left suprarenal vein. The right renal vein is typically lower than the left and enters the right lateral wall of the IVC.

Common Iliac Veins

The common iliac veins drain venous blood from the lower limbs and pelvis into the inferior vena cava. Unlike most regions of the body these veins are more posterior and inferiorly situated than the adjacent common iliac arteries. These veins are formed by the union of the external and internal iliac veins at the L5–S1 joint space.

ABDOMEN PROCEDURES

CT had been utilized extensively as a tool for the evaluation of abdominal masses with the visual ability of differentiating tumors from other solid masses. Physicians order abdominal/pelvic studies for tumor staging, to pinpoints the size, and location of the tumor, and to determine whether the tumor is infringing upon adjacent structures. This information is critical patients undergoing radiation therapy and chemotherapy. With the onset of trauma emergency rooms, CT scanning is a typical trauma protocol for assessing the extent of trauma-related injuries. The results of the studies conclude whether immediate surgical intervention is warranted. Because it is noninvasive, CT is the preferred method for determining cause of acute abdominal pain related to infection and inflammation. Its only disadvantage is patient radiation dose.

Indications for Routine CT Abdominal Examinations
Abdominal/pelvic survey for patients with cancer or trauma
Abdominal/pelvic trauma
- lacerations
  - liver, spleen, and/or kidney
Lymph node pathologic processes
Abscesses
Hematomas
Abdominal pain
Right lower quadrant (appendicitis)
Left lower quadrant (diverticulitis)
Retroperitoneal bleed
Prostate, cervical, ovarian, urinary bladder carcinomas
Soft tissue masses
- disease of the pelvic muscles

Patient Preparation
All metallic objects removed
Patient should be NPO
- 3 to 4 hours prior to study if receiving IV contrast
- purpose is to avoid aspiration if patient vomits
Patients receiving oral contrast
- should arrive 1 to 1½ hours prior to study

They should be positioned feet-first supine
- this allows the technologist to have full visualization of the patient's face
  - claustrophobic patients
  - patients with difficulty in breathing and those who require head elevation
  - trauma patients in whom the extent of injury is unknown
Arms should be raised above head (if physically possible)
- avoids artifact noise
Immobilization may be necessary
- prevents motion achieving high-quality images
Trauma patients arriving on restraint boards and neck braces
- should be kept on these devices
Most importantly
- explains the procedure to the patient
- alleviates stress and concern on the patients part
- ensures full cooperation of the patient
- produces high-quality images

Routine abdominal studies require the patient to drink oral contrast (300 mL), 30 minutes prior to the start of the examination, while a routine abdominal/pelvic examination necessitates the patient to drink (450 mL), 60 to 90 minutes prior to the commencement of the examination. In order to fill the stomach and the beginning of the small bowel, a "top-off" dose of 150 mL of oral contrast is required. This will ensure the rugae within the lining of the stomach are opacified. When the area of interest is the distal large bowel or rectum a delay time of 4 to 6 hours is necessary. When this delay time is impossible to wait, rectal contrast may be employed.

As long as the patient's renal functions are normal and there is no contraindication for the use of IV contrast the choice of the type, concentration, amount, method of administration, and scanning delay should be determined.

Abdominal/Pelvic Acquisition Parameters
Slice thickness
- 5 to 7 mm
Increments
- 5 to 7 mm
DFOV
- 320 to 480 mm (skin to skin)
Kernel (algorithm)
- standard/soft tissue
IV contrast
- 100 cc with 50 cc saline flush
Flow rate
- 2 to 3 cc/s
  - ideally

Scan delay
- 70 to 90 seconds

R/O RLQ pain delay 80 to 95 seconds
- if injection rate varies from standard imaging
  - remember to calculate length of injection and length of scan, so as not to have significant contrast left upon scan completion

Retrospective reconstruction
- slice thickness/intervals
- ≤3 mm
  - ensures artifact elimination on reformatted images

Reformation
- sagittal
- coronal

It is important to remember, when scanning for hemorrhage, an unenhanced scan is appropriate. The use of oral contrast is used for the evaluation of postsurgical bowel leaks.

Liver CT Examinations

Contrast enhance CT imaging can accurately characterize lesion enhancement patterns. The use of different phases of injection significantly improves the specificity of diagnosis. Liver masses enhance during the period between when contrast arrives in the hepatic artery and when it enters the porta hepatis—in conjunction with the noncontrast scan. Hypervascular tumors enhance during the arterial phase, while hypovascular tumors visualize during the portal venous phase of injection. Enhancement of the normal liver is homogeneous throughout the parenchyma on all enhancement phases. The three phases of contrast enhancement entail:

Bolus Phase (Arterial)
- Refers to the timing immediately following an IV injection
- Defined by density difference at least a 30 HU between the abdominal aorta and the inferior vena cava (IVC)
- This phase usually occurs within 25 seconds after initiation

Nonequilibrium Phase (Portal Venous)
- Refers to the timing shortly after an IV injection
- Defined by a density difference a 10 to 30 HU between the abdominal aorta and the inferior vena cava (IVC)
- This phase usually occurs within 70 to 90 seconds after initiation

Equilibrium Phase
- Refers to the timing usually a few minutes after an IV injection
- Defined by a density difference less than 10 HU between the abdominal aorta and the inferior vena cava (IVC)

Delayed Phase
- Refers to the timing usually 10 to 20 minutes after an IV injection

Indications for Dedicated Liver Examinations

Detection and characteristics of mass
Hemangioma
Hepatoma
Focal nodular hyperplasia
Abnormal liver function
Hepatitis and cirrhosis
Kaposi's sarcoma
Hypervascular tumors
- breast
- colon

Liver transplants
- donor and recipient

Liver Acquisition Parameters

Unenhanced Scan

Anatomical coverage
- dome of the diaphragm to the iliac crest

Slice thickness
- 5 mm

Increments
- 5 mm

Kernel (algorithm)
- standard/soft tissue

IV contrast
- none

Unenhanced scans provide a baseline for degree of lesion enhancement. Unenhanced images are superior to postcontrast scans for the diagnosis of fatty infiltrates and other alterations of parenchymal attenuation.

Bolus/Arterial Phase

Anatomical coverage
- dome of the diaphragm to the iliac crest

Slice thickness
- 5 mm

Increments
- 5 mm

Kernel (algorithm)
- standard/soft tissue

IV contrast
- 100 cc with 50 cc saline flush

Flow rate
- 4 to 5 cc/s

Scan delay
- tracking bolus at celiac trunk
- manual timing
- 25 to 30 seconds from start of injection

The bolus/arterial phase acquisition is ideal for imaging hypervascular lesions supplied by the hepatic artery. These lesions include hepatomas, carcinoid metastases, and focal nodular hyperplasia. These lesions are noted because they enhance more than the surrounding parenchyma.

Nonequilibrium/Portal Venous Phase

Anatomical coverage
- dome of the diaphragm through the ischial tuberosities

Slice thickness
- 5 mm

Increments
- 5 mm

Algorithm
- standard/soft tissue

Scan delay
- 70 to 90 seconds from start of injection

The nonequilibrium phase demonstrates the greatest lesion detection, since the parenchyma enhancement is maximized during this phase. Lesions are detected because they are low in attenuation within the background of maximally enhanced liver parenchyma.

Delayed Phase

Anatomical coverage
- dome of the diaphragm to the iliac crest

Slice thickness
- 5 mm

Increments
- 5 mm

Kernel (algorithm)
- standard/soft tissue

Scan delay
- 10 to 20 minutes from start of injection

The delayed phase is utilized to demonstrate delayed contrast fill-in of hemangiomas and to detect fibrotic tumors such as chalangiocarcinomas.

Retrospective reconstructions require the acquisition date to be reconstructed with 2- to 3-mm slice thicknesses and an overlap in increments. As stated above, these images provide the best data for image reformations of sagittal and coronal planes. If there is an interest in the hepatic arterial system, data should be reconstructed into 0.5- to 1.25-mm slices and reformatted into MIP 3D images.

Pancreas Acquisition Parameters

Imaging the pancreas is similar to imaging the liver with a few exceptions. Oral contrast may be limited to water instead of positive oral contrast. Water will dilate the duodenum, which will aid in the delineation of the duodenum from the head of the pancreas. The unenhanced scan is generally not necessary, but is mainly performed to identify the position of the pancreas and to identify bile duct or pancreatic duct stones in patients with known chronic pancreatitis. The bolus/arterial phase of injection occurs approximately 30 to 40 seconds post injection. This phase is considered the parenchymal phase of pancreatic enhancement, since the contrast between the parenchyma and the lesion is the highest and there is still visual enhancement of the arteries in order to evaluate vascular tumor involvement. The nonequilibrium/portal venous phase covers the liver and pancreas requiring a 60- to 100-second delay. In order to increase spatial resolution, the images may be reconstructed with a smaller DFOV centering on the pancreas.

Adrenal CT Examination

Adrenal adenomas have two properties that differentiate them from nonadenomas. Seventy percent of adenomas contain high intracellular fat (lipid-rich adenomas) and will be of low attenuation on unenhanced CT. A number of these adenomas however can be differentiated from malignant masses on the basis of their fast "wash-out" of contrast. The way of measuring contrast enhancement "wash-out" depends on the scanning protocol, either an absolute or relative percentage "wash-out" can be calculated from densitometry measurements. They are as follows:

Relative Wash Out

Enhanced CT $_{(HU)}$ − Delayed CT $_{(HU)}$ ÷ Enhanced CT $_{(HU)}$ ×100%

Absolute Wash Out

Enhanced CT $_{(HU)}$ − Delayed CT $_{(HU)}$ ÷ Enhanced CT $_{(HU)}$ − Unenhanced CT $_{(HU)}$ × 100%

The interpretation of the wash-out is as follows:

Unenhanced CT with a <10 HU
- Lipid-rich adenoma

Wash-out >60%
- Lipid-poor adenoma

Wash-out <60%

- Undetermined—biopsy required

Indications for Dedicated Adrenal Gland Examinations

- Cushing's disease
- Conn's syndrome
- Pheochromocytoma
- Adrenal carcinoma
- Adrenal metastasis

Adrenal Acquisition Parameters

Unenhanced Scan

Anatomical coverage

- adrenal glands

Oral contrast

- water

Slice thickness

- 1 to 3 mm

Slice increments

- 1 to 3 mm

Kernel (algorithm)

- standard/soft tissue

Get images checked by radiologist before continuing: to determine HU of lesion. If lesion is <10 HU, study is complete; otherwise an enhanced and delayed series are required.

Nonequilibrium/Portal Venous Phase

Anatomical coverage

- abdomen
  - dome of the diaphragm to the ischial tuberosities
- pelvis
  - dome of the diaphragm to the iliac crest

Slice thickness

- 1 to 3 mm

Slice increments

- 1 to 3 mm

If pelvis is ordered

- 5 mm × 5 mm through rest of abdomen

IV contrast

- 100 cc with 50 cc saline flush

Flow rate

- 2.5 cc/s

Scan delay

60 to 90 seconds from start of injection

Delayed Scan

Coverage

- adrenal glands

Slice thickness

- 1 to 3 mm

Slice increments

- 1 to 3 mm

Kernel (algorithm)

- standard/soft tissue

Scan delay

- 15 minutes from start of injection

Kidney CT Examination

Kidney imaging as with the liver and pancreas requires multiple series to delineate pathological conditions. Coronal reformats should be employed to optimally demonstrate the extent and location of lesions. To improve coronal images, thick MPR sections (3 mm) should be performed. Maximum intensity projections aid in the diagnosis of renal calculi and to illustrate the urinary tract during the excretory phase.

Indications for Kidney Examinations

- Indeterminate lesion
- Ureteral lesion
- Pyelonephritis
- Abscess
- Urinary track stone
- Trauma
- Vascular injury

Kidney Acquisition Parameters

Unenhanced Scan

Anatomical coverage

- dome of the diaphragm to the ischial tuberosities

Oral contrast

- water/positive contrast

Slice thickness

- 3 mm

Increments

- 3 mm

Kernel (algorithm)

- standard/soft tissue

This scanning protocol is good for defining baseline measurement for renal lesions and separate high-density renal cysts from hypovascular lesions. It must be noted, if the examination is performed for the detection of renal stone, an unenhanced series is performed. Once the radiologist reviews the images, a nephrographic phase of injection may be required.

Corticomedullary Phase

Coverage

- kidneys

Slice Thickness
- 3 mm

Slice Increments
- 3 mm

Kernel (algorithm)
- standard/soft tissue

IV contrast
- 100 cc with 50 cc saline flush

Scan delay
- tracking bolus
  - ROI on the aorta at the level of the renal arteries

The purpose of this scanning series is to detect acute hemorrhage in patients with suspected renal injuries. It also aids in distinguishing small hypervascular tumors from pseudoenhancing cysts. The arterial phase best diagnosis renal cell carcinoma.

Nephrographic Phase

Coverage
- dome of the diaphragm through the ischial tuberosities

Slice thickness
- 3 mm

Slice increments
- 3 mm

Kernel (algorithm)
- standard/soft tissue

Scan delay
- 100 to 180 seconds from start of injection

The nephrographic phase is considered the parenchyma phase; since the renal cortex and medulla show equal enhancement while lesions appear hypo-attenuating to the renal parenchyma. This phase of injection is especially helpful for detecting renal tumors. It may only be necessary to perform a nephrographic phase series for patients with known renal tumors, in order to save the patient radiation dose.

Excretory Phase

Coverage
- kidneys

Slice thickness
- 3 mm

Slice increments
- 3 mm

Kernel (algorithm)
- standard/soft tissue

Scan delay
- 5 minutes from the start of injection

The purpose of the excretory phase is to define the collecting system. If the entire urinary tract is of interest then a delayed excretory scan must be performed. This scan commences 15 minutes after the start of injection and the entire abdomen and pelvis compartments are scanned. This phase aids in the detection of contrast retention in the renal tubules that is characteristic of acute inflammatory processes.

CT Urogram Examinations

A CT Urogram examination is used as a primary imaging techniques to evaluate patients with blood in the urine (hematuria), follow patients with prior history of cancers of the urinary collecting system and to identify abnormalities in patients with recurrent urinary tract infections.

Urogram Acquisition Parameters

Unenhanced Scan

- All technical parameter are the same as for kidney acquisition

Combined Nephrographic & Excretion

Compression band
- place at the level of the 5th vertebra

Anatomical coverage
- kidneys to above compression band

Slice thickness
- 2.5 mm

Increments
- 2 mm

Kernel
- standard/soft tissue

First injection
- 90 cc with 110 cc of saline

Flow rate
- 2.5 cc/s

Delay time
- 6 minutes
  - no scanning is performed at this time

Inflate compression band

Second injection
- 60 cc with 140 cc of saline
- begin scanning 180 seconds after start of second injection

Excretion Phase

Anatomical coverage
- 2 cm above iliac crest through bladder

Slice thickness
- 2.5 mm

Increments
- 2 mm

Remove compression band

Delay time
- pelvis is scanned at approximately 12 minutes after start of first injection

In addition to imaging the urinary tract, CT urography can provide valuable information about other abdominal and pelvic structures and diseases that may affect them.

Peritoneal and Retroperitoneal Pathology

Ascites

Ascites is the common term for the collection of serous fluid in the peritoneal cavity. Its usual cause is from cirrhosis, hypoproteinema, congestive heart failure, or venous obstruction. Exudative ascites is the result of an inflammatory process that can be due to pancreatitis, peritonitis, and bowel perforation. Serous ascites has a CT attenuation value between -10 to a $+15$ HU and has the tendency to accumulate in the greater peritoneal space. Due to its isodensity, unenhanced CT studies will suffice. Ample bowel opacification aids in the detection of small amounts of fluid in the infracolic spaces.

Abscess

Majority of abscesses appear as loculated fluid collections, often with internal debris, fluid levels, and sometimes air–fluid levels and have a definable wall with irregular thickening. On an enhanced CT examination of the abdomen, the nearby fascia is thickened and fat places are obliterated because of inflammation. Once identifies, a CT percutaneous aspiration confirms the diagnosis and provides material for culture.

Hemorrhage

Abdominal trauma from a sharp or blunt force most often results in intra-abdominal hemorrhage. Other sources of hemorrhage are from bowel perforation, tumor rupture, ectopic pregnancy, or anticoagulant medication. CT imaging for the detection of active abdominal/pelvic hemorrhage is performed in the arterial phase, since it appears as a hyperdensity with attenuation values in the range of 85 to 370 HU and is usually within 20 HU of the aorta. Such finding indicates a life threatening situation and requires immediate surgical intervention.

Peritonitis

Peritonitis commonly occurs from an infection of the abdominal cavity as a result of peritoneal injury or bacterial seepage through the peritoneum. This process may be localized or may involve the entire peritoneum. It is characterized on CT images by ascites with dilation of mesenteric vascular structures and a hazy increase of attenuation of the mesenteric fat. Following the administration of IV contrast, the peritoneal layers appear smoothly thickened and display enhancement. The ideal oral contrast administration for suspected peritonitis is a water soluble solution.

Lymphoma

Lymphoma is divided into two categories: Hodgkin's and non-Hodgkin's type. CT has become the imaging modality of choice, since staging of the disease is based on the number of nodal groups affected, their location in relation to the diaphragm and the involvement of the spleen and extralymphatic organs. A CT scan in the nonequilibrium phase (portal/venous) of injection will enhance vessels distinguishing them from the surrounding lymph nodes.

Soft Tissue Sarcoma (Fig. 2.38)

Soft tissue sarcomas are a group of malignant tumors that originate in the connective tissues. These sarcomas account for approximately 1% of malignant tumors discovered in adults. It is unknown how these sarcomas develop, but there is evidence to support that genetics and occupational exposure to certain chemicals may be the culprit. In studies performed by the American Cancer Society, of farmers and agricultural workers, the results showed an increase in soft tissue sarcomas, which may relate to herbicide exposure. Soft tissue sarcomas have also been linked to dioxin (by-product of Agent Orange) exposure in some chemical manufacturing workers and Vietnam War veterans.

Kidney Pathology

Angiomyolipoma

Angiomyolipoma is a benign tumor composed of blood vessels, smooth muscle, and fat. The imaging appearance depends on the proportional component of each tissue element. The vascular and smooth muscle portions will enhance with the administration of IV contrast. These tumors are sometimes indistinguishable from renal cell carcinoma (RCC) if they present with very little fat content. Hemorrhage is common with these benign tumors because of the weak wall of the tumor blood vessels.

Pyelonephritis

Pyelonephritis is an inflammation of the kidney parenchyma and renal pelvis caused by a bacterial infection. This pathological process on the parenchymal phase of

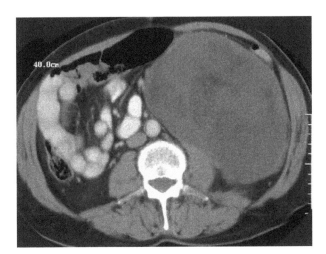

Figure 2.38. Contrast-enhanced axial CT image of the abdomen demonstrating a large malignant soft tissue sarcoma within the abdomen resulting in shifting of the bowel loops to the right. Sarcomas are usually named according to the type of tissue they involve. (Reproduced, with permission, from Grey ML, Ailinani JM. *CT and MRI Pathology: A Pocket Atlas*. 2nd ed. New York, NY: McGraw-Hill; 2012.)

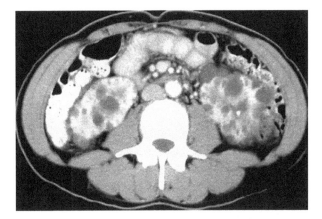

Figure 2.39. Contrast-enhanced axial CT image of the abdomen demonstrating bilateral polycystic kidney disease. Note the heterogeneous densities and the enlargement of both kidneys. (Reproduced, with permission, from Grey ML, Ailinani JM. *CT and MRI Pathology: A Pocket Atlas*. 2nd ed. New York, NY: McGraw-Hill; 2012.)

contrast enhancement appears as rounded, linear, or wedge-shaped areas of diminished enhancement with a typical radially oriented pattern across the corticomedullary boundary. When delayed imaging is performed the pattern is reversed. Symptoms usually resolve within 72 hours following the administration of the appropriate antibiotic therapy.

Polycystic Kidney Disease

Adult polycystic kidney disease is a hereditary autosomal dominant disorder categorized with multiple hypodense or cystic masses involving one or both kidneys (Fig. 2.39). It is associated with hepatic cysts, pancreatic cyst, and an increased rate of arteriovenous malformation and aneurysms.

Renal Cell Carcinoma

RCC is the most common malignancy affecting the kidneys. These tumors are heterogeneous and multilobulated. It is not uncommon for the tumors to contain internal hemorrhage, cystic necrosis, and coarse and irregular calcifications. Unenhanced studies an exhibit hypodense or isodense renal mass, while the post contrast images show an enhancing mass.

Renal Stones

The exact is unknown, but these stones may form anywhere throughout the urinary tract. Most stones develop in the renal pelvis or the calyces of the kidney. Majority of the stones are composted of calcium salts, but a percentage

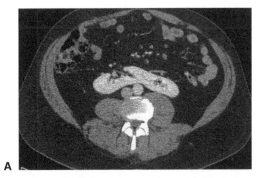

A

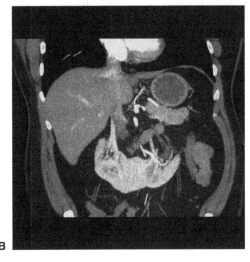

B

Figure 2.40. Contrast-enhanced axial CT image demonstrating a common fusion abnormality of the kidneys known as a horseshoe kidney. The renal pelvis is usually rotated anteriorly with one or both kidneys have two to three renal arteries. (Reproduced, with permission, from Grey ML, Ailinani JM. *CT and MRI Pathology: A Pocket Atlas*. 2nd ed. New York, NY: McGraw-Hill; 2012.)

are forms from excessive uric acid within the system. CT imaging usually consist of an unenhanced series to demonstrate the calcified stones in the kidney or ureter. A percentage of patients may have hydronephrosis and hydroureter with perinephric soft tissue stranding.

Horseshoe Kidney

Horseshoe kidney is a congenital anomaly (found in about 1 in every 500 patients), characterized by the fusion of the lower (90%) or upper (10%) poles of the kidney. This produces a horseshoe-shaped structure continuous across the midline and anterior to the great vessels (Fig. 2.40). The disorder is usually asymptomatic but some complications can arise such as ureteropelvic junction obstruction, infection, and stone formation.

Renal Artery Stenosis

The most common cause of renal artery stenosis is hypertension. Hypertension of the renal artery can occur as a result of either atherosclerosis or fibromuscular dysplasia. CT imaging includes a bolus injection with the tracking ROI on the aorta at the L1 level utilizing a 4 to 5 cc/s flow rate. Coronal MPR is the preferred plane to demonstrate the stenosis.

CROSS-SECTIONAL ANATOMY OF THE PELVIS

Urinary Bladder

The urinary bladder is a pyramid-shaped muscular organ that rest on the pelvic floor, immediately posterior to the symphysis pubis. It functions as a temporary reservoir for the storage of urine. An empty bladder has four surfaces and four angles.

Superior surface
- covered by peritoneum, allowing loops of ileum and sigmoid colon to rest on it

Posterior surface
- known as the fundus or base of the bladder

Inferolateral surface
- consists of two surfaces and are in contact with the fascia covering the levator ani muscles

Angles of the Bladder

Inferior angle
- funnel-shaped narrowing formed by the junction of the inferolateral and posterior surface
  - it is termed as the neck of the bladder and is continuous with the urethra

Posterolateral angles
- marks the point where the ureters enter the bladder

Anterior angle
- is joined by the superior and inferolateral surface and is referred to as the apex

Urethra

The urethra in both genders passes through the urogenital diaphragm, which contains the urethral sphincter muscle. This muscle is responsible for the voluntary closure of the bladder. The female urethra is a short muscular tube that drains urine from the bladder. The male urethra subdivides into three regions:

Prostatic urethra
- passes through the middle of the prostate gland

Membranous urethra
- is the shortest and narrowest section of the urethra, which penetrates the external urethral sphincter

Penile urethra
- is the longest portion that extends from external urethral sphincter to the tip of the penis

Rectum

The rectum is the terminal part of the large intestine found behind the bladder. It extends between the distal part of the sigmoid colon and the anal canal. The upper third of the rectum is an area termed the rectal ampulla. This section has considerable distensibility and as fecal material accumulates in the area it triggers the urge to defecate. The anus is the exit of the anal canal and is controlled by involuntary and voluntary sphincter muscles.

Reproductive Organs

Female Organs

The female reproductive system (Fig. 2.41) is responsible for producing sex hormones and ova. Its function is to protect and the support of the developing fetus. It principal organs are:

Uterus
- pear-shaped muscular organ located in the anterior portion of the pelvis cavity
- located between the bladder and rectum
- the walls are composed of the:
  - endometrium—inner glandular tissue
  - myometrium—the thickest middle muscular tissue
  - perimetrium—outer layer consisting of serous membrane

Ovaries
- paired, small almond-shaped organs located on either side of the uterus

- they produce ova as well as hormones partly responsible for regulating the reproduction cycle

Fallopian tubes
- the fallopian tubes are slender, muscular tubes that extend laterally from the body of the uterus to the peritoneum near the ovaries
- they are supported by the broad ligament at the distal end
- they are only visible on CT images when there is an abnormality

Cervix
- narrow inferior third part of the uterus, which communicates with the vagina

Vagina
- narrow muscular tube located within the third part of the uterus, connecting the uterine cavity with the exterior
- this organ is termed a hollow organ, but a tampon is necessary to delineate the vaginal margins in sectional imaging
- ascites may be present in the cul-de-sac, which is an area posterior to the uterus and ovaries in woman suspected of malignancy

Ligaments of the Uterus

The ligaments of the uterus stabilize the uterus within the peritoneum. There are three main ligaments:

- Round
  - This ligament keeps the body of the uterus flexed anteriorly (anteversion) preventing posterior movement of the uterus
- Broad
  - This ligament encloses the ovaries, uterine tubes, and uterus, extending from the sides of the uterus to the walls of the posterior floor of the pelvis
  - Prevents side to side movement
- Cardinal
  - Aids is suspending the uterus above the bladder
  - Prevents downward displacement

Male Organs

The principal structures of the male reproductive system (Fig. 2.42) consist of:

Scrotum

The scrotum is a musculotendinous pouch that encloses the testes, epididymis, and lower portion of the spermatic cord. It facilitates sperm formation by distending the testes outside the peritoneum in a cooler environment in effect regulating the temperature of the testes.

Testes

The testes are paired organs suspended in the fleshy, pouch-like scrotal sacs. The purpose of the testes is to produce sperm and male sex hormones.

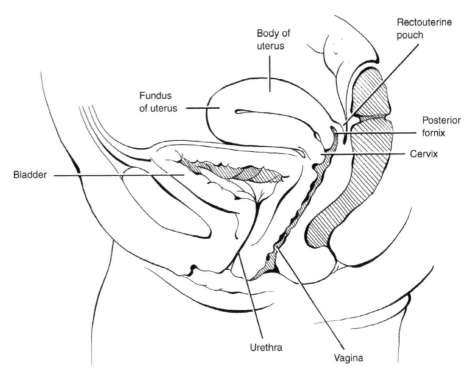

Figure 2.41. Sagittal illustration of the female pelvis. (Reproduced, with permission, from Madden ME. *Introduction to Sectional Anatomy*. 3rd ed. Philadelphia, PA: Wolters Kluwer; Lippincott Williams & Wilkins; 2013.)

Epididymis

The epididymis is a tightly coiled tubular structures located on the superoposterior surface of each testis. It is divided into head, body, and tail. Sperm is transmitted from the testis to the epididymis where they are stored as they undergo the final stage of maturation.

Vas Deferens (Ductus)

The vas deferens continues from the tail of the epididymis and is a long muscular tube that ascends in the posterior portion of the spermatic cord. Each vas deferens along with the testicular artery and vein is surrounded by the tough connective tissue and muscle of the paired spermatic cord.

Spermatic Cord

Each vas deferens along with the testicular artery and vein is surrounded by tough connective tissue and muscle of the paired spermatic cord

Seminal Vesicles

The seminal vesicles are located above the prostate gland and the rectum on either side of the vas deferens. The vesicles ducts join with the vas deferens intersecting the prostatic urethra. During ejaculation the vesicles secrete an alkaline fluid rich in sugar that contributes to sperm viability.

Prostate Gland

The prostate gland is the largest accessory gland of the male reproductive system. It is located inferior to the bladder and anterior to the rectum. It is one of the densest glands consisting of a high concentration of connective tissue and smooth muscle. It secretes a thin, slightly alkaline fluid during ejaculation into the prostate urethra contributing to sperm motility. In sectional imaging can be divided into zonal anatomy.

Central—base comprising 25%
Peripheral—largest comprising 70%
• 70% to 80% cancers originate in this section
Transitional—comprises 5%
• this section enlarges due to benign prostatic hypertrophy
Periurethral—less than 1%

Bulbourethral Gland

The bulbourethral gland also known as Cowper's gland are two small glands that lie, posterolateral to the membranous urethra, embedded in the urogenital diaphragm.

Their function is to secrete an alkaline fluid into the membranous urethra that forma a portion of the seminal fluid.

Penis

The penis is the external reproductive organ. It is divided into two sections, the root, which attaches to the pubic arch via suspensory ligaments and the body, which remains free. There are three masses of erectile tissue composing the root of the penis; two corpora cavernosa and the corpus spongiosum. The corpora cavernosa is erectile tissue surrounded by a strong fibrous capsule which attaches to the ischiopubic rami. The corpus spongiosum has an irregularly shaped bundle of erectile tissue that contains the penile urethra.

Imaging Procedures of the Pelvis

CT Colonoscopy

CT colonoscopy is becoming a viable alternative to optical colonoscopy to screen for colorectal cancer. The goal of this technique is to detect polyps of greater than 10 mm in diameter. Virtual colonoscopy is not only utilized as a screening technique, but has become a procedure for high-risk patients in which conventional colonoscopy or barium enemas were not successfully completed due to torturous colons. Proper bowel preparation is the most important aspect for a successful study. The procedure begins with a localizer image checking to ensure the colon has been fully cleaned out that ensures residual fecal material is not misinterpreted for an abnormality. The next step is to insert a rectal tube then the colon is insufflated with carbon dioxide or room air in order to distend the colon. The patient is scanned in the supine and prone positions using a low dose technique with thin collimations and reconstruction intervals. It is not uncommon for a decubitus scan to be obtained to allow for accurate diagnosis.

Once the images have been reconstructed, they are networked to reading station that has the capability of performing endoluminal display and "fly-through" along with 3D volume rendering processing. Standard interpretation includes the two-dimensional axial images and the 3D volume rendering imaging.

CT Cystography

CT cystography may be performed for bladder trauma. Nearly every patient with visible hematuria should have a prompt CT cystography. The CT cystogram will demonstrate bladder injury only if completed properly. The procedure involves placing a urinary catheter into the bladder and infusing at least 350 cc of diluted contrast

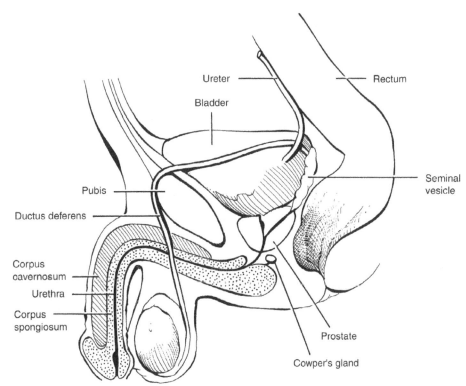

Figure 2.42. Sagittal view of the male pelvis. (Reproduced, with permission, from Madden ME. *Introduction to Sectional Anatomy.* 3rd ed. Philadelphia, PA: Wolters Kluwer; Lippincott Williams & Wilkins; 2013.)

media for distension of the bladder and accurate diagnosis. A routine abdomen and pelvis scan is obtained followed by postvoid images concentrating just on the bladder.

Pathology of the Pelvis

Appendicitis
Appendicitis is the inflammation of the vermiform appendix due to obstruction and is the most common acute surgical ailment of the abdomen. Patients present with pain and/or tenderness in the right lower quadrant. CT examinations may be performed with or without IV contrast and a number of institutions do not utilize oral contrast. CT imaging demonstrates a fluid-filled appendix due to inflammation and may also contain calcification (appendicolith). On CT enhanced images there may be a ring-like enhancement associated with periappendiceal abscess (Fig. 2.43).

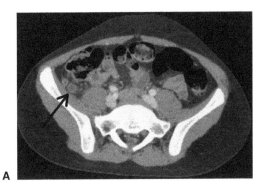
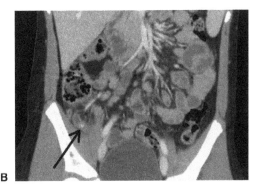

Figure 2.43. Contrast-enhanced axial CT image of a patient with an acute appendicitis. There is a rim enhancement of the appendix with bordering fat staining. (Reproduced, with permission, from Grey ML, Ailinani JM. *CT and MRI Pathology: A Pocket Atlas.* 2nd ed. New York, NY: McGraw-Hill; 2012.)

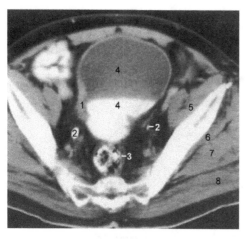

Figure 2.44. Contrast-enhanced axial image depicting bladder cancer. Observe the thickened bladder wall (1) and the filling defect in the left lateral wall of the urinary bladder (4), (2) ureters, (3) sigmoid colon, (5) iliac muscle, (6) gluteus minimus, (7) gluteus medius, (8) gluteus maximus. (Reproduced, with permission, from Seeram E. *Computed Tomography: Physical Principles, Clinical Applications, and Quality Control.* 3rd ed. St. Louis, MO: Saunders Elsevier; 2009.)

Bladder Cancer

Bladder is usually superficial and confined to the mucosa, but if invasion of the bladder musculature wall occurs risk for spread to regional and distant nodes increases. On CT imaging, the primary tumor appears as focal thickening of the bladder wall or as a soft tissue mass projecting into the bladder lumen (Fig. 2.44). Approximately 95% of malignant bladder tumors are transitional cell carcinomas. These tumors tend to spread into the ipsilateral ureter and renal collecting system.

Crohn's Disease

Crohn's disease is characterized by submucosal edema with ulcerations involving a thickened segment of distal ileum. The disease can occur at any age, but usually presents itself in adolescents between the ages of 15 and 35. On an enhanced CT image the bowel wall shows marked enhancement. Patients present with persistent or recurrent diarrhea, abdominal pain with cramping, weight loss, and fever.

Diverticulitis

Diverticulitis is a complication of diverticulosis. It is an abscess or inflammation initiated by the rupture of the diverticula into the pericolic fat. On CT imaging diverticulitis shows a colon segment with wall thickening hyperemic contrast enhancement and inflammatory changes that extend into the pericolic fat (Fig. 2.45).

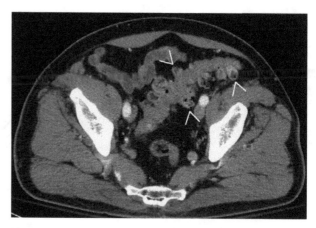

Figure 2.45. Contrast-enhanced axial CT projection of the abdomen showing diverticulitis. There is an infiltration of pericolonic fat at the level of the descending colon. (Reproduced, with permission, from Grey ML, Ailinani JM. *CT and MRI Pathology: A Pocket Atlas.* 2nd ed. New York, NY: McGraw-Hill; 2012.)

Colorectal Carcinoma

Colon cancer is the second leading cause of cancer death in the United States. The primary tumors may be a colon polyp nearly always larger than 1 cm. They appear as soft tissue masses that narrow the lumen of the colon. Flat lesions appear as focal lobulated thickening of the bowel wall (Fig. 2.46).

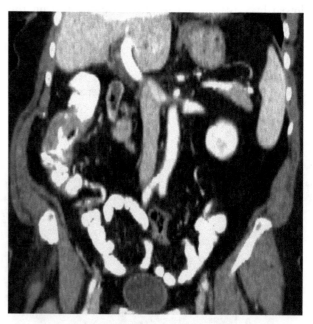

Figure 2.46. Contrast-enhanced coronal CT reformation of the abdomen in a patient with colon cancer. Take notice to the thickening bowel wall of the mid ascending colon. (Reproduced, with permission, from Grey ML, Ailinani JM. *CT and MRI Pathology: A Pocket Atlas.* 2nd ed. New York, NY: McGraw-Hill; 2012.)

Pelvic Inflammatory Disease (PID)

Pelvic inflammatory disease is an infection and inflammation of the endometrium, fallopian tubes, and ovaries. This infection is usually caused by gonorrhea or chlamydia. PID is seen on CT images as thickening of the fallopian tubes, edema and abnormal enhancement of the ovaries. This disease may integrate adjacent small or large bowel, obstruct the ureters, and inflame and thicken the bladder wall.

Ovarian Cyst

Ovarian cysts are small fluid-filled sacs that develop in a woman's ovaries. Most cysts are harmless, but some may rupture causing bleeding and pain. Ovarian cysts affect women of all ages and are considered functional. They occur normally and are not part of a disease process. On CT images these benign cysts appear as well-defined mass with fluid density usually in the range of ± 15 HU (Fig. 2.47).

Benign Prostatic Hyperplasia

Benign Prostatic Hyperplasia is a nodular enlargement with urethral construction and obstructing of the bladder while emptying. BPH on CT imaging shows bladder wall thickening with the prostate raised upward into the bladder. There will be high- and low-density areas within the prostate with some variable enhancement and calcifications.

CROSS-SECTIONAL ANATOMY OF THE MUSCULOSKELETAL SYSTEM

Upper Extremity (Fig. 2.48)

Humerus

The humerus is the longest and largest bone of the upper extremity that articulates with the scapula superiorly and the radius and ulna inferiorly. The head of the humerus is the most proximal section consisting of a round surface that forms an articulation with the glenoid process. The two tubercles, the lesser and greater tubercles, provide attachment sites for tendons and ligaments and are separated by the bicipital groove. The surgical neck is the constricted part of the humerus inferior to the two tubercles. This area is important because it is a frequent site for fracture. At the distal end of the humerus are the medial and lateral epicondyles. Lying just below the medial epicondyle is the trochlea. The trochlea articulates with the trochlear notch of the ulna. The capitulum is the small prominence of bone located inferior to the lateral epicondyle that articulates with the fovea on the head of the radius. On the posterior aspect of the distal humerus is the olecranon. It is a depression between the medial and lateral epicondyles that allows a space for the olecranon

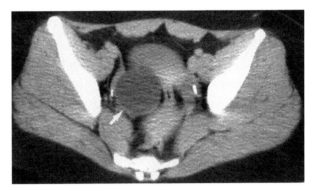

Figure 2.47. Contrast-enhanced axial CT image of a female pelvis exhibiting a large 5 cm round ovarian cyst (*arrow*). This is a low-density lesion located in the right adnexal region. (Reproduced, with permission, from Grey ML, Ailinani JM. *CT and MRI Pathology: A Pocket Atlas*. 2nd ed. New York, NY: McGraw-Hill; 2012.)

process of the ulna. The coronoid fossa is the depression on the anterior surface of the distal humerus between the medial and lateral epicondyles for the coronoid process of the ulna to glide smoothly during arm movement.

Scapula

The scapula forms the posterior part of the bony shoulder. The bone is flat and triangular shaped having four projections: scapular spine, acromion, coracoid process, and glenoid process. The scapular spine is located on the upper posterior surface of the scapula, which protrudes laterally and oblique to form the flattened acromion process. This process articulates with the acromial end of the clavicle. The coracoid process is situated on the anterolateral surface of the scapula arising medial to the glenoid process and functions to protect the shoulder joint. The glenoid fossa is the largest of the four projections. This process forms the lateral angle of the scapula and ends in a depression known as the glenoid fossa. The glenoid fossa also known as the glenoid cavity resembles a cup that houses the head of the humerus. Together they form the glenohumeral joint.

Glenohumeral Joint

The glenohumeral joint is a multiaxial synovial ball and socket joint and involves articulation between the glenoid fossa of the scapula and the head of the humerus. The fluid within the joint space acts like an oil, so that the smooth surfaces of the glenoid fossa and head of the humerus glide easily during movement.

Glenoid Labrum

The glenoid labrum is a fibrocartilaginous ring surrounding the edge of the glenoid fossa. Its function is to deepen the articular surface of the glenoid fossa.

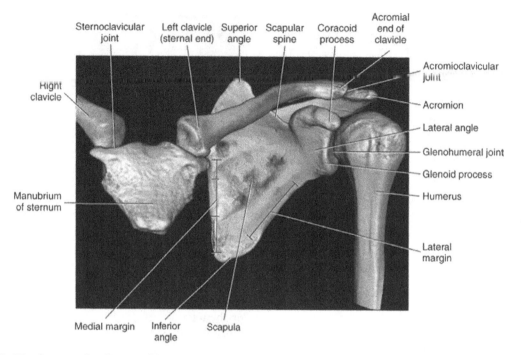

Figure 2.48. 3D volume-rendered image of the shoulder girdle. (Reproduced, with permission, from Kelley LL, Petersen CM. *Sectional Anatomy for Imaging Professionals*. 3rd ed. St. Louis, MO: Mosby Elsevier; 2013.)

Sternum

The sternum is anterior boundary of the bony thorax that functions to protect the organs of the chest (Fig. 2.49). The sternum consists of three main components: manubrium, body, and xiphoid process. The manubrium is the most superior section which articulates with the first two ribs and the clavicle. Within the superior surface of the manubrium is the jugular notch. This notch is a common radiology landmark at the T2–T3 vertebral level. The body is the long slender section having depressions on both sides for the articulation with the cartilages of the third through seventh ribs. The sternal angle is located at the T4–T5 vertebral level formed by the manubrium and the body of the sternum. The xiphoid process is the inferior section of the sternum and is the site for muscle attachments.

Brachial Plexus

The brachial plexus is an arrangement of nerve fibers, running from the spine, formed by the ventral rami of the lower cervical and upper thoracic nerve roots, specifically from above the fifth cervical vertebra to underneath the first thoracic vertebra (C5–T1). Symptoms of a brachial plexus injury include:

- Limp or paralyzed arm
- Lack of muscle control in the arm, hand, or wrist
- Lack of feeling or sensation in the arm or hand
- Injuries that happen mostly during birth

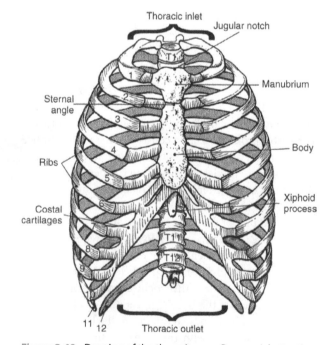

Figure 2.49. Drawing of the thoracic cage. Pay special attention to the contour of the sternum. (Reproduced, with permission, from Kelley LL, Petersen CM. *Sectional Anatomy for Imaging Professionals*. 3rd ed. St. Louis, MO: Mosby Elsevier; 2013.)

- The baby's shoulders may become impacted during the birth process causing the brachial plexus nerves to stretch or tear

Musculature of the Upper Extremity (Figs. 2.50 and 2.51)

Scapular Musculature

Deltoid Muscle

The deltoid muscle originates on the clavicle, acromion, and scapular spine to blanket the shoulder joint. Its insertion point is the deltoid tuberosity of the humerus. This muscle forms the contour of the shoulder and functions primarily to abduct the arm medial and laterally.

Teres Major

The teres major muscle is a flat rectangular muscle originating at the inferior angle of the scapula. It attaches to the greater tubercle of the humerus with the function of rotating the arm laterally and to abduct the arm. It is important not to confuse this muscle with the teres minor muscle, which is part of the rotator cuff.

Rotator Cuff Muscles

An easy way to remember the architecture is the word SITS:

- Supraspinatus
- Infraspinatus
- Teres minor
- Subscapularis

Supraspinatus Muscle

The supraspinatus lies in the supraspinatus fossa of the scapula and inserts on the greater tubercle of the humerus. The attachment tendon is the most frequently injured tendon of the rotator cuff due to possible impingement as it extends under the acromioclavicular joint and continues over the humeral head. This occurs at approximately 1 cm from the insertion site referred to as the critical zone. The function of this muscle is to abduct the arm.

Infraspinatus Muscle

The infraspinatus muscle is a triangular muscle that lies below the scapular spine in the infraspinatus fossa. This muscle also inserts in the greater tubercle. Its action is to laterally rotate the arm and give stability to the glenohumeral joint.

Teres Minor Muscle

The teres minor muscle lies along the inferior boarder of the infraspinatus muscle. This is the only posterior muscle of the rotator cuff muscles that has an insertion point at the lesser tubercle. The purpose of this muscle is to abduct, extend, and medially rotate the arm.

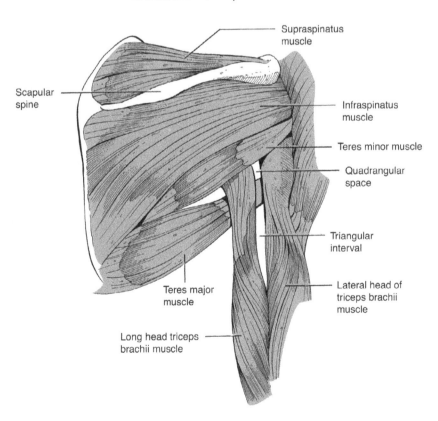

Figure 2.50. Posterior view of the shoulder muscles. (Reproduced, with permission, from Madden ME. *Introduction to Sectional Anatomy.* 3rd ed. Philadelphia, PA: Wolters Kluwer; Lippincott Williams & Wilkins; 2013.)

Subscapularis Muscle

The subscapularis muscle is the only muscle located on the anterior surface of the scapula. It lies within the subscapular fossa then inserts on the lesser tubercle of the humerus. This rotator cuff muscle stabilizes the glenohumeral joint and medially rotates the humerus.

Ventral Muscular Group of the Upper Extremity

Biceps Brachii Muscle

The biceps brachii muscle gets its name because of its two expanded heads: the long and short head. The long head originates on the supraglenoid tubercle of the scapula and inserts on the radial tuberosity. The short head begins at the coracoid process of the scapula to join the long head to terminate into two tendons, the radial tuberosity and fascia of the forearm. These muscles function to supinate and flex the forearm.

Brachialis Muscle

The brachialis muscle originates in the distal anterior humerus then attaches to the ulna tuberosity and coronoid process. The purpose of this muscle is for flexion of the forearm.

Dorsal Muscle Group

Triceps Muscle

This muscle is named triceps because it is associated with three heads of proximal attachment: the long, medial, and lateral heads. The long head attaches the infraglenoid tubercle of the scapula to the olecranon process of the ulna. The medial head's proximal attachment is the posterior surface of the humerus below the radial grove, while the lateral head attaches the posterior surface of the humerus just below the greater tubercle. The three heads join at a common tendon inserting at the proximal end of the olecranon process of the ulna. The main purpose of these muscles is to extend the forearm. The long head steadies the head of the humerus when abducted.

Anconeus Muscle

The anconeus muscle provides joint stability due to its crossing nature. The muscle's proximal attachment is the lateral epicondyle of humerus and inserts on the olecranon process of the ulna. This muscle aids the triceps brachii in extending the elbow.

Forearm

The forearm consists of two bones—the radius and ulna. The radius is shorter and lateral, while the ulna is longer and located medial in the body. The proximal part of the radius is the head, consisting of a large flattened area that articulates with the capitulum of the humerus. The fovea is the pitted part of the head of the radius. The radial neck is located between the head and the radial tuberosity. The area of the radius that provides attachment for the biceps muscle is the radial tuberosity. This area is located at the proximal radius recognized as a projection of bone jutting

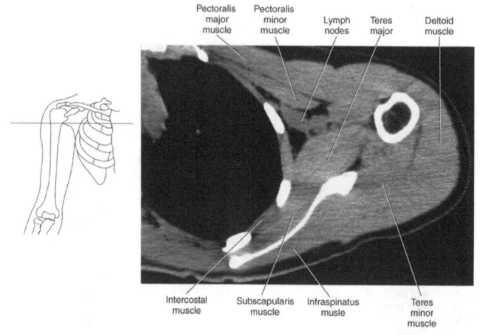

Figure 2.51. Axial CT image of the shoulder muscles. (Reproduced, with permission, from Kelley LL, Petersen CM. *Sectional Anatomy for Imaging Professionals*. 3rd ed. St. Louis, MO: Mosby Elsevier; 2013.)

out from the shaft. At the proximal ulna is the olecranon process located on the posterior distal humerus, while the coronoid process is seen on the anterior distal humerus. The trochlear notch is situated between the olecranon process and the coronoid process. The ulna nerve, because of its superficial location, is the most frequently injured nerve of the body. It passes between the medial epicondyle of the humerus and the olecranon process. The nerve is very superficial and easily palpable. The elbow joint is considered a ginglymus or hinged joint giving the upper extremity the ability for flexion and extension.

Ligaments of the Elbow

Stability of the elbow joint primarily depends on the collateral ligaments, which are woven into the lateral portions of the joint capsule. They are the ulnar and radial collateral ligaments.

Ulnar Collateral Ligament

The ulnar collateral ligament consists of three components, the anterior, transverse, and posterior band. This ligament is also known as the ligament of Cooper. The anterior band expands from the medial epicondyle of the humerus to the coronoid process and is the strongest of the three ligaments. The posterior band comes off the anterior band and inserts on the medial aspect of the olecranon process. These bands together form a triangular plate. The weakest band, the transverse band spans the medial surfaces of the coronoid and olecranon process to unite the anterior and posterior bands.

Radial Collateral Ligament

The radial collateral ligament reinforces the lateral side of the arm. It originates from the lateral epicondyle of the humerus and stretches distally to insert on the annular ligament and the anterior and posterior surface of the radial notch of the ulna.

Annular Ligament

The annular ligament forms a fibrous ring that encircles the radial head. The narrow portion tightens around the radial neck to prevent inferior displacement of the radius. This ligament is an important structure of the elbow joint because it allows the radius to rotate freely.

Muscles of the Forearm

The main muscles of the forearm are the flexor and extensor muscles.

- Flexors carpi radialis
- Palmaris longest
- Flexors carpi ulnaris

Their main function is to flex and abduct the hand.

- Extensor carpi radialis longus
- Extensor carpi radialis brevis

Their major actions are to extend and abduct the hand at the wrist.

Wrist

The wrist is an interwoven group of bones located between the forearm and hand. Known as the carpal bones they articulate with the radius, ulna, and metacarpal bones to provide great amount of movement. The wrist is comprised of eight bones, four in the proximal row articulating with the radius and ulna and four in the distal row next to the metacarpal bones.

Proximal Row

Scaphoid
- largest and most lateral
- articulates with the radius
- most wrist fractures occur within this bone

Lunate
- also called the semilunar
- articulates with the radius

Triquetrum
- also called the triangular or cuneiform
- articulates with the pisiform

Pisiform
- most medial
- articulates with the triquetrum
- flexor carpi ulnaris muscle inserts on this bone

Distal Row

Trapezium
- most lateral
- also called the greater multangular
- articulates with the first metacarpal

Trapezoid
- also called the lesser multangular
- smallest of the distal row
- articulates with the second metacarpal
- appearance on cross-sectional images
  - oblique deep groove

Capitate
- also called the magnum bone
- largest of the carpal bones
- articulates with the third metacarpal
- due to its unique shape and location
  - forms the foundation of the carpal tunnel

Hamate
- also called the unciform

- most medial articulates with the fourth and fifth metacarpal
- distinguished by its hook-like process
  - hamulus

Vascular System of the Upper Extremity

Arterial Supply

The axillary artery is a continuation of the subclavian artery beginning at the lateral boarder of the first rib and ending at the inferior boarder of the teres major muscle. At this point it passes through the upper extremity to become the brachial artery. The brachial artery runs inferiorly on the medial side of the humerus and then continues anteriorly to the cubital fossa of the elbow. This artery is very superficial and palpable and is the main arterial blood supply to the arm. As it descends from the cubital fossa it divides into the radial and ulna arteries.

Venous Supply

The brachial veins are two veins that lie on either side of the brachial artery and ascend the arm from the joining of the radial and ulna veins then ending as the axillary vein. The basilic vein is the superficial vein that arises from the ulnar side of the dorsal venous arch of the hand, passes up the forearm, and joins with the brachial veins to form the axillary vein. The cephalic vein courses along the radial side of the elbow and give rise to the median cubital vein creating an anastomosis between the basilic and cephalic veins.

IMAGING PROCEDURES OF THE UPPER EXTREMITY

Indications
- Trauma
- Fractures
- Dislocation
- Tumor
- Evaluating cortical integrity
- Articular involvement
- Defining extraosseous extension
- GH joint arthropathy and intra-articular bodies
- Rotator cuff (CT arthrography)
- Infection

Shoulder

Technical Factors
- Anatomical coverage

- above the acromioclavicular joint to below the scapular tip
- affected arm supinated, unaffected arm above head
- Slice thickness
  - ≤5 mm
- Slice increments
  - ≤5 mm
- DFOV
  - 250 mm
    - include entire deltoid muscle
- Kernel
  - standard/soft tissue
- IV contrast
  - unenhanced images only
    - except when infection or abscess is of concern
      - radiologist preference
- Retrospectives reconstruction
  - slice thickness
    - ≤1 mm
  - slice increments
    - overlap
  - kernel
    - standard/soft tissue
    - bone/detail
- Reformats
  - MPR
    - sagittal
      - prescribe sagittal plane off axial images which lies parallel to bony glenoid
        - image from scapular wing through deltoid muscle
    - coronal
      - prescribe coronal plane off of axial images parallel to supraspinatus muscle
    - 3D
      - volume rendered

Elbow

Technical Factors
Anatomical coverage
- proximal third of humerus through 2 cm below the radius tuberosity
Slice thickness
- ≤3 mm
Slice increments
- ≤3 mm
DFOV
- 150 to 180 mm
  - include entire area of interest
Kernel

- standard/soft tissue

IV contrast
- unenhanced images only
  - except when infection or abscess is of concern
    - radiologist preference

Retrospective reconstruction
- slice thickness
  - ≤1 mm
- slice increments
  - overlap
- kernel
  - standard/soft tissue
  - bone/detail

Reformats
- MPR
  - sagittal
    - prescribe plane perpendicular to coronal plane.
  - coronal
    - prescribe plane parallel to anterior humerus at condyles
      - scan through entire elbow

Hand and Wrist

Technical Factors

Anatomical coverage
- distal third of the radius and ulna through the fingers

Slice thickness
- ≤3 mm

Slice increments
- ≤3 mm

DFOV
- 120 to 180 mm
  - cover the entire wrist and hand

Kernel
- standard/soft tissue

IV contrast
- unenhanced images only
  - except when infection or abscess is of concern
    - radiologist preference

Retrospective reconstruction
- slice thickness
  - ≤1 mm
- slice increments
  - overlap
- kernel
  - standard/soft tissue
  - bone/detail

Reformats
- sagittal
  - prescribe plane perpendicular to coronal plane

- coronal
  - prescribe plane parallel to line drawn from ulnar styloid through radial styloid
- 3D
  - volume rendered

PATHOLOGY OF THE UPPER EXTREMITY

Shoulder Instability

Approximately 96% of all great joint dislocations occur in the shoulder. These dislocations are mostly anterior and can be reduced by indirect forces, such as abduction and extension. Patients experiencing chronic shoulder dislocations are commonly diagnosed as having Hill–Sachs lesions, which is a depressed fracture on the posterolateral aspect of the humeral head. CT arthrography is the modality of choice for the evaluation of chronic instability. CT images should include the coracoid process to avoid confusion with the normal flattening of the humeral head contour that is visible at lower levels.

Tennis Elbow

Tennis elbow is typically known as lateral epicondylitis. It is a degenerative condition of the tendon fibers that attach on the lateral epicondyle caused by excessive strain to the dorsal muscles: palmaris longus, extensor carpi radialis, and the extensor carpi ulnaris. Pain occurs when the extensor carpi radialis muscles are strained.

Golfer's Elbow

Golfer's elbow is also referred to as medial epicondylitis. It causes pain and inflammation on the inner side of the elbow, where the tendons of the forearm muscles attach to the medial epicondyle. The pain may spread into the forearm and wrist and is caused by excessive strain to the ventral superficial muscles: the flexor carpi-ulnaris, flexor carpi-radialis, and the palmaris.

Carpal Tunnel Syndrome

The carpal tunnel is created by the concave arrangement of the carpal bones. There is a thick ligamentous band called the flexor retinaculum that stretches across the carpal tunnel to create the enclosure for the passage of tendons and the median nerve. Carpal tunnel syndrome occurs when there is compression of the median nerve and is associated with repetitive activity, such as typing. Injections of hydrocortisone may be very beneficial to most patients, but surgery may be needed to release the flexor retinaculum.

CROSS-SECTIONAL ANATOMY OF THE LOWER EXTREMITY (FIG. 2.52)

Hip

The hip is a strong ball-and-socket joint that provided strength to support the body in the erect position. The joint is created by the articulation of the femoral head to the acetabulum of the pelvis. The acetabulum is formed by the ilium, pubis, and the ischium bones of the pelvis.

Ilium

The ilium is the largest and most superior bone of the pelvis made up of the body and ala (wing-like structure). On the superior surface of the ala is a section called the iliac crest. As the crest descends it gives rise to the superior and inferior iliac spines. The ilium and the sacrum join, in the posterior aspect of the body. This union forms the right and left sacroiliac joints. The body of the ilium is important for it contribution to the superior portion of the acetabulum.

Pubis

The pubis is the inferior and anterior section of the pelvic girdle, which is divided into three parts: the body, the inferior ramus, and the superior ramus. The body is the most medially section. The two sections join together at the symphysis pubis joint. This joint is a fibrocartilagenous joint known as amphiarthroses joint. These joints can move slightly but not a lot. The symphysis pubis acts to absorb shock to the body when a person walks around. This shock absorbing capability is due to the flexibility and toughness of the fibrocartilage of the joint. The movement that occurs is a gliding motion, where each side of the pubic bone can move up or down relative to the other. The inferior ramus joins the ischium to form the inferior boundary for the obturator foreman, while the superior ramus forms the superior section of the obturator forearm and the anterior part of the acetabulum.

Ischium

The ischium is the inferior and posterior portion of the pelvic girdle made up of a body and two rami. The body of the ischium forms the inferior posterior section of the acetabulum. The ischial tuberosity is an enlarged rounded area that supports the body in the seated position. The ischial spine projects posteriorly forming the inferior border of the greater sciatic notch. The two notches are bridged by ligaments creating foramina for the passage of nerves and vessels.

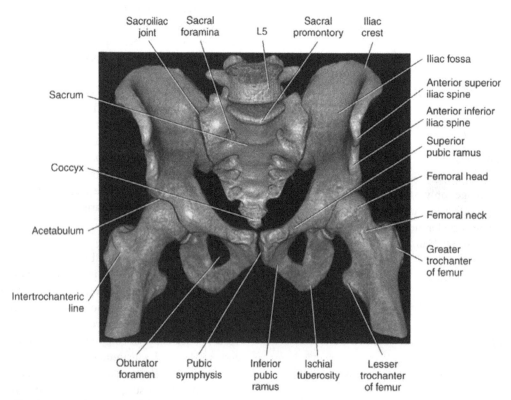

Figure 2.52. 3D volume-rendered image of the pelvic girdle. (Reproduced, with permission, from Kelley LL, Petersen CM. *Sectional Anatomy for Imaging Professionals.* 3rd ed. St. Louis, MO: Mosby Elsevier; 2013.)

Femur

The femur is located within the thigh and is the longest, strongest, and heaviest bone in the body. The proximal end of the bone consists of a head, neck, and two large processes, the greater and lesser trochanter. The head of the femur is covered by articular cartilage with the exception of a small depression called the fovea capitis. The capitis is the attachment site for the ligamentum teres, which provides the major arterial blood supply to the femoral head. The femoral neck extends obliquely from the head in an inferolateral direction to meet the shaft. The 120- to 125-degree obliquity results in an increased of movement within the hip joint.

Acetabular Fossa

The acetabular fossa is a centrally located nonarticulating depression formed by the ischium and filled with fat. On cross-sectional CT images, this area will appear hypodense with an HU number between −80 and −100.

Acetabular Labrum

The acetabular labrum or cotyloid ligament creates a fibrocartilagenous rim attached to the brim of the acetabulum. The labrum surrounds the femoral head and aids in keeping it in place by pressing it against the acetabular fossa. The labrum's other function is to deepen the joint and provide increased stability to the joint.

Muscles of the Hip and Thigh

Iliopsoas

The iliacus muscle spans across the iliac fossa to join the psoas muscle forming the iliopsoas muscle. This muscle inserts on the lesser trochanter of the femur with the function of flexing and rotating the thigh laterally. This muscle makes walking possible.

Gluteal Compartment (Fig. 2.53)

Gluteus Maximus Muscle

The gluteus maximus muscle is the largest of and most superficial muscle the group. The proximal attachment is the ilium, sacrum, and coccyx then travels distally to the greater trochanter. Its major function is to extend the hip and preserve an erect body position.

Gluteus Medius Muscle

The gluteus medius muscle is situated on the lateral and upper buttock originating at iliac crest spreading distally to the greater trochanter, lateral to the gluteus maximus muscle. Its purpose is to abduct and medially rotate the thigh.

Gluteus Minimus Muscle

The gluteus minimus muscle, like its name is the smallest of the gluteal group. It is located inferior to the gluteus medius muscle beginning at the gluteal surface of the ilium then distally inserting on the greater trochanter. Similar to the gluteus medius muscle, its function is to abduct and medially rotate the thigh.

Piriformis Muscle

The piriformis muscle originates on the inner surface of the sacrum traveling laterally and anteriorly to insert on the superior boundary of the greater trochanter. Its action is to laterally rotate and abduct the thigh.

Obturator Internus Muscle

The obturator internus muscle originates at the inner boarder of the obturator foreman traveling through the lesser sciatic foramen for its distal attachment on the

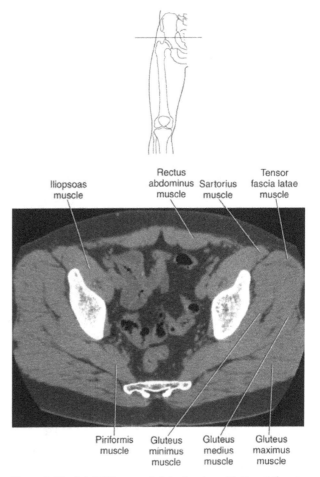

Figure 2.53. Axial CT image of gluteal region with the piriformis muscle. (Reproduced, with permission, from Kelley LL, Petersen CM. *Sectional Anatomy for Imaging Professionals*. 3rd ed. St. Louis, MO: Mosby Elsevier; 2013.)

greater trochanter. Its purpose is to laterally rotate and abduct the thigh.

Obturator Externus Muscle

The obturator externus muscle stem from the outer boarder of the obturator foramen, which then mirrors the obturator internus muscle. Its pathway is from the posterior side of the neck of the femur to insert into the medial side of the greater trochanter. Its action is to laterally rotate the thigh.

Anterior Thigh Muscles

Psoas Major

The psoas major muscle arises from the transverse processes of the lumbar vertebrae and course inferiorly within the pelvis. As it leaves the pelvis, it travels under the inguinal ligament to enter the thigh distally at the lesser trochanter. Its main purpose is to flex the thigh at the hip and for stabilization of the hip.

Quadriceps Femoris Muscle

The quadriceps femoris muscle is the largest muscle in the body. It covers almost all of the anterior surface and sides of the femur (Fig. 2.54). It originates as four heads: rectus femoris, vastus lateralis, vastus medialis, and vastus

intermedius, to create a powerful extensor of the knee. The rectus femoris has its proximal attachment at the anterior inferior iliac spine. The vastus lateralis originates at the greater trochanter and lateral lip of the linea aspera (raised ridge on the proximal posterior end of the femoral shaft). The vastus medialis originates at the intertrochanteric line and medial lip of the linea aspera, while the vastus intermedius is situated on the anterior and lateral surface of the femoral body. All four muscles have their distal insertion on the patellar ligament.

Adductor Muscles

The adductor muscles are composed of three muscles: the adductor longus, adductor brevis, and adductor magnus. The abductor muscle group originates at the pubic bone. The longus has its distal insertion at the middle third of the linea aspera, the brevis ends at the superior linea aspera, while the distal insertion of the magnus is the linea aspera and abductor tubercle of the medial condyle of the knee. The adductor muscle group, as name states, acts to adduct the thigh.

Hamstring Muscles

The hamstring muscles are composed of the semitendinosus, semimembranosus, and biceps femoris. They

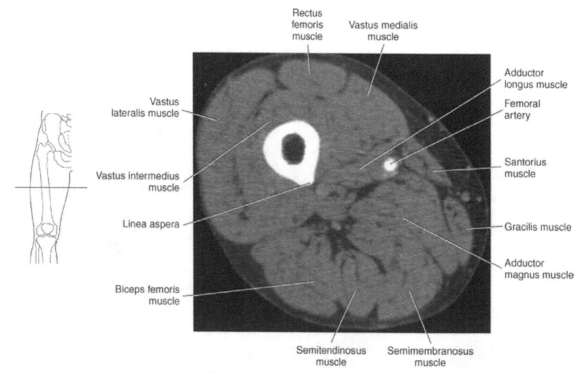

Figure 2.54. Axial CT projection of the quadriceps femoris muscle. (Reproduced, with permission, from Kelley LL, Petersen CM. *Sectional Anatomy for Imaging Professionals.* 3rd ed. St. Louis, MO: Mosby Elsevier; 2013.)

make up the large mass of muscles that can be palpated on the posterior aspect of the thigh. The proximal attachment of the semitendinosus and semimembranosus is located at the ischial tuberosity. The distal attachment of the semitendinosus is the anterior medial side of the tibia, while the semimembranosus is the posterior aspect of the medial condyle of the tibia. The biceps femoris is composed of two heads: the long and short head. Both heads have their distal insertion on the lateral surface of the fibular head. The long head originates on the ischial tuberosity, while the short head is seen on the lateral lip of the linea aspera.

Knee

Located on either side of the knee joint are the medial and lateral condyles forming the distal part of the femur. Since these condyles are in direct contact with the tibia, they are covered with a layer of articular cartilage serving as a smooth surface to protect the underlying bone.

Tibia

The tibia is the second longest bone of the body also known as the shin bone. In the lower leg, it is located on the medial aspect of the leg. The superior articular surface of both condyles has a flattened surface, called the tibial plateaus, for articulation with the femoral condyles. The tibial condyles are separated by the intercondylar eminence, also called the tibial spine, ending in two peaks called the medial and lateral intercondylar tubercles. The eminence is the place where ligaments attach to the tibia. The distal tibia has a flattened articular end with a medial extension that forms the medial malleolus.

Fibula

The fibula is located on the lateral aspect of the lower leg. The bone is rather thin with expanded proximal and distal ends. The proximal aspect of the bone articulated with the lateral condyle of the tibia creating the tibiofibular joint. The distal end of the bone articulates with the talus forming a section of the ankle joint.

Patella

The patella is a subcutaneous, flat, triangular-shaped bone with the broad base facing proximally and the pointed apex facing distally. It is the largest of the sesamoid bones. The rough anterior surface of the bone provides attachment for the quadriceps femoris tendon. The femoropatellar joint is formed by the junction of the medial and lateral articular facets on the posterior surface of the patella and the femur.

Ligaments of the Knee

Anterior Cruciate Ligament

The anterior cruciate is a round ligament extending from the anterior part of the tibial spine and attaching to the posterior part of the medial surface of the lateral femoral condyle. Its purpose is to prevent hyperextension and anterior displacement of the tibia.

Posterior Cruciate Ligament

The posterior cruciate ligament is the stronger of the two ligaments extending from the posterior tibial spine to the anterior portion of the medial femoral condyle. It functions to prevent hyperflexion and posterior displacement of the tibia.

Medial Meniscus

The medial meniscus is a crescent-shaped ligament attaching the tibia, in front, to the anterior cruciate ligament, and the posterior intercondylar fossa. The function of this meniscus is to deepen the medial tibial condyle.

Lateral Meniscus

The lateral meniscus is a circular ligament connecting the tibia in front, to the anterior cruciate ligament, and behind the intercondylar eminence. The purpose of this ligament is to deepen the lateral tibial condyle.

Medial Collateral Ligament

The medial collateral ligament (also called the tibial collateral ligament) is a flattened triangular-shaped ligament that originates from the medial femoral epicondyle and extends to the medial tibial condyle, continuing to the medial shaft of the tibia, fusing with the medial meniscus. Its action is to prevent lateral bending and checks extension, hyperflexion, and lateral rotation.

Lateral Collateral Ligament

The lateral collateral ligament is also called the fibular collateral ligament is shorter with a rounded cord appearance. It originates from the lateral femoral condyle to the head and styloid process of the fibula. This ligament prevents hyperextension.

Patellar Ligament

The patellar ligament is the largest ligament of the knee. The patellar ligament and the patellar retinaculum strengthen the anterior joint capsule. The point of attachment is the patella and inserts on the tibial tuberosity being a continuation of the quadriceps femoris tendon below the patella. Its function is to maintain the position of the patella within the knee joint and extend the lower leg.

Infrapatellar Fat Pad

Posterior to the patella is a collection of fatty tissue known as the Infrapatellar fat pad. The purpose of this fat pad is to protect the underlying femur and tibia during patellar movement.

Foot and Ankle

The anatomical articular region between the lower leg and the foot is termed the ankle. The joint is formed by the distal tibia and fibula articulating with the talus. This type of joint is known as a ginglymus or hinged joint. The ankle joint allows for dorsiflexion and plantar flexion. Movement within the foot is caused by the articulation of the tarsal bones. The joint is called an arthrodial joint, since it allows the tarsal bones to possess a gliding movement, but with limited rotation.

Tarsal Bones

The tarsal bones are as follows:

Calcaneus
- known as the heel or os calcis
- articulates with the talus and cuboid bone
- carries 25% of the bodies weight in the standing position

Talus
- most proximal tarsal bone
- articulates with the tibia and fibula
- transmits 50% of the bodies weight to the calcaneus and the navicular

Cuboid
- located on the lateral side of the foot
  - between the calcaneus and the base of the 4th and 5th metatarsals

Navicular
- known as the scaphoid bone
- located on the medial side
  - between the talus and the three cuneiform bones

Cuneiforms
- three bones located medially
  - between the navicular and the first three metatarsals
  - referred to medial, intermediate and lateral
    - the lateral situated next to the navicular

Metatarsals
- numbered one through five
  - medial to lateral
- articulate with the cuboid and cuneiform bones
- each foot bears 25% of the bodies weight in the standing position
  - first metatarsal accounts for 10% of this weight

Vascular System of the Lower Extremity

Arterial System

Femoral Artery

The external iliac artery becomes the femoral artery as it enters the anterior section of the thigh behind the inguinal ligament. The artery is rather superficial and easily palpable supplying all the compartments of the thigh and the skin of the anterior abdominal wall, inguinal region, and external genitalia. As it descends the thigh through the adductor muscles it becomes the popliteal artery.

Popliteal Artery

The popliteal artery courses deep within the knee joint descending through the popliteal fossa. It passes distally over the popliteus muscle and divides into the anterior and posterior tibial arteries.

Anterior Tibial Artery

The anterior tibial artery runs anteriorly, at the level of the fibular head, descending into the anterior section of the lower leg. It courses distally through the anterior side of the ankle, where it becomes the dorsalis pedis artery.

Posterior Tibial Artery

As its name states the posterior tibial artery runs distally to the posterior medial side of the lower leg. This artery is usually larger than the anterior tibial artery. The posterior tibial artery divides into the medial and lateral plantar arteries of the foot.

Fibular Artery

The fibular artery arises from the posterior tibial artery below the distal border of the popliteal muscle. It runs posteriorly down the medial aspect of the fibula and ends on the lateral surface of the calcaneal tuberosity.

Venous System

Great Saphenous Vein

The great saphenous vein ascends the medial aspect of the leg and thigh to drain into the femoral vein near the hip joint.

Popliteal Vein

The popliteal vein, located on the posterior aspect of the knee, becomes the femoral vein in the thigh.

Femoral Vein

The femoral vein courses medial to the femoral artery and continues deep to the inguinal ligament as the external iliac vein.

Imaging Procedures of the Upper Extremity

Indications

- Trauma
- Fractures
- Dislocation
- Tumor
- Evaluating cortical integrity
- Articular involvement
- Defining extraosseous extension
- Labrum integrity (CT arthrography)
- Infection

Hip

Technical Factors

Anatomical coverage

- 2 cm above the iliac crest through the proximal third of the femur
  - through the fracture or prosthesis
- patient position
  - supine
  - feet first
  - adduct the legs (pigeon toed)
  - arms above head

Slice thickness

- ≤3 mm

Slice increment

- ≤3 mm

DFOV

- 320 to 400 mm
  - encompass bilateral hips including muscle and skin surfaces

Kernel

- standard/soft tissue

IV contrast

- unenhanced images only
- except when infection or abscess is of concern
  - radiologist preference

Retrospective reconstruction

- unilateral
- slice thickness
  - ≤2 mm
- slice increments
  - overlap
- DFOV
  - 200 to 220 mm
- make sure all muscular and skin structures are included
- Kernel
  - standard/soft tissue
  - bone/detail

- Reformats
- MPR
  - sagittal
    - prescribe plane perpendicular to coronal plane
    - scan from acetabulum through greater trochanter
  - coronal
    - prescribe plane parallel to femoral heads
    - scan from ischium through pubic
- 3D
  - volume rendered

Knee

Technical Factors

Anatomical coverage

- unilateral/bilateral—distal femur to proximal tibia
- supine
- feet first
- knee position
  - 30-degree angle
    - open the joint

Slice thickness

- ≤3 mm

Slice increment

- ≤3 mm

DFOV

- encompass area of interest

Kernel

- standard/soft tissue

IV contrast

- unenhanced images only
- except when infection or abscess is of concern
  - radiologist preference

Retrospective reconstruction

- slice thickness
  - ≤1 mm
- slice increments
  - overlap
- kernel
  - standard/soft tissue
  - bone/detail

Reformats

- MPR
  - sagittal
    - prescribe plane perpendicular to coronal plane
    - scan from the medial to the lateral femoral condyle
  - coronal
    - prescribe plane with line parallel to femoral condyles
    - image entire knee

- 3D
  - volume rendered

Foot and Ankle

Technical Factors

Anatomical coverage

- mid-shaft tibia/fibula to 2 cm posterior of the foot
- patient position
  - unilateral
    - affected leg extended with foot dorsiflexed
    - opposite leg, bent at knee with foot flat on table
  - bilateral
    - both legs extended with both feet dorsiflexed
    - make sure both feet are symmetrical

Slice thickness

- ≤ 3 mm

Slice increment

- ≤ 3 mm

DFOV

- 200 to 220 mm
  - encompass entire foot

Kernel

- standard/soft tissue

IV contrast

- unenhanced images only
  - except when infection or abscess is of concern
  - radiologist preference

Retrospective reconstruction

- slice thickness
  - ≤ 1 mm
- slice increments
  - overlap
- kernel
  - standard/soft tissue
  - bone/detail

Reformats

- MPR
  - sagittal
    - prescribe plane with line bisecting calcaneus
    - scan through entire foot
  - coronal
    - prescribe plane perpendicular to axial imaging plane
    - scan ankle from calcaneus through metatarsal bases

CT Arthrography

CT arthrography is declining in the number of examinations due to the onset of MR arthrography, but is utilized when MR is impossible. It is most commonly utilized in the shoulder for the evaluating the labrum and joint capsule, when joint instability is suspected (Fig. 2.55). The examination commences with the injection of 2 to 3 mL of nondiluted contrast material and 12 to 15 mL of air into the

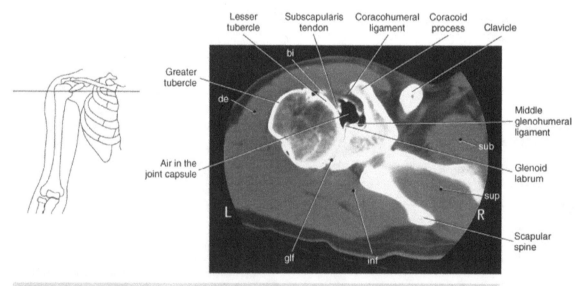

Lesser tubercle · Subscapularis tendon · Coracohumeral ligament · Coracoid process · Clavicle · Greater tubercle · Air in the joint capsule · Middle glenohumeral ligament · Glenoid labrum · Scapular spine

KEY: de, Deltoid; **bi,** biceps tendon; **sub,** subscapularis; **sup,** supraspinatus tendon; **inf,** infraspinatus; **glf,** glenoid fossa.

Figure 2.55. Axial CT image of a shoulder arthrogram. This study requires a mixture of air and contrast for the diagnosis of labrum tears. (Reproduced, with permission, from Kelley LL, Petersen CM. *Sectional Anatomy for Imaging Professionals.* 3rd ed. St. Louis, MO: Mosby Elsevier; 2013.)

inferior third of the joint capsule from the AP approach. The arm is placed in the abduction external rotation (ABER) position with the arm abducted greater than 90 degrees, and the elbow flexed. The hand placed over head. The study is then preceded using the institutions routine shoulder protocol. For diagnostic examinations, lidocaine, or long-acting anesthetic can be injected.

A single injection of a nonionic contrast media is employed for arthrograms of the hip and knee for most indications. When assessing the acetabular labium, a weight can be applied as traction in order to open up the joint.

PATHOLOGY OF THE LOWER EXTREMITY

Acetabular Fractures

Acetabular fractures are usually caused by axial or lateral forces that are transmitted through the femoral head. Multislice CT is the modality of choice when classifying acetabular fractures for appropriate treatment. It is difficult to diagnosis these fractures on axial images alone, so reformation of 3D imaging is employed. Volume-rendered images with the femoral head subtracted gives a direct view of the acetabulum.

Osteochondral Dissecans (OCD)

Osteochondral dissecans (OCD) occurs when a small segment of bone begins to separate from its surrounding region due to a lack of blood supply. As a result, the small piece of bone and the cartilage covering it begin to crack and loosen. It usually occurs in conjunction with a history of chronic stress. It is sometimes also known as an osteochondral fracture of the talus, chip fracture of the articular surface or a chondral fracture of the talus.

Avascular Necrosis (Osteonecrosis)

Avascular necrosis occurs as an interruption of the blood flow within the bone resulting in death of the cells within the bone. The cause of this disease is usually trauma, corticosteroids, and deep sea diving. It occurs in patients between the ages of 30 and 70. In 50% of the cases, bilateral involvement may occur. The hip is the most common site for the development of avascular necrosis.

Osteosarcoma

The most common malignant primary bone tumor is osteosarcoma. Its etiology is unknown, but individuals exposed to radiation have a predisposition linked to bone cancer. The tumors are commonly located in the knee, distal femur, or the proximal tibia and mostly seen the younger population (early teens to twenties). It generally

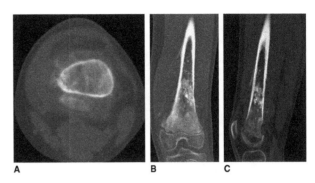

A   B   C

Figure 2.56. CT image in the axial projection with coronal and sagittal reformations of the femur demonstrating a malignant osteosarcoma. Notice the heterogeneous densities within the distal femur extending into the soft tissue. (Reproduced, with permission, from Grey ML, Ailinani JM. *CT and MRI Pathology: A Pocket Atlas.* 2nd ed. New York, NY: McGraw-Hill; 2012.)

affects male more than females. Osteosarcoma is rare, but approximately 400 to 500 cases are reported annually. A patient will first undergo plain x-rays, but CT imaging is excellent to demonstrate the bony destruction of the affected area, while MRI is utilized for the evaluation of the soft tissue (Fig. 2.56). The treatment plan involves surgical resection followed by chemotherapy. Prognosis is dim, if metastatic disease has already occurred.

Liposarcoma of the Thigh

Liposarcomas are a malignant tumor that develops from fat cells. They account for approximately 18% of all soft tissue sarcomas and can occur in any part of the body, but more than half of all these cases develop in the thigh. The cause of the disease is not known then again they have been noticed following a patient experiences an injury. Liposarcomas are diagnosed by physical examination and radiology imaging. On CT images, they appear as hypodensities within the muscle (Fig. 2.57). Treatment of these tumors is by surgical intervention and in some cases these tumors can grow back. Prognosis depends on the grade of the tumor.

Patellar Fracture

Patellar fractures are rare accounting for only approximately 1% of reported skeletal fractures. Over 50% of the fractures are classified as transverse. CT imaging with multiplanar reformations is the standard modality for the evaluation of these fractures (Fig. 2.58).

Tibial Plateau Fracture

A tibial plateau fracture involves the proximal end of the tibia bone that carries the weight of the body across it. A fracture in the proximal end of the tibia can have an acute effect on the functioning of the knee joint, since this part of the tibia has important ligaments attached to it that

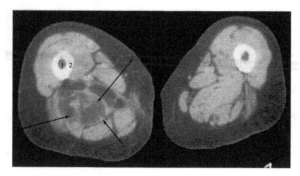

Figure 2.57. Bilateral axial CT image of the femur depicting a liposarcoma of the right femur affecting the adductor magnus muscle. The hypodensities (*black arrows*) within the upper femur are the fatty tumors. (Reproduced, with permission, from Seeram E. *Computed Tomography: Physical Principles, Clinical Applications, and Quality Control.* 3rd ed. St. Louis, MO: Saunders Elsevier; 2009.)

helps to maintain the stability of the knee joint. CT imaging employing 3D volume-rendered or sagittal and coronal multiplanar reformations is a useful tool to evaluate the bony fragments and degree of displacement (Fig. 2.59). Surgery is the treatment of choice.

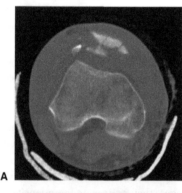

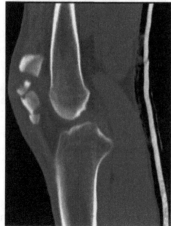

Figure 2.58. CT axial and reformatted sagittal image of the knee depicting a severe patellar fracture. (Reproduced, with permission, from Grey ML, Ailinani JM. *CT and MRI Pathology: A Pocket Atlas.* 2nd ed. New York, NY: McGraw-Hill; 2012.)

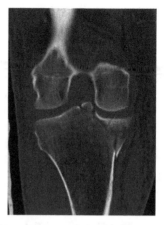

Figure 2.59. CT coronal image of the lower leg reformatted in the bone/detail convolution kernel. The image shows a distinct tibial plateau fracture. (Reproduced, with permission, from Grey ML, Ailinani JM. *CT and MRI Pathology: A Pocket Atlas.* 2nd ed. New York, NY: McGraw-Hill; 2012.)

CROSS-SECTIONAL ANATOMY OF THE SPINE

Vertebral Structure

The vertebral column is a bony structure composed of individual vertebrae and fibrocartilaginous pads, called intervertebral discs. Their classifications are as follows:

- 7 Cervical vertebra
- 12 Thoracic vertebra
- 5 Lumbar vertebra
- 5 Sacrum—fused
- 3–4 Coccyx

The structure of the vertebral column consists of a body or centrum which is the thick, anterior, weight-bearing portion of a vertebra. The vertebral arch, resembling a ring, is the posterior curved portion formed by pedicles, laminae, transverse process, spinous processes, and the inferior and superior articular processes. This arch creates a space termed the vertebral foramen. Lying within the vertebral foramen is the vertebral canal. The transverse processes project laterally from the vertebral arch, while the spinous process is in the posterior midline. These processes are places for muscle attachment. The portion of the vertebral arch adjacent to the body between the body and the transverse process is the pedicle. The vertebral notch is the concave surface on the upper and lower margins of the pedicles. The openings formed by the inferior notch of one vertebra and superior notch of another vertebra are termed as intervertebral foramina. The lamina is the portion between the transverse process and the spinous process. The superior and inferior articular processes are smooth areas on the vertebral arch for the articulation of one vertebra over another.

Intervertebral Disc

The intervertebral discs are located between the vertebral bodies. They are fibrocartilaginous pads classified as symphysis joints.

Anatomy of the Intervertebral Disc

Nucleus pulpous—central core
- acts as a shock absorber and as a ball bearing during flexion, extension, and lateral bending of the vertebral column

Annulus fibrosis—outer ring
- composed of rings of fibrocartilage that run obliquely from one vertebra to another to form strong bonds between the vertebrae

Ligaments of the Vertebral Column

There are two major ligaments supporting the spinal column, the anterior longitudinal, and the posterior longitudinal ligaments. These ligaments are composed of dense connective tissue tightly attached to the anterior and posterior surface of the vertebral column. Several accessory ligaments circle the vertebral column to maintain stability and help protect the spinal cord (Fig. 2.60).

Anterior Longitudinal Ligament

The anterior longitudinal ligament consists of a layer of dense connective tissue. This tissue is firmly attached to the anterior surface of the vertebral bodies and intervertebral disc. The ligament extends from C2 to the sacrum. Its functions are to maintain vertebral column stability and prevent hyperextension.

Posterior Longitudinal Ligament

The posterior longitudinal ligament lies within the vertebral canal extending along the posterior surface along the length of the canal starting at C2. This ligament is narrower and weaker than the anterior longitudinal, with the purpose of preventing hyperflexion and hyperextension of vertebral the column and protrusion of the nucleus pulpous.

Transverse Ligament

The transverse ligament extends across the ring of C1 to form a sling over the posterior surface of the odontoid process. This ligament contains longitudinal fibers that attach to the anterior margin of the foramen magnum and insert on the body of the axis. The function of this ligament is to hold the odontoid process against the anterior arch of C1. It is also known as the cruciform ligament due to its cross-like appearance.

Ligamentum Flava

The ligamentum flava is located on either side of the spinous process consisting of strong yellow elastic tissue. Its purpose is to join the laminae of adjacent vertebral arches to preserve the normal curvature of the spine.

Interspinous Ligament

The interspinous ligament is a thin membranous ligament connecting adjoining spinous processes that extends from the root to the apex of each spinous process. They are slightly developed in the cervical region, narrow and elongated in the thoracic region, and broader, thicker, and quadrilateral in the lumbar region. Their action is to limit flexion of the spine.

Supraspinous Ligament

The supraspinous ligament is a strong fibrous cord running over and connecting the tips of the spinous processes from C7 through the sacrum. This ligaments function is to limits flexion along with other ligaments of vertebral column. The supraspinous ligament serves as a midline attachment for some important muscles and helps maintain the upright position of the head.

Spinal Cord and Nerve Roots

Spinal Cord

The spinal cord resides within the vertebral foramen extending from the foramen magnum to approximately the L1 level, ending as it tapers into the conus medullaris (Fig. 2.61). Large nerve roots travel within the vertebral foramen, exiting at specific levels at each interspace. These groups of nerves have an appearance referred to as the cauda equina (horse's tail). The spinal cord is centrally located containing cerebral spinal fluid and is continuous with the ventricles of the brain. It is composed of gray matter and white matter. The gray matter is made up of nerve cells that run the full length of the cord, while the white matter covers the external borders of the cord and is more abundant.

Spinal Nerve Root

Each spinal nerve is connected to the spinal cord by a dorsal root and a ventral root. The dorsal root ganglion can be recognized by an enlargement, of the dorsal root, which contains the cell bodies of afferent (sensory) neurons that

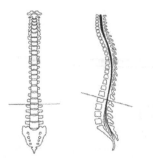

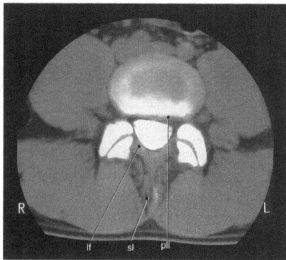

KEY: lf, Ligamentum flava; **sl,** supraspinous ligament; **pll,** posterior longitudinal ligament.

Figure 2.60. Axial CT image of the lumbar spine illustrating the ligamentum flava, the supraspinous, and the posterior longitudinal ligament. (Reproduced, with permission, from Kelley LL, Petersen CM. *Sectional Anatomy for Imaging Professionals.* 3rd ed. St. Louis, MO: Mosby Elsevier; 2013.)

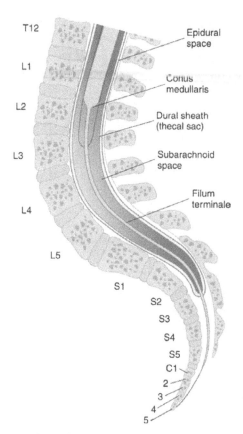

Figure 2.61. Sagittal illustration of the spinal cord, conus medullaris, and thecal sac. (Reproduced, with permission, from Kelley LL, Petersen CM. *Sectional Anatomy for Imaging Professionals.* 3rd ed. St. Louis, MO: Mosby Elsevier; 2013.)

transmit impulses from the peripheral of the body to the nervous system. Cell bodies of efferent (motor) neurons are in the ventral horns of the gray matter. These nerve roots exit the spinal cord by way of the ventral root to supply motor skills throughout the body. On the outer side of the intervertebral foramen, the dorsal and ventral nerve root join to form the 31 pairs of spinal nerves.

Nerve Plexuses

The nerve plexuses are a network of intersecting nerves that serve the motor and sensory needs of the muscles and skin of the extremities. These plexuses include:

Cervical
- C1–C4 located under the sternocleidomastoid muscle

Brachial
- C5–T1 runs between the anterior and middle scalene muscle

Lumbar
- L4–L5 formed within the psoas major muscle

Sacral
- S1–S4 anterior surface of the piriformis muscle

Muscles of the Vertebral Column

Superficial Muscle Group (Fig. 2.62)

Splenius Muscles

The splenius muscles are located on the posterior and lateral aspect of the cervical and upper thoracic spine. They are divided into a cranial segment, the splenius capitis and the cervical segment, the splenius cervicis. The splenius capitis is the cranial portion originating on the spinous processes of C7 through T3 and inserting on the mastoid process of the temporal bone. Splenius cervicis is the cervical portion attached to the spinous process of T3 through T6 and appending on the transverse process of C1 through C4. The functions of these muscles are to extend the head and neck.

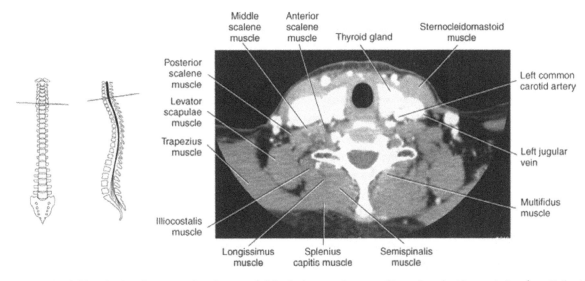

Figure 2.62. Axial CT projection demonstrating the superficial splenius muscle group. (Reproduced, with permission, from Kelley LL, Petersen CM. *Sectional Anatomy for Imaging Professionals.* 3rd ed. St. Louis, MO: Mosby Elsevier; 2013.)

Intermediate Muscle Group

Erector Spinae Muscle

The erector spinae muscles are the group of muscles forming the prominent bulge on each side of the vertebral column. These muscles are divided into three columns: the iliocostalis muscles, the longissimus muscles, and the spinalis muscle group. Their function is for the extension of the spine, for lateral flexion (side-bending) of the spine.

Deep Muscle Group

Transversospinal Muscles

The transversospinal muscle groups are several short muscles located in the groove between the transverse and spinous processes of the spine. Their fibers run obliquely from the transverse process of one vertebra to the spinous process of the vertebra above. Their role is to flex and rotate the vertebral column. They are divided into the semispinalis muscles, the multifidus muscles, and the rotatores.

Semispinalis
- largest muscle mass in the posterior portion of the neck
- arise from the cervical and thoracic spine

Multifidus
- span the entire length of the spine
- most prominent in lumbar

Rotators
- insert on the lamina of one vertebra to the transverse process of the vertebra below
- poorly developed in the cervical and lumbar region

IMAGING PROCEDURES OF THE VERTEBRAL COLUMN

Indications
- Trauma
- Fractures
- Dislocation
- Degenerative disease
- Herniated disc
- Osteoporosis
- Radiculopathy
- Stenosis
- Tumor
- Infection (osteomyelitis)/abscess

Cervical Spine

Technical Factors

Anatomical coverage
- 1 cm above the atlanto-occipital joint through the body of T1

Slice thickness
- 2 mm

Slice increments
- 2 mm

DFOV
- 120 to 150 mm

Kernel
- standard/soft tissue

Retrospective reconstruction
- slice thickness
  - ≤2 cm
- slice increments
  - overlap
- kernel
  - standard/soft tissue
  - bone/detail

Reformats
- MPR
  - sagittal
  - coronal
- 3D
  - volume rendered

IV contrast
- R/O infection or abscess
- Flow rate
  - 2 cc/s
- Delay time
  - 60 to 120 seconds
  - radiologist preference

Thoracic Spine

Technical Factors

Anatomical coverage
- above the body of C7 through the body of L1

Slice thickness
- 2 mm

Slice increments
- 2 mm

DFOV
- 150 to 180 mm
- Remember to take into consideration the curvature of the spine

Kernel
- standard/soft tissue

Retrospective reconstruction
- slice thickness
  - ≤2 cm
- slice increments
  - overlap
- kernel
  - standard/soft tissue
  - bone/detail

Reformats
- MPR
  - sagittal
  - coronal
- 3D
  - volume rendered

IV contrast
- R/O infection or abscess
- Flow rate
  - 2 cc/s
- Delay time
  - 60 to 20 seconds
    - radiologist preference

Lumbar Spine

Technical Factors

Anatomical coverage
Above the body of T12 through the sacroiliac joints

Slice thickness
- ≤3 mm

Slice increments
- ≤3 mm

DFOV
- 150 to 180 mm
- Remember to take into consideration the width of the sacrum

Kernel
- standard/soft tissue

Retrospective reconstruction
- slice thickness
  - ≤2 cm
- slice increments
  - overlap
- kernel
  - standard/soft tissue
  - bone/detail

Reformats
- MPR
  - sagittal
  - coronal

3D
- volume rendered

IV contrast
- R/O infection or abscess
- Flow rate
  - 2 cc/s
- Delay time
  - 60 to 120 seconds
  - radiologist preference

Post Myelogram

A post myelogram is performed following injection of intrathecal contrast. The patient should be scanned within 2 hours of injection to sustain the density of contrast in spinal cord. Imaging parameters are the same as routine imaging of the spine. The patient should perform a complete 360° roll onto the table in order to mix the contrast within the spinal cord. The institutions routine scanning parameters should be used.

Discogram

A discogram is a diagnostic test performed to view and assess the internal structure of a disc and determine if it is the source of pain. Under fluoroscopy a needle is placed into the disc of interest. Saline solution and nonionic contrast media are injected into the disc or discs if more than one disc is being examined. The purpose of the examination is to demonstrate annular tears, scarring, disc bulges, and changes in the nucleus of the disc. The expected results include: recreation of painful symptoms if the disc/discs is abnormal and the confirmation of a diagnosis and/or determination of which disc/discs is the source of pain.

Technical Factors

Scan mode
- step and shoot

Anatomical coverage
- vertebral endplate above the disc of interest to the vertebral endplate of the disc below

Gantry angle
- parallel to the disc/discs of interest

Slice thickness
- 3 mm

Slice increments
- 3 mm

Kernel
- standard/soft tissue
- bone/detail

PATHOLOGY OF THE VERTEBRAL COLUMN

C1 Fracture

A C1 fracture is usually the cause of direct pressure on the top of the head. This can be due to swimming or diving related accident. C1 fractures can be categorized as follows:

Posterior arch fracture
- occurring at the posterior arch and the lateral mass

Anterior arch fractures (Fig. 2.63)
- occurring at the anterior arch and the lateral mass
  - solitary anterior arch fracture is usually caused by the propelling force of the odontoid through the anterior arch

Lateral mass fracture
- occurs unilaterally having the fracture line passing through the articular surface or inferior to the anterior and posterior lateral mass on one side

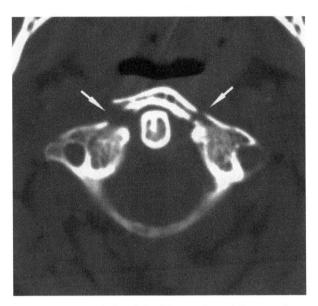

Figure 2.63. Detailed axial CT of C1 anterior arch fracture also known as a plough fracture. (Reproduced, with permission, from Grey ML, Ailinani JM. *CT and MRI Pathology: A Pocket Atlas*. 2nd ed. New York, NY: McGraw-Hill; 2012.)

Burst fracture
- in the cervical spine
  - known as the Jefferson fracture
- occurs as two fractures in the anterior arch and two in the posterior arch

These fractures are either nondisplaced or displaced with the latter causing various degrees of encroachment of the spinal cord. An unenhanced CT is utilized for the diagnosis of these fractures due to its high resolution, (ability to show bony and soft tissue related injuries), and its quickness in completing the study (elimination of motion). Trauma to the spine happens in the cervical more than in any other area of the spine.

C2 Fracture

A C2 fracture is a fracture of the laminae, articular facets, pedicles or pars interarticularis of C2 with disruption of C2–C3 junction. Its common etiology is from a fall, diving, or a motor vehicle collision. The mechanism of the injury is forcible hyperextension of the head. When there is a break in the posterior element of the cervical vertebrae with dislocation of C2 it is known as a Hangman's fracture or traumatic spondylolisthesis.

Burst Fracture

A burst fracture is a fracture of the spine in which the vertebral body is severely compressed. Fractures of the vertebral body, pedicles, and lamina are seen (Fig. 2.64).

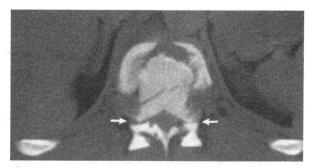

Figure 2.64. Axial CT in the bone/detail algorithm demonstrating a burst fracture of the T12. Notice how the vertebral body is compressed with bilateral fractures of the pedicles. The *white arrows* are pointing out a small paraspinal hematoma and spinal cord compression. (Reproduced, with permission, from Grey ML, Ailinani JM. *CT and MRI Pathology: A Pocket Atlas.* 2nd ed. New York, NY: McGraw-Hill; 2012.)

They typically occur from severe trauma, such as a motor vehicle accident or a fall from a height, when there is a great deal of vertical force onto the spine. These fractures mostly occur in the thoracic and lumbar regions. The treatment of choice is surgical fusion of the damaged vertebra in order to stabilize the spine.

Spondylolysis

A spondylolysis is a defect (usually fracture) of the vertebral arch in between the superior and inferior facet joints (specifically, the pars interarticularis), occurring on one or both sides. The great majority of cases occur in the lowest of the lumbar vertebra (L5), but it can also be seen in other vertebrae. Spondylolysis can be present with or without spondylolisthesis. CT imaging utilizing the sagittal reformations is the most common entity for identifying pars defects. It has been noted that reviewing the midvertebral body in the axial plane is also useful.

Spondylolisthesis

Spondylolisthesis is an abnormal slip (anteriorly or posterity) of one vertebra with respect to the vertebra immediately below. It affects the region of the pars interarticularis, which is roughly the region of the junction of the pedicle and lamina, where the articular and transverse processes of the vertebrae arise. The cause of this disease may be a result of acute trauma, congenital, or due to spinal instability from degenerative changes of the facet joints or discs. They are classified into four types:

Type 1
- 25% involve vertebral displacement of one vertebra over another inferior to it

Type 2
- 50% involve vertebral displacement of one vertebra over another inferior to it

Type 3
- 75% involve vertebral displacement of one vertebra over another inferior to it

Type 4
- anything >75% involve vertebral displacement of one vertebra over another inferior to it

Sagittal reformatted CT imaging is superior in the demonstration of the shifting of a vertebra over an inferior vertebra in addition to demonstrating the pars interarticularis.

Ankylosing Spondylitis

Ankylosing spondylitis is an inflammatory disease that can cause some of the vertebrae in your spine to fuse together. Fusing makes the spine less flexible and can result in a hunched-forward posture. If ribs are affected, it may be difficult to breathe deeply. This disease affects males more often than females.

Spinal Stenosis

Spinal stenosis is a condition where the spinal canal is sufficiently reduced in size from a variety of causing, such as, nerve root impingement, osteophyte formation, disc herniation. This disorder can be categorized as congenital or acquired. The congenital form may be due to achondroplasia or idiopathic. The acquired form is probably due to one of the following:

- Degenerative disc disease
- Ligamentum flava hypertrophy
- Spondylolisthesis
- Disc bulging
- Trauma

This disease process is a frequent cause of low back and leg pain. MRI is the modality of choice, since it has a greater sensitivity rate in demonstrating the spinal cord and the soft tissue surrounds. When MRI cannot be utilized, CT myelography is the next best choice.

Disc Herniation

The term herniated nucleus pulposus and bulging annulus fibrosis are mentioned together as contained extruded and sequestered discs. When disc material migrates from the parent disc it is termed sequestered or free fragment which can press against neural tissue causing pain, numbness, or weakness of the leg. Disc protrusions may or may not be symptomatic.

Review Questions

1. What is described as a tear in the wall of the aorta that causes blood to flow between the layers of the wall of the aorta and force the layers apart?

   (A) aortic aneurysm
   (B) aortic dissection
   (C) embolism
   (D) thrombosis

2. Which chamber of the heart consists of the strongest cardiac muscle?

   (A) pericardium
   (B) epicardium
   (C) myocardium
   (D) endocardium

3. What structure is adjacent to the head of the caudate nucleus?

   (A) thalamus
   (B) anterior horn of the lateral ventricle
   (C) pons
   (D) posterior horn of the lateral ventricle

4. What organ of the body is considered the largest lymph node and highly vascular?

   (A) spleen
   (B) gallbladder
   (C) stomach
   (D) liver

5. Which of the following is the longest and largest bone of the upper extremity?

   (A) scapula
   (B) humerus
   (C) radius
   (D) ulna

6. In the female pelvis what soft tissue structure is located posterior to the urinary bladder and anterior to the rectum?

   (A) uterus
   (B) ovaries
   (C) urethra
   (D) symphysis pubis

7. Which of the following is a funnel-shaped fibro-muscular tube 12 cm in length that acts as an opening for both the respiratory and digestive systems?

   (A) epiglottis
   (B) auditory tube
   (C) palatine tonsil
   (D) pharynx

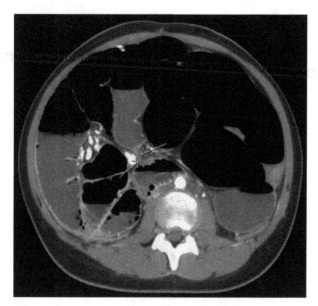

Figure Q2.1. Reproduced, with permission, from Grey ML, Ailinani JM. *CT and MRI Pathology: A Pocket Atlas.* 2nd ed. New York, NY: McGraw-Hill; 2012.

8. Figure Q2.1 demonstrates a mechanical or functional obstruction of the intestines, preventing the normal transit of the products of digestion. It can occur at any level distal to the duodenum of the small intestine and is a medical emergency. What is this pathological condition called?

   (A) small bowel obstruction
   (B) Crohn's disease
   (C) pelvic inflammatory disease
   (D) diverticulitis

9. What structures make up the brain stem?

   (A) cerebellar tonsils and thalamus
   (B) thalamus, midbrain, and the medulla oblongata
   (C) thalamus, midbrain, and the pons
   (D) midbrain, pons, and the medulla oblongata

10. What dome-shaped muscular sheet forms a convex floor for the chest and serves a septum between the thoracic and abdominal cavities?

    (A) diaphragm
    (B) costomediastinal recess
    (C) costodiaphragmatic recesses
    (D) intercostal muscle

11. The abdominal aorta divides into the right and left common iliac arteries at what lumbar vertebrae?

    (A) L2
    (B) L4
    (C) S1
    (D) S2

12. What vessel branches off the aortic arch and extends to the right and divides into the right subclavian and the right common carotid?

    (A) ascending aorta
    (B) descending aorta
    (C) brachiocephalic artery
    (D) right vertebral artery

13. What duct traverses the length of the pancreatic gland to join with the common bile duct at the hepatopancreatic ampulla?

    (A) cystic duct
    (B) left and right intrahepatic ducts
    (C) duct of Wirsung
    (D) duct of Santorin

14. Which of the following neck structures are directly responsible for voice production?

    (A) vestibular folds
    (B) glottic space
    (C) true vocal cords
    (D) infraglottic space

15. What blood vessel is considered responsible for major strokes?

    (A) coronary arteries
    (B) femoral arteries
    (C) carotid arteries
    (D) jugular veins

16. What is the name of the largest foramen found in the body?

    (A) foramen magnum
    (B) obturator foramen
    (C) rotundum foramen
    (D) foramen ovale

17. What is the pyramid-shaped muscular organ that rest on the pelvic floor immediately posterior to the symphysis pubis?

    (A) bladder
    (B) uterus
    (C) prostate gland
    (D) seminal vesicles

18. When an adrenal lesion measures less than −20 HU, it is said to be what kind of lesion?

    (A) cystic lesion
    (B) adenoma
    (C) metastatic
    (D) lymphoma

19. The carina of the trachea is where the trachea bifurcates into the right and left main stem bronchi, what is the vertebral location of this bifurcation?

    (A) C6
    (B) T1
    (C) T5
    (D) T12

20. Which of the following pathological conditions is characterized by a soft tissue homogeneous mass with focal bone destruction of the middle ear?

    (A) cholesteatoma
    (B) cavernous hemangioma
    (C) acoustic neuroma
    (D) glomus tumor

21. What abdominal wall muscle compresses the abdominal viscera when the trunk bends and its insertions are the xiphoid process, linea alba, and the pubis?

    (A) longissimus capitis
    (B) psoas
    (C) external oblique
    (D) transverse abdominis

22. Which of the following salivary glands are seen as hypodense structures on cross-sectional images?

    (A) parotid gland
    (B) subbuccal gland
    (C) submandibular gland
    (D) sublingual gland

23. What is the formation development, or existence of a clot within the vascular system?

    (A) embolus
    (B) thrombosis
    (C) hematoma
    (D) dissection

24. Which of the following ligaments is referred to as the cruciform ligament?

    (A) ligamentum flava
    (B) supraspinous ligament
    (C) anterior longitudinal ligament
    (D) transverse ligament

25. Which of the following pathological conditions must be performed in two planes, the axial and the coronal, due to the pyramidal shape of their bony structure?

    (A) mandibular fracture
    (B) orbital imaging
    (C) temporal bone imaging
    (D) sinus imaging

26. What is the landmark for the terminal part of the large intestine (rectum)?

    (A) L5
    (B) L4
    (C) S3 to the tip of the coccyx
    (D) S1

27. On an unenhanced abdominal CT, what is the range of CT attenuation values of a normal liver?

    (A) −10 to 0 HU
    (B) 10 to 40 HU
    (C) 55 to 65 HU
    (D) 125 to 165 HU

28. What abdominal arteryies lies at approximately L3 and supplies blood to the distal half of the large intestines?

    (A) superior renal arteries
    (B) inferior mesenteric artery
    (C) superior mesenteric artery
    (D) superior rectal artery

29. How many valves are there in the heart?

    (A) 1
    (B) 2
    (C) 3
    (D) 4

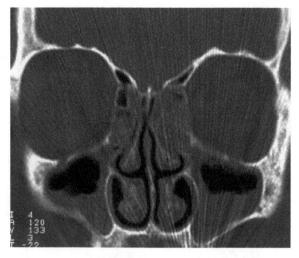

Figure Q2.2. Reproduced, with permission, from Grey ML, Ailinani JM. *CT and MRI Pathology: A Pocket Atlas.* 2nd ed. New York, NY: McGraw-Hill; 2012.

30. What pathological condition is demonstrated in Figure Q2.2?

    (A) orbital fracture
    (B) acoustic neuroma
    (C) sinusitis
    (D) Le Fort III fracture

31. The small intestine is divided into three parts, what is the name of the distal portion?

    (A) ileum
    (B) duodenum
    (C) jejunum
    (D) cecum

32. What muscle is not associated with rotator cuff injury?

    (A) supraspinatus
    (B) infraspinatus
    (C) subscapularis
    (D) teres major

33. Injection flow rate is a pertinent aspect when scanning, which of the following flow rates will deliver a higher concentration of contrast to the desired area when the scan commences?

    (A) 1 cc/s
    (B) 3 cc/s
    (C) 5 cc/s
    (D) drip infusion

34. What artery located in the supra aortic mediastinum is most posterior and is situated adjacent to the left side of the trachea?

    (A) left common carotid artery
    (B) right common carotid artery
    (C) left subclavian artery
    (D) brachiocephalic trunk

35. What are the white matter tracts that connect the two cerebral hemispheres?

    (A) anterior commissure
    (B) posterior commissure
    (C) septum pellucidum
    (D) corpus callosum

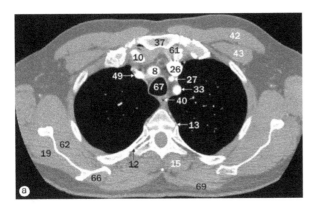

Figure Q2.3. Reproduced, with permission, from Weir J, Abrahams PH, Spratt JD, et al. *Imaging Atlas of Human Anatomy.* 4th ed. St. Louis, MO: Mosby Elsevier; 2011.

Use figure Q2.3 to answer questions 36-38.

36. In Figure Q2.3, label #27 represents which anatomical structure?

(A) brachiocephalic trunk

(B) left subclavian artery

(C) left common carotid artery

(D) left internal carotid artery

37. Label #49 in figure Q2.3 represents which of the following structures?

(A) right brachiocephalic vein

(B) brachiocephalic trunk

(C) SVC

(D) right subclavian vein

38. Which of the following is demonstrated by label #40 in figure Q2.3?

(A) trachea

(B) esophagus

(C) thymus gland

(D) pericardial fat

39. Which of the following pathological conditions appear as hypodense interior masses with a ring of enhancement in its peripheral?

(A) salivary gland abscess

(B) goiter

(C) thymus CA

(D) carotid stenosis

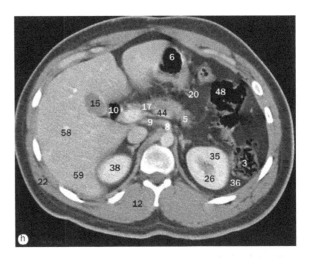

Figure Q2.4. Reproduced, with permission, from Weir J, Abrahams PH, Spratt JD, et al. *Imaging Atlas of Human Anatomy.* 4th ed. St. Louis, MO: Mosby Elsevier; 2011.

40. What muscle is the largest and most important of the pelvic floor?

(A) coccygeus muscle

(B) levator ani

(C) gluteus maximus

(D) obturator externus

Use Figure Q2.4 to answer questions 41-43

41. Label #8 in figure Q2.4 represents which of the following structures?

(A) superior mesenteric vein

(B) celiac artery

(C) left hepatic artery

(D) splenic artery

42. What number in figure Q2.4 illustrates the pancreas?

(A) 44

(B) 17

(C) 15

(D) 5

43. Label #15 in figure Q2.4 represents what anatomical structure?

(A) liver

(B) gall bladder

(C) hepatic flexure

(D) pancreas

44. What is the scanning range when performing an abdominal survey that includes all the abdominal compartments and pelvis?

    (A) diaphragm to the iliac crest
    (B) lung bases to the iliac crest
    (C) diaphragm to the ischial tuberosities
    (D) kidneys through the bladder

45. Which of the following vessels does **not** contribute to the vascular supply to the brain?

    (A) posterior cerebral artery
    (B) anterior communicating artery
    (C) vertebral artery
    (D) internal carotid artery

46. How many carpal bones are there in the wrist?

    (A) 2
    (B) 4
    (C) 6
    (D) 8

47. Which of the following structure is not surrounded by perirenal fat?

    (A) superior poles of both kidneys
    (B) renal arteries
    (C) renal vein
    (D) inferior mesenteric artery

Use Figure Q2.4 to answer questions 48-50

48. In figure Q2.5, which of the following illustrates the superior vena cava?

    (A) 57
    (B) 4
    (C) 46
    (D) 65

49. In figure Q2.5, which of the following illustrates the left superior pulmonary vein?

    (A) 14
    (B) 35
    (C) 32
    (D) 55

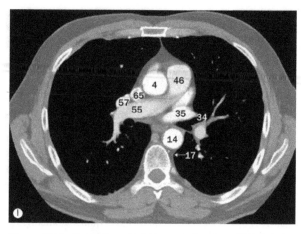

Figure Q2.5. Reproduced, with permission, from Weir J, Abrahams PH, Spratt JD, et al. *Imaging Atlas of Human Anatomy.* 4th ed. St. Louis, MO: Mosby Elsevier; 2011.

50. What number in figure Q2.5 illustrates right pulmonary artery?

    (A) 55
    (B) 46
    (C) 32
    (D) 63

51. The common bile duct is formed by the union of which two ducts?

    (A) common hepatic duct and the cystic duct
    (B) intrahepatic duct and the pancreatic duct
    (C) cystic duct and the left intrahepatic ducts
    (D) porta hepatic duct and the cystic duct

52. Which of the following paranasal sinuses is most posterior?

    (A) cavernous sinus
    (B) sphenoid sinus
    (C) mastoid sinus
    (D) maxillary sinus

Use figure Q2.6 to answer question 53

53. What pathological condition is demonstrated in Figure Q2.6?

    (A) lymphangioma
    (B) mesenteric pseudocyst
    (C) abscess
    (D) Crohn disease

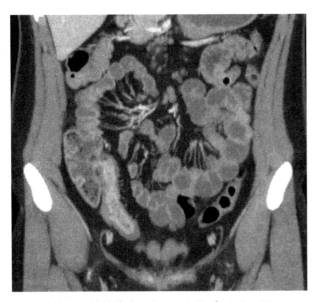

Figure Q2.6. Reproduced, with permission from Gray ML, Ailinani JM, *CT and MRI Pathology: A Pocket Atlas*, 2nd ed. New York, NY: McGraw-Hill; 2012.

54. What is the largest division of the acetabulum?

    (A) ilium
    (B) ischium
    (C) pubis
    (D) sacrum

55. What structure forms the lower portion of the brain stem containing white matter verve fibers communicating between the brain stem and the spinal cord?

    (A) pons
    (B) medulla oblongata
    (C) lenticular nucleus
    (D) extreme capsule

56. In most institutions what is the preferred oral contrast administered to patients undergoing a CT scan of the pancreas?

    (A) barium sulfate
    (B) VoLumen
    (C) water-soluble iodinated
    D) water

57. What ligament extends downward from C2 along the anterior surface of the vertebral surface to the sacrum?

    (A) transverse ligament
    (B) anterior longitudinal ligament
    (C) posterior longitudinal ligament
    (D) supraspinatus ligament

58. During what phase of renal enhancement do the renal cortex and medulla show equal levels of enhancement?

    (A) precontrast
    (B) nephrographic phase
    (C) corticomedullary phase
    (D) excretory phase

59. Which of the following muscles of the neck originates on the sternum and clavicle and inserts onto the mastoid tip?

    (A) sternocleidomastoid
    (B) levator scapulae muscle
    (C) trapezius muscle
    (D) anterior scalene muscle

60. Give the name of this primary cancer that has an etiology of unknown origin, mostly diagnosed in the younger population, but individuals exposed to radiation have a predisposition linked to this cancer.

    (A) kidney cancer
    (B) lung cancer
    (C) brain cancer
    (D) bone cancer

61. The use of flow control mechanical pressure injectors are recommended for CT studies of the abdomen and pelvis due to which of the following characteristics?

    (A) there is a reduced risk of extravasation of the contrast media into the soft tissue
    (B) side effects such as heat and nausea re reduced
    (C) contrast media dose and timing can be easily regulated and reproduced in subsequent studies
    (D) the risk of air embolism is eliminated

62. Which chamber of the heart pumps blood into the pulmonary trunk through the pulmonary semilunar valve?

    (A) left ventricle
    (B) left atrium
    (C) right ventricle
    (D) right atrium

63. What are the structures located around the base of the brain where the subarachnoid space becomes widened?

    (A) lentiform nucleus
    (B) red nucleus
    (C) cisterns
    (D) quadrigeminal plate

64. The liver has a dual blood supply. What percent of the hepatic artery supplies blood to the liver?

    (A) 25%
    (B) 35%
    (C) 50%
    (D) 80%

65. Which ligament in the upper extremity forms a ring that encircles the radial head?

    (A) radial collateral ligament
    (B) annular ligament
    (C) supraspinatus ligament
    (D) ulna collateral ligament

66. In the male pelvis, what musculotendinous pouch encloses the testes, epididymis, and lower portion of the spermatic cord?

    (A) tunica albuginea
    (B) vas deferens
    (C) scrotum
    (D) corpora cavernosa

67. Which of the following pathological conditions appear as a loculated fluid collection with irregular thickening and fat planes due to inflammation?

    (A) cyst
    (B) abscess
    (C) ascites
    (D) hemorrhage

68. What major vein is formed by the junction of the right and left brachiocephalic vein?

    (A) internal jugular
    (B) superior vena cava
    (C) external jugular
    (D) retromandibular vein

69. Which of the following carpal bones is the most frequently fractured?

    (A) triquetral
    (B) scaphoid
    (C) trapezoid
    (D) trapezium

70. During what phase of renal enhancement demonstrates the vascular anatomy of the kidneys?

    (A) precontrast
    (B) nephrographic phase
    (C) corticomedullary phase
    (D) excretory phase

71. What branch of the Circle of Willis originates from the basilar artery to supply blood to the occipital lobe?

    (A) anterior communicating
    (B) middle cerebral
    (C) posterior cerebral
    (D) internal carotid

72. What space separates the upper and middle lobes from the lower lobe of the right lung?

    (A) pleural cavity
    (B) oblique fissure
    (C) horizontal fissure
    (D) hilum

73. What mater is located in the innermost layer of the meninges?

    (A) dura mater
    (B) pia mater
    (C) arachnoid mater
    (D) falx cerebri

74. What veins are located in the thigh that passes over the pubic bone to enter the pelvis?

    (A) common iliac veins
    (B) femoral veins
    (C) internal iliac veins
    (D) gluteal veins

75. Which of the following muscles is named because it is associated with three heads of proximal attachment of the upper extremity?

    (A) deltoid muscle
    (B) brachialis muscle
    (C) subscapularis muscle
    (D) triceps muscle

Answers and Explanations

1. **(B)** An aortic dissection occurs when blood enters the wall of an artery separating the vascular layer creating a cavity or false lumen in the vessel wall. *(Grey, 2nd ed., p. 202)*

2. **(C)** The myocardium is the middle layer of the three layers of the heart. This layer is composed of a thick muscular muscle that contracts with each heartbeat. Ten percent of the total cardiac blood volume of each heartbeat is required solely for supply to the heart muscle. *(Kelley, 3rd ed., p. 336)*

3. **(B)** The anterior horn of the lateral ventricles are part of the lateral ventricles found within the frontal lobe. The roof is formed by the corpus callosum, the floor and lateral wall are formed by the head of the caudate nucleus, and the medial wall is formed by the septum pellucidum. *(Madden, 3rd ed., p. 17)*

4. **(A)** The spleen is the largest lymph organ in the body composed of lymphoid tissue. It is a highly vascular organ that functions to produce white blood cells, filter abnormal blood cells, store iron, and initiate immune responses. *(Kelley, 3rd ed., p. 441)*

5. **(B)** The humerus is the longest and largest bone of the upper extremity that articulates with the scapula superiorly and the radius and ulna inferiorly. The head of the humerus is the most proximal section consisting of a round surface that forms an articulation with the glenoid process. *(Madden, 3rd ed., p. 233)*

6. **(A)** The uterus is a pear-shaped organ located between the bladder and the rectum. The parts of the uterus are the fundus, body, and the cervix. *(Madden, 3rd ed., p. 397)*

7. **(D)** The pharynx is the fibromuscular tube located within the neck. It is divided into three sections, the nasopharynx, oropharynx, and the laryngopharynx. *(Kelley, 3rd ed. p. 251)*

8. **(A)** The image demonstrates markedly distended loops of small bowel with air fluid levels. Surgical intervention is the usual treatment of choice. *(Grey, 2nd ed., pp. 246–248)*

9. **(D)** The brain stem is the posterior part of the brain, adjoining the structurally continuous with the spinal cord. The brain stem provides the main motor and sensory distribution of nerves to the face and neck by way of the cranial nerves. It regulates the central nervous system and is imperative in maintaining consciousness and regulating the sleep cycle. *(Kelley, 3rd ed., p. 120)*

10. **(A)** The diaphragm is a dome-shaped muscle that spans the entire thoracic outlet separating the thoracic cavity from the abdominal cavity. It is the chief muscle of inspiration with the purpose of enlarging the cavity vertically as the dome moves inferiorly and flattens. *(Kelley, 3rd ed., p. 389)*

11. **(B)** Common iliac arteries are bilateral arising from the abdominal aorta at the level of the fourth lumbar vertebrae. They diverge laterally as they enter the pelvis. *(Madden, 3rd ed., p. 328)*

12. **(C)** The brachiocephalic artery is the first major branch off the aorta on the right side. It divides into the right subclavian and right common carotid artery. It should be noted that there is not a left brachiocephalic artery, since the aorta arches to the left side of the body. *(Madden, 3rd ed., p. 239)*

13. **(C)** The duct of Wirsung is the main pancreatic duct that carries enzymes to the duodenum. The duct runs the length of the pancreas gland to the ampulla of Vater. *(Kelley, 3rd ed., p. 437)*

14. **(C)** The true vocal cords are named accordingly for their production of sound. When the cords are relaxed they create an opening between them called the glottis, which is part of the larynx most directly involved with voice production. *(Madden, 3rd ed., pp. 175–176)*

15. **(C)** The common carotid arteries divide into the internal and external carotid arteries with the internal carotid extending into the brain to supply blood to the middle cerebral and anterior cerebral artery. An emboli or thrombus in the internal carotid arteries are major reasons for strokes. *(Kelley, 3rd ed., p. 300)*

16. **(B)** The union of the pubic rami and the ischium surrounds a large opening in the pelvis, known as the obturator foramen. It is enclosed by the obturator muscles. *(Kelley, 3rd ed., pp. 495–497)*

17. **(A)** The bladder is roughly pyramid shaped with the apex pointing downward between the pubis and vagina, in females, and the rectum, in males. *(Madden, 3rd ed., p. 396)*

18. **(B)** An adrenal adenoma is a common benign tumor arising from the cortex of the adrenal gland. These lesions are characterized as being well-circumscribed, homogeneous masses consisting of intracellular fat, which accounts for the low attenuation number. *(Grey, 2nd ed., p. 320)*

19. **(C)** The trachea bifurcates into the left and right main stem bronchi at an area called the carina. This bifurcation occurs at the T5 vertebral level. *(Madden, 3rd ed., p. 14)*

20. **(A)** Cholesteatoma appears as a soft tissue homogeneous density in the middle ear with thickening of the tympanic membrane. High-resolution CT imaging is the preferred modality to evaluate this mass-like lesion. *(Grey, 2nd ed., pp. 140–141)*

21. **(D)** The transverse abdominis muscle extends transversely to provide support for the abdominal viscera. Its function is to compress the abdominal viscera. *(Kelley. 3rd ed., p. 493)*

22. **(A)** The parotid gland contains a fair amount of fat, which displays as hypodense structures on cross-sectional CT images. *(Kelley, 3rd ed., p. 270)*

23. **(B)** A thrombosis is the formation of a blood clot inside a blood vessel, obstructing the flow of blood through the circulatory system. When a thrombus is significantly large enough to reduce the blood flow to a tissue, hypoxia can occur and metabolic products such as lactic acid can accumulate. *(Webb, 3rd ed., pp. 203–204)*

24. **(D)** The transverse ligament is also termed the cruciform ligament due to its cross-like appearance. It extends across the ring of C1 to form a sling over the posterior surface of the odontoid process. This ligament contains longitudinal fibers that attach to the anterior margin of the foramen magnum and insert on the body of the axis. It functions to hold the odontoid process against the anterior arch of C1. *(Kelley, 3rd ed., p. 193)*

25. **(B)** Orbital imaging should be performed in both the axial and coronal planes due to the pyramidal shape of the bony orbit. These planes provides the radiologists the ability to see bony fragments and if these fragments are impinging on the rectus muscle. *(Seeram, 3rd ed., p. 398)*

26. **(C)** The rectum is the terminal part of the large intestine which extends from S3 to the tip of the coccyx. It is approximately 15 cm in length and follows the curve of the sacrum and coccyx ending at the anus. *(Kelley, 3rd ed., p. 523)*

27. **(C)** Normal liver parenchyma has a CT attenuation of 55 to 65 HU, which is slightly higher in attenuation when comparing to other soft tissue organs. This higher attenuation accounts for the glycogen content of the liver. *(Prokop, p. 411)*

28. **(B)** The inferior mesenteric artery originates from the aorta at approximately L3 and supplies blood to the left half of the transverse colon, descending colon, sigmoid colon, and upper rectum. *(Madden, 3rd ed., p. 3)*

29. **(D)** The four valves in the heart maintain one-way directional blood flow throughout the heart. The valves can be divided into atrioventricular (AV) and semilunar valves. The two AV valves are the tricuspid and bicuspid (mitral) valves, and the two

semilunar valves are the pulmonary semilunar and aortic semilunar valves. (*Kelley, 3rd ed., p. 346*)

30. **(C)** Sinusitis is a bacterial, viral, or fungal inflammation of the paranasal sinuses. The CT coronal plane in the image demonstrates mucosal thickening of the maxillary sinuses and opacification of the ethmoid sinuses. (*Grey, 2nd ed., pp. 156–157*)

31. **(A)** The ileum is the distal portion of the small intestines approximately 3.5 m in length, located in the RLQ. The loops of ileum terminate at the ileocecal valve, a sphincter that controls the flow of material from the ileum into the cecum of the large intestines. (*Kelley, 3rd ed., p. 458*)

32. **(D)** The teres major muscle is a flat rectangular muscle originating at the inferior angle of the scapula. It attaches to the greater tubercle of the humerus with the function of rotating the arm laterally and to abduct the arm. It is important not to confuse this muscle with the teres minor muscle, which is part of the rotator cuff. (*Madden, 3rd ed., p. 529*)

33. **(C)** When performing spiral scanning, contrast injection rates as high as 5 cc/s provides excellent opacification of arterial structures. (*Webb, 3rd ed., p. 6*)

34. **(C)** The left subclavian artery is the third major branch of the aorta. This artery is located more laterally ascending through the upper thorax to exit through the thoracic inlet thus forming the left axillary artery. (*Madden, 3rd ed., p. 240*)

35. **(D)** The corpus callosum is the largest and densest bundle of white matter in the cerebrum. The midline structure forms the roof of the lateral ventricles and connects the right and left cerebral hemispheres. (*Madden, 3rd ed., p. 14*)

36. **(C)** The carotid arteries supply arterial blood to the head and neck. They are located on either side of the trachea. Even though both arteries have the same structure, the left common carotid artery is the second branch off the aorta when viewing from left to right. (*Madden, 3rd ed., p. 176*)

37. **(A)** The brachiocephalic veins originate at the junction of the internal jugular and subclavian veins. In cross-sectional images, the right brachiocephalic vein is more vertical than the left and will

be seen as a circular structure to the right of the brachiocephalic trunk. (*Madden, 3rd ed., p. 240*)

38. **(B)** The esophagus is found at the terminal end of the pharynx at the approximate level of C6. It descends through the thoracic cavity ending at the stomach. On cross-sectional images, the esophagus is seen between the trachea and the vertebral bodies near the medial plane of the body. (*Kelley, 3rd ed., p. 268*)

39. **(A)** Submandibular salivary gland abscesses are mucous-filled cysts caused by trauma or obstruction. On unenhanced CT images, stones may be visualized along Wharton's duct, while the enhanced images show these abscesses as hypodense interior masses with hyperdensity in their peripheral. (*Grey, 2nd ed., p. 152*)

40. **(B)** The two levator ani muscles are the largest and most important of the pelvic floor originating from the symphysis pubis and ischial spines to form wing-like arches that attach to the coccyx. These muscles along with the coccygeus muscle provide support for the pelvic content. (*Kelley, 3rd ed., p. 510*)

41. **(B)** The celiac trunk is a very short vessel that leaves the anterior wall of the aorta just after the aorta passes through the diaphragm at approximately T12/L1. This vessel divides into three branches: left gastric artery, common hepatic artery, and the splenic artery. (*Madden, 3rd ed., p. 327*)

42. **(D)** The pancreas is a long narrow retroperitoneal organ lying posterior to the stomach and medial to the spleen. It is located in LUQ and RUQ between the 12th thoracic and 3rd lumbar vertebra. It is a collection of glandular tissue with little connective tissue having both exocrine and endocrine functions. (*Madden, 3rd ed., p. 325*)

43. **(B)** The gallbladder is located in RUQ, on the anterior aspect of abdomen under the inferior surface of the liver—associated with the main lobar fissure. It can be seen medial to the stomach between the 12th thoracic and 3rd lumbar vertebra. (*Kelley, 3rd ed., pp. 431–434*)

44. **(C)** Longitudinal coverage should encompass the diaphragm through the ischial tuberosities. Standard protocols usually require 5- to 7-mm slice thickness, but the evaluation of individual organs, intra and retroperitoneal disease should be examined with thinner slices. (*Prokop, p. 601*)

45. **(C)** The vertebral arteries are a branch of the subclavian arteries and join to form the basilar artery. They run bilaterally through the transverse foramina from C7 through C1. *(Madden, 3rd ed., p. 21)*

46. **(D)** There are eight carpal bones divided into proximal and distal rows. There are many mnemonics for remembering the order of these bones from lateral in the proximal row to medial in the distal row. Here is an example, Send Letter to Peter To Tell (him to) Come Home. *(Madden, 3rd ed., pp. 545–546)*

47. **(D)** The kidneys are retroperitoneal bean-shaped organs, located in RUQ and LUQ between the levels of T12 and L4. The kidneys along with the renal arteries and veins are embedded in perirenal fat in an attempt to prevent bumps and jolts to the body from injuring the kidneys. *(Kelley, 3rd ed., p. 446)*

48. **(D)** The superior vena cava is the major vein located on the superior aspect of the right side of the heart posterior to the ascending aorta. It is formed by the junction of the right and left brachiocephalic veins. On cross-sectional imaging, it is visible anterior and to the right of the trachea and is usually oval in shape. *(Madden, 3rd ed., p. 240)*

49. **(B)** The left superior pulmonary vein collects blood from the left upper lobe of the lung. It runs anterior and inferior to the left main bronchus as it enters the left atrium. *(Kelley, 3rd ed., p. 350)*

50. **(A)** The right pulmonary artery arises from the pulmonary trunk located posterior to the ascending aorta and SVC and anterior to the esophagus and right main stem bronchus to enter the hilum of the right lung. *(Madden, 3rd ed., p. 240)*

51. **(A)** The common bile duct transports bile from the gall bladder via the cystic duct and the liver via the hepatic duct to the duodenum. *(Madden, 3rd ed., p. 325)*

52. **(B)** The sphenoid sinuses occupy the body of the sphenoid bone directly below the sella turcica. This group is present at birth and continues to grow until the age of 12. On cross-sectional images they are the most posterior. *(Kelley, 3rd ed., pp. 25–27)*

53. **(D)** Crohn's disease is characterized by submucosal edema with ulcerations involving a thickened segment of distal ileum. The coronal reformatted image depicts the mesenteric hypervascularity, known as the comb sign. *(Grey, 2nd ed., p. 228)*

54. **(A)** The ilium is the largest and most superior bone of the pelvis made up of the body and ala (wing-like structure). The body of the ilium is important for it contribution to the superior portion of the acetabulum. *(Kelley, 3rd ed., p. 655)*

55. **(B)** The medulla oblongata is located in the lower brain stem just below the pons. It is the communication between the brain and the spinal cord and controls the vital functions of the body, such as respirations, heart rate, and blood pressure. The motor nerve fibers crossover causing one side of the brain to control the motor functions on the opposite side of the body. *(Kelley, 3rd ed., pp. 124–126)*

56. **(D)** Water may be the preferred oral contrast utilized for CT examinations of the pancreas. Positive contrast is too dense and may obscure small stones near the ampulla and detail in the pancreatic head. *(Webb, 3rd ed., p. 247)*

57. **(B)** The anterior longitudinal ligament consists of a layer of dense connective tissue. This tissue is firmly attached to the anterior surface of the vertebral bodies and intervertebral disc. The ligament extends from C2 to the sacrum. Its functions are to maintain vertebral column stability and prevent hyperextension. *(Madden, 3rd ed., p. 129)*

58. **(B)** The nephrographic or parenchymal phase of injection occurs at approximately 100 to 180 seconds from the start of injection. This phase is best for distinguishing renal tumors, since the lesions appear hypoattenuating. *(Prokop, p. 645)*

59. **(A)** The sternocleidomastoid muscle is a broad strap-like muscle that originates on the sternum and clavicle and inserts onto the mastoid tip. It function is to turn the head from side to side and turn the neck. Due it this muscles superficial position, it provides landmarks for identifying structures within the neck. *(Madden, 3rd ed., p. 180)*

60. **(D)** The most common malignant primary bone tumor is osteosarcoma. Its etiology is unknown, but individuals exposed to radiation have a predisposition linked to bone cancer. The tumors are commonly located in the knee, distal femur, or the proximal tibia and mostly seen the younger population (early teens to twenties). *(Grey, 2nd ed., p. 398)*

61. **(C)** Modern contrast injectors' volume and flow rates can be easily programed into the injector.

Documenting the examinations volume, flow rate, and delay time for individual patients will enable the technologist to reproduce the exact protocol on subsequent studies. *(Prokop, pp. 96–97)*

62. **(C)** The right ventricle lies on the diaphragm and is the largest portion of the anterior surface of the heart. It receives deoxygenated blood from the right atrium and forces it into the pulmonary trunk via the semilunar valves. *(Kelley, 3rd ed., pp. 336–337)*

63. **(C)** Cisterns are locations primarily around the base of the brain where the subarachnoid space becomes widened. They are generally named after the brain structure it borders. It is important to recognize these cisterns so as not to misinterpret them as abnormalities. *(Kelley, 3rd ed., p. 100)*

64. **(A)** The liver has a dual blood supply from the hepatic portal vein and hepatic arteries. The hepatic arteries supply arterial blood to the liver, accounting for 25% of its blood flow. *(Kelley, 3rd ed., p. 426)*

65. **(B)** The annular ligament forms a fibrous ring that encircles the radial head. The narrow portion tightens around the radial neck to prevent inferior displacement of the radius. This ligament is an important structure of the elbow joint because it allows the radius to rotate freely. *(Kelley, 3rd ed., p. 607)*

66. **(C)** The scrotum is a musculotendinous pouch encloses the testes, epididymis, and lower portion of the spermatic cord. It facilitates sperm formation by distending the testes outside the peritoneum in a cooler environment in an effort to regulate the temperature of the testes. *(Kelley, 3rd ed., pp. 535–536)*

67. **(B)** Majority of abscesses appear as loculated fluid collections, often with internal debris, fluid levels, and sometimes air–fluid levels and have a definable wall with irregular thickening. On an enhanced CT examination of the abdomen, the nearby fascia is thickened and fat places are obliterated because of inflammation. *(Webb, 2nd ed. p. 180; Prokop, p. 604)*

68. **(B)** The superior vena cava is the major vein located on the superior aspect of the right side of the heart. It is formed by the junction of the brachiocephalic veins and its function is to drain blood from the upper trunk into the right atrium. *(Madden, 3rd ed., p. 19)*

69. **(B)** Approximately 70% of all carpal bone fractures involve the scaphoid bone. In most cases, these fractures are unstable when the fracture is complete. On CT images, scaphoid fractures are best demonstrated in the oblique long axis plane with the addition of ulnar deviation. Fracture lines are transverse or oblique. *(Prokop, p. 960)*

70. **(C)** The corticomedullary phase of injection occurs at approximately 20 to 25 seconds post injection. This phase enhances the arterial flow of the kidneys, which is especially useful for transplant surgery and depicts hypervascular tumors. *(Prokop, p. 645)*

71. **(C)** The posterior cerebral artery originates from the basilar artery. It is located along the upper border of the pons and extends above the tentorium cerebelli supplying blood to the occipital lobe. As the posterior cerebral leaves the basilar artery, the posterior communicating artery connects to the internal carotid artery. *(Kelley, 3rd ed., p. 131)*

72. **(C)** The lungs are divided into lobes by fissures that are lined by pleura. The horizontal fissure is the division of the upper and middle lobes from the lower lobe of the right lung. Since the left lung only has two lobes; therefore, the left lung does not have a horizontal fissure. *(Kelley, 3rd ed., p. 313)*

73. **(B)** The pia mater is the innermost layer of the meninges surrounding the brain and spinal cord. *(Madden, 3rd ed., p.18)*

74. **(B)** The femoral veins originate from smaller vessels within the thigh that extend through the thigh to terminate in the external iliac vein as it passes over the pubic bone to enter the pelvis. *(Madden, 3rd ed., p. 393)*

75. **(D)** This muscle is named triceps because it is associated with three heads of proximal attachment: the long, medial, and lateral heads. The three heads join at a common tendon inserting at the proximal end of the olecranon process of the ulna. These muscles' main purpose are to extend the forearm. The long head steadies the head of the humerus when abducted. *(Kelley, 3rd ed., p. 600)*

Subspecialty List

QUESTION NUMBER AND SUBSPECIALTY
correspond to subcategories in each of the ARRT
examination specification sections.

1. Pathology—Abdomen Vascular
2. Anatomy—Heart
3. Anatomy—Brain
4. Anatomy—Spleen
5. Anatomy—Upper Extremity
6. Anatomy—Reproductive Organs
7. Anatomy—Larynxv
8. Procedures—GI Track
9. Anatomy—Brain
10. Anatomy—Mediastinum Muscular
11. Anatomy—Abdomen Vascular
12. Anatomy—Chest Vascular
13. Anatomy—Biliary
14. Anatomy—Larynx
15. Anatomy—Brain Vascular
16. Anatomy—Lower Extremity
17. Anatomy—Bladder
18. Anatomy—Adrenal Glands
19. Anatomy—Airway
20. Pathology—Internal Auditory Canal
21. Anatomy—Abdomen Muscles
22. Anatomy—Neck Soft Tissue
23. Pathology—Abdomen
24. Anatomy—Spine
25. Procedure—Orbits
26. Anatomy—Colorectal
27. Anatomy—Liver
28. Anatomy—Abdomen Vascular
29. Anatomy—Heart
30. Anatomy—Sinuses
31. Anatomy—GI Track
32. Anatomy—Upper Extremity Muscular
33. Procedures—Abdomen
34. Anatomy—Chest Vascular
35. Anatomy—Brain
36. Anatomy—Chest
37. Anatomy—Chest
38. Anatomy—Chest
39. Pathology—Soft Tissue
40. Anatomy—Pelvis
41. Anatomy—Abdomen Vascular
42. Anatomy—Pancreas
43. Anatomy—Biliary
44. Procedures—Abdomen
45. Anatomy—Brain Vascular
46. Anatomy—Upper Extremity
47. Anatomy—Kidney/Ureters
48. Anatomy—Chest Vascular
49. Anatomy—Chest Vascular
50. Anatomy—Chest Vascular
51. Anatomy—Biliary
52. Anatomy—Sinuses
53. Pathology—Abdomen
54. Anatomy—Lower Extremity
55. Anatomy—Posterior Fossa
56. Procedures—Abdomen
57. Anatomy—Spine
58. Procedures—Kidney
59. Anatomy—Soft Tissue Muscular
60. Pathology—Lower Extremity

61. Procedures—Abdomen
62. Anatomy—Heart
63. Anatomy—Brain
64. Anatomy—Liver
65. Anatomy—Upper Extremity
66. Anatomy—Reproductive Organs
67. Pathology—Abdomen
68. Anatomy—Chest Vascular

69. Pathology—Lower Extremity
70. Procedures—Kidney
71. Anatomy—Brain Vascular
72. Anatomy—Lungs
73. Anatomy—Brain
74. Anatomy—Pelvis Vascular
75. Anatomy—Upper Extremity

CHAPTER 3

Physics and Instrumentation

RADIATION PHYSICS

Radiation Interaction with Matter

At the atomic level, x-ray photons are created by the interaction of energetic electrons with matter. The photons' energy deceases by transferring their energy to electrons in matter. Photons react in matter in three possible ways:

- penetrate matter without interacting;
- interact with matter and are completely absorbed by depositing its energy;
- interact with matter and are scattered or deflected from its original direction and deposit part of its energy.

There are two types of photon interactions with electrons; the Photoelectric interaction in which the photon loses all its energy and the Compton scatter in which a portion of its energy is lost and the remaining energy is scattered.

Photoelectric Interaction

Photoelectric interaction typically transpires when an incident x-ray photon transfers all its energy to a firmly bound electron located in the inner shell electron (usually the K or L shell) of the atom. When the electron is ejected from the atom, it quickly loses energy and moves only a relatively short distance from its original location and deposits its energy close to the site of the interaction. The loss of the electron in the K or L shell creates a vacancy forcing an electron from an outer shell to move down and fill it in. The drop in energy of the filling electron frequently produces a characteristic photon. This interaction can only take place when the electron binding energy is only somewhat less than the energy of the photon. The photoelectric effect is a two divisional process: the first step is its loss of energy to the binding electron, while the second step involves the depositing of its energy to the

surrounding matter. In other words, the photoelectric effect occurs when low energy photons interact with high atomic number materials, such as bone or iodinated contrast media.

Compton Scatter

Compton scatter occurs when an incident x-ray photon interacts with an electron in the atom's outer shell resulting in ionization of the target atom. A portion of the photon's energy is absorbed (attenuation), and a new photon is produced with reduced energy. This photon is deflected in a direction different from the original photon. Due to its change of direction, this type of interaction is classified as a scattering process. The wavelength of the scattered x-ray is greater than that of the incident x-ray. As opposed to the photoelectric effect, Compton scatter utilizes high energy (i.e., 120 kVp) x-ray photons in order to penetrate the body and produce attenuated intensities at the detectors.

Acquisition Geometry

Data Acquisition

Data acquisition refers to a technique by which the patient is systematically scanned by the x-ray tube and detectors to collect enough information to produce a computed tomography (CT) image path. The mechanisms that encompass the data acquisition schema are the beam geometry, which denotes the size, shape, and the motion of the x-ray beam, and the physical components that shape and define the beam measure its transmission through the patient and convert the data into digital data for computer input. The data acquisition geometries have changed dramatically through the modernization of technology. CT has evolved through the generations with the primary concern involving: the beam geometry, the scanning motion (how the x-ray tube and detectors work together), and the number of detectors.

Data Acquisition Geometries

Acquisition geometries can be categorized by the parallel or pencil beam, which is defined by a set of parallel rays that generates data to produce an image, the fan beam is described as a small fan whose apex originates at the x-ray tube, while the spiral/helical is the most recently developed geometry that is referred to the type of acquisition with continuous scanning.

First Generation

The first generation scanner, developed by Hounsfield, utilized pencil-shaped x-ray beam known as translate–translate principle with the capabilities of:

Slice thickness
- 13 mm

Display field-of-view (DFOV)
- 24 cm

Scan time
- up to 5 minutes to complete scan

Reconstruction
- 2.5 hours

Algebraic reconstruction technique based on the parallel beam geometry

Detector type
- single

Linear array
- NaCl crystal/photomultiplier

Acquiring 180 parallel readings through 180 angles each 1-degree apart

Total number of samples: 28,800

Disadvantages
- produce only tomographic sections of the brain
- required use of a water-filled Perspex tank with a preshaped "head cap" which enclosed the patient's head (water bath)
- used to filter out the long wavelength x-rays
- images were relatively low resolution
- matrix size of 80 × 80
- spatial resolution of 3 line pairs/cm
- visualize an object 1.6 mm
  - today's scanners can visualize objects as small as 0.6 mm

Electric and Musical Industries (EMI) scanner
- first installed in Atkinson Morley's Hospital
- Wimbledon, England

First patient scanned in 1972
- woman suspected with a brain lesion
- images showed a detailed dark circular cyst

First scanner installed in the United States
- Mayo Clinic

Second Generation

The second generation scanner became the first scanner to become a head and body imager. Its scanning geometry, like the first generation scanner, employed translate–translate principle with the beam geometry of a fan. This generation's scanning capabilities were similar to the first generation with the exception of:

Detector type consisted of linear array
- 5–30 detectors constituted the linear array assembly

Single translation resulted in same number of data points as several translations with the first generation
- 10-degree rotation increment
- resulted in only 18 translations required for 180-degree image acquisition

Imaging time of 30 seconds
- shorter scanning time than first-generation scanners

Time decease is inversely proportional to the number of detectors
- more the detectors shorter the scan time

Disadvantages
- increased scatter radiation
- affects the final image as in conventional radiography
- increased intensity toward the edges of beam
  - due to body shape

Compensation method
- use of a "bow tie" filter
  - equalized the radiation intensity reaching the detector array

Translate–Translate Principle

The x-ray beams of the first- and second-generation scanners were not designed wide enough to cover the entire width of the slice of interest; therefore, a mechanical arrangement was required to move the x-ray source and detectors horizontally across the field-of-view (FOV). Following the initial sweep, the source and detector assembly would be rotated a few degrees (1-degree for first/10-degrees for second) and another sweep would be performed. This process would be repeated until the entire 180-degrees were covered.

Third Generation

The third generation CT employed the rotate–rotate scanning geometry principle with the fan beam geometry. This principle allowed the x-ray tube and detectors to make a complete 360-degree rotation around the patient in order to collect a large set of data samples for the reconstruction process. This is referred to as continuously rotating fan beam scanning. The capabilities of this generation scanner included:

Sub-second imaging time
- 0.4 to 10 seconds
  - increases patient throughput and limits the production of artifacts caused by respiratory motion

Detector configuration
- several hundred detectors are incorporated into the curvilinear detector array with an arc of 30- to 40-degrees from the apex of the fan
  - curvilinear detector array results

Constant source-to-detector path length

Advantages
- good image reconstruction
- allows for better x-ray beam collimation
- reduces the effect of scatter radiation
- employs the introduction of gas ionization detectors

Disadvantages
- highly sensitive to detector performance which results in the appearance of ring artifact
- fixed relationship of a detector to specific part of the beam
- any miscalibration or malfunction of an individual detector will appear as a ring in the final reconstructed image
  - software corrected image reconstruction algorithms minimize such artifacts

These scanners offered better scatter suppression and require less detectors than the 4th generation scanners; and for this reason, multislice CT scanners use this type of technology.

Fourth Generation

The fourth generation scanners were developed principally to suppress ring artifacts that the third generation scanners were subjected to. Its scanner geometry consisted of a rotating fan beam within a circular stationary ring of detectors. The principal working of a circular detector array is as follows:

Tube is positioned within a stationary, circular detector array

Beam geometry describes a wide fan

Apex of the fan now originates at each detector

As the tube moves from point to point within the circle, single rays strike a detector

Scan times are short
- 1 to 5 seconds

Image reconstruction algorithm
- used the fan beam geometry

Spiral/Helical Geometry

The spiral/helical geometry was developed in 1989 due to the need for faster scan times and to improve 3D and multi-planar reformations (MPRs). The data acquisition involves:

X-ray tube is in continuous motion while the patient is transported through the gantry aperture
- resulting in volume data
- made possible by slip-ring technology
  - electromechanical device constructed with circular electrical conductive rings and brushes
  - transmit electrical energy across a rotating interface

Single slice scanner
- use the fourth generation geometry

Multislice scanners
- use the third generation geometry
- scanners possessing 16 or more detector rows
  - based on cone beam geometries rather than fan-beam geometries

Fifth Generation

The fifth generation scanners were classified as high-speed CT scanners also known as the Electron Beam CT scanner. They acquired their data by means of an electron gun instead of an x-ray beam. The process of acquiring data for reconstruction is as follows:

Electrons are accelerated, focused, and deflected at a prescribed angle to hit one of the four tungsten targets located beneath the patient to produce an x-ray beam

Detector array consists of two separate rings in a 260-degree arc

Arrangement allows for two to four image slices

Scanner does not have any moveable parts

Scan time
- milliseconds

Application purpose is for cardiovascular scanning

Sixth Generation

The sixth generation scanners are known as dual source CT scanners. These scanners were introduced in 2006 by Siemens Medical in an effort to produce images with:

Increased spatial and temporal resolution
- especially imperative for cardiac imaging

To deal effectively with artifacts created by IV contrast during CT angiography (CTA)

To decrease the rotation time of the x-ray tube and detectors

To eliminate mechanical disruptions

The design concept of the scanner is based on the use of two x-ray tubes coupled to two detector systems

Technical components
- two Data Acquisition Systems (DAS) offset by 90-degrees

- detector A system has a scan field-of-view (SFOV) of 50 cm
- detector B system has an SFOV of 26 cm

Cone beam geometry

Allows dual-energy imaging

- tube A can operate at 80 kVp
- tube B can operate at 140 kVp

Image reconstruction involves

- subtraction method
- eliminate beam hardening streaking artifact
  - caused by the high concentration of IV contrast in the arteries

Physical Principles of Attenuation

Attenuation

Attenuation is the reduction of the intensity of a beam of radiation as it passes through an object. The x-ray photons are either absorbed or scattered. Attenuation depends on the electrons per gram of tissue, the atomic number Z (# of protons), the tissue density (mass/volume), and the energy of the photons. Since attenuation depends on the energy of the photons, it is important to discuss the types of radiation beams.

Homogenous Beam

In a homogenous beam, all the photons have the same energy. This type of beam is also known as a monochromic or monoenergetic beam. The homogeneous beams like the gamma rays that Hounsfield used for his first CT device satisfied the requirements of the Lambert–Beer law for image reconstruction. This law defines what happens to the photons as they travel through tissues according to the following attenuation equation:

$$I = I_0 e^{-\mu x}$$

I = transmitted intensity
I_o = original intensity
e = natural logarithm
$-\mu$ = attenuation coefficient
x = thickness of the object

The complete goal of CT is to find the values of μ for each voxel in the patient. The unit μ is denoted in inverse length (cm^{-1}), hence the term "linear" attenuation coefficient. If I_0, I, and x are known or can be measured in CT, then the linear attenuation coefficient μ can be calculated.

Heterogeneous Beam

CT utilizes an x-ray beam, which is heterogeneous, as an x-ray beam passes through an absorber, the quantity (number of photons) is reduced by absorber (tissue).

Equal thickness of absorber now reduces a smaller percentage of photons as photons pass through absorber, causing the quality (mean energy) of the photons to be altered by the absorber (tissue). The lower energy photons are absorbed, causing the mean photon energy to increase, thus increasing the penetrating power of the beam. This phenomenon is termed as "beam hardening." As stated earlier, a homogeneous beam satisfies the Lambert–Beer law to calculate the linear attenuation coefficient, but CT utilizes a heterogeneous beam; therefore, it is necessary to make the heterogeneous beam approximate a homogeneous beam to satisfy the equation. X-ray beams can be attenuated due to absorption (photoelectric effect) and scattering (Compton Effect); hence, the total attenuation can then be calculated by the following equation:

$$I = I_0 e^{-\left(\mu_p + \mu_c\right)}$$

In this calculation, μ_p represents the linear attenuation from the photoelectric absorption, while μ_c represents the linear coefficient resulting from the Compton Effect.

CT SYSTEM PRINCIPLES, OPERATIONS, AND COMPONENTS

X-Ray Tube

Modern CT x-ray scanner having continuous rotation must be able to sustain higher power levels. The new technical component design of these scanners is made to deal with the problem of heat generation, heat storage, and heat dissipation. The x-ray tubes now are encased in a metal envelop instead of the glass envelop, which solves the problem of electrical arcing resulting from tungsten deposits caused by vaporization. The tube is equipped with ceramic insulators in order to isolate the metal envelope from the anode and cathode voltage.

Anode

The anode is the positive terminal and part of the tube where the target material is located. The spiral/helical scanners employ a 200 mm diameter rotating anode disk allowing for the use of higher tube currents in the range of 120 to 140 kVp. The heat storage capacity with these disks is increased with an improvement in heat dissipation. The assembly of the anode entails the disk, rotor stud, and hub, rotor, and bearing assembly. This disk is thicker than conventional disks. The three basic disk designs are as follows:

Conventional All-Metal Disk
- base body made of titanium, zirconium, and molybdenum

- focal track layer consists of 10% rhenium and 90% tungsten
  - transfers heat from the focal track very rapidly
- limitations
  - cannot meet the needs of spiral/helical CT imaging due to its weight

Brazed Graphite Disk

- consists of a tungsten–rhenium focal track brazed to a graphite base body
- graphite increases the heat storage capacity
  - high thermal capacity, $10\times$ greater than tungsten
- material used in the brazing process
  - influences the operating temperature of the tube
  - higher temperatures result in higher heat storage capacity
  - faster cooling of the anode
- these attributes contribute to the use of this disk in spiral/helical CT scanners

CVD Graphite Disk

- graphite base body with a tungsten–rhenium layer deposited on the focal track
  - CVD—chemical vapor deposition
- accompanies large, lightweight disks with large heat storage capacity and fast cooling
- suitable for spiral/helical CT scanners

Cathode

The cathode is the negative terminal and part of the tube where the negatively charged electrons flow into the tube from the high-voltage generator. The cathode construction consists of one or two filaments, each of a different length, and placed in a focusing cup. The focusing cup forces the electrons to form a small stream as they move toward the target material. The dual filaments sizes are 0.5 mm and 1.2 mm in CT scanners. Smaller focal spots produce thinner slice with high spatial resolution.

Scanning Parameters

Tube current (mA)

- determines the number of x-ray photons produced (quantity)
- greater the mA more the photons are produced

Tube voltage (kV)

- determines the energy level of x-ray photons produced (quality)
- greater the kV more the penetration

Tube window

- opening is in the tube housing that allows the passage of photons

Warm-up procedure

- performed daily or when scanner has been idle for a period of time

- purpose
  - to warm the filament up
  - which prolongs the life of the tube
    - the warm-up technique is part of each vendor's software package
      - procedure employs the use of a low mA with both the small and large focal spot, low kVp, and a long exposure time
      - then gradually increases until the tube hits maximum heat units
  - this procedure will heat the anode uniformly so that higher subsequent exposures will not damage it

Generator and Transformers

Modern CT scanners use high-frequency generators because they are small, compact, and more efficient than conventional generators. Once high-voltage rectification and smoothing are performed, the voltage ripple is less than 1% making these generators more efficient at x-ray production. Current CT generators can have a maximum power rating of about 50 kilowatts allowing kVp settings in the range of 80 to 140 and tube currents in the range of 100 to 400 mA depending on the vendor. The advantages of utilizing high-frequency generators include: the use of high kVp to minimize the photoelectric absorption which in turn reduces radiation dose, reduces bean attenuation relative to soft tissue permitting a wider dynamic range of the image, and finally it increases the intensity of the photons at the detector array in turn reducing tube loading. These compact generators are located inside the CT gantry. Some CT manufacturers mount them on the rotating frame with the x-ray tube and are considered a low-voltage slip-ring design. In this design, the AC power and control signals are transmitted to the slip-rings via low-voltage brushes, the slip-ring then provides power to the high voltage transformer which provides high voltage to the tube and detectors. Other vendors place the high frequency generators in the corner of the gantry; therefore, they do not rotate with the tube and are termed high-voltage slip-ring design. In this type of system, AC is distributed to the high-frequency generator, then it transmits the high voltage to the slip ring. The slip-ring in turn transfers the high voltage to the x-ray tube and detectors.

Detector Characteristics

The purpose of detectors is to capture the radiation beam from the patient and convert it into electrical signals; thus converting this information into binary coded information. Each detector must exhibit several characteristics to produce good quality CT images. One of the most important features is the detectors efficiency. Its efficiency can be defined as its ability to capture, absorb, and convert x-ray photons to electrical signals and can be broken down into two categories, capture and absorption efficiency. Capture efficiency is described as the effectiveness with which the detectors can obtain photons transmitted from the patient, the size of the detector area facing the beam, and the distance between two detectors. Absorption efficiency is referred to the number of photons absorbed by the detector, which is dependent on atomic number, physical density, size, and thickness of the detector face. Since the goal of CT is to calculate the linear attenuation coefficient the geometric efficiency of the detectors is imperative. Another attribute the detector must exhibit is stability. Stability refers to the steadiness of the detectors' response. Instability causes a signal not to be useful. This can occur when a detector falls out of alignment. This happened somewhat frequently with third generation scanners causing ring artifacts. Corrective measures such as frequent calibrations would correct the problem. When performing spiral/helical scanning the response time of the detector is imperative. Response time indicates the speed with which the detector can detect the x-ray event and then recover to detect another event. Response time should be short (100 milliseconds) to avoid problems such as afterglow (energy emitted after removal of a source of energy) or detector "pile-up" (photons arriving at the detector within a time-interval shorter than the time after the arrival of a photon, during which the system is busy). Another property of the detector is its dynamic range. This is the ratio of the largest signal to be measured to the precision of the smallest signal to be discriminated. In other words it can be described as the range of voltage or input signals that results in a digital output. The dynamic range for many modern CT scanners today is a million to one.

Detector Types

The conversion of x-rays to electrical energy depends on two fundamental types: scintillation and gas ionization detectors. Scintillation detectors convert x-ray energy into light, and then the light is converted into electrical energy by means of crystal plates coupled to a solid-state photodiode semiconductor. Photodiode is a semiconductor whose p–n junction allows current flow when exposed to light. The light produced from the crystal is directly proportional to the amount of current. The gas ionization detectors convert x-ray energy directly into electrical energy. These detectors are based on the principle of ionization and are configured in a series of individual gas chambers separated by tungsten plates. The gas employed in these detectors was xenon due to its relative lightness. As a photon enters the channel it ionizes the gas. The ions produced are accelerated and amplified by the electric field between the plates. The collected charge produces an electric current and this current is processed as raw data. These detectors were introduced in the third generation CT scanners, but are obsolete due to their low quantum detector efficiency (QDE). QDE is a measure of the percentage (%) of x-rays that hit the detector and are absorbed. It is a way of measuring the system's ability to produce images with high signal-to-noise ratios (SNR) relative to the detector. It is especially useful for the measurement of radiation dose efficiency of a detector. It is safe to say as the QDE increases, radiation dose and its biological effects decrease. All modern CT scanners are based on the third generation geometry, but utilize the solid-state detector array systems.

Detector Configuration

Detector configuration is defined as the number of data collection channels and the effective section thickness determined by the data acquisition system settings. Multi-detector or multi-slice CT detectors can be configured in several ways by combining various detector elements electronically (binning) to produce the desired slice thickness required for the examination at the isocenter. Multi-detector computed tomography (MDCT) z-axis resolution can be preserved or even improved in multiple-row detector designs (Fig. 3.1). MDCT configurations improve spatial resolution and decrease partial volume averaging. The detector aperture size (d) and the x-ray beam collimation (D) have the following relationship:

$$d(\text{mm}) = D(\text{mm}) \div N$$

where N = number of detector rows.

This equation can be further explained by: if the beam collimation is 20 mm and the scanner has a 4 row detector array the detector aperture size is 5 mm:

$$d(\text{mm}) = 20 \text{ mm} \div 4$$

d (mm) or aperture size equals 5 mm.

The goal of MDCT is to improve the volume coverage and speed performance. This technology opened new opportunities to improve the quality of care for patients by offering a new range of clinical applications. The dual-slice spiral CT scanner was introduced in 1991 by Elscint with technological improvements with detector configurations as high as 320 detector row systems manufactured by Toshiba today.

Detector Array

The detector row configuration depends on the manufacturer's preference. High geometric efficiency is a require-

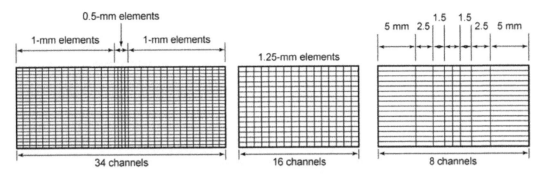

Figure 3.1. Different detector row designs, diagram on the left showing the hybrid design with narrow elements in the center and wider towards the outer rows, middle diagram depicts the matrix array with all detectors being the same size, while the diagram on the right demonstrates the nonuniform detector array system. (Reproduced, with permission, from Seeram E. *Computed Tomography: Physical Principles, Clinical Applications, and Quality Control*. 3rd ed. St. Louis, MO: Saunders Elsevier; 2009).

ment for detectors in MDCT. Geometric efficiency is determined by the amount of radiation that actually hits the detector elements relative to the amount of radiation that leaves the patient. This efficiency mainly depends on the detector width, the spatial orientation, and the absorption of the septa (collimator) that separates each single detector (Fig. 3.1). MDCT detectors fall into the following categories:

Matrix or Uniform Array
- several solid state small detectors of the same dimension are arranged in rows of identical thickness
- image acquired depends on the beam width, selection of detector rows, and how the two are coupled

Adaptive, Variable, or Nonuniform Array
- detector width gradually increases in thickness as it moves away from the center of axis rotation
- two detector rows in the center of the array are 1 mm each
- detectors adjacent to the central rows are of increasing thickness, with the outmost detector row of 5 mm thick

Hybrid Element Array
- incorporated the features of uniform and nonuniform design
- detector array is composed of thin detectors at the center and thick detectors on either side of the central detectors

Data Acquisition System (DAS)

The data acquisition system is a group of detector electronics positioned between the detector array and the computer. Its main functions are to measure the transmitted radiation beam, encode these measurements into binary data, and finally to transmit the binary data to the computer (Fig.3.2). Each detector's photodiode measures the transmitted beam from the patient and converts it into electrical energy.

The energy is proportional to the light striking the diode. At this point, the electrical energy is so weak that it must be amplified by the preamplifier before it can be analyzed further. The transmission measurement data must then be transformed into attenuation and thickness data through a process known as the logarithmic conversion. Following the conversion, the data are sent to the analog-digital-converter (ADC). The purpose of the ADC is to divide the

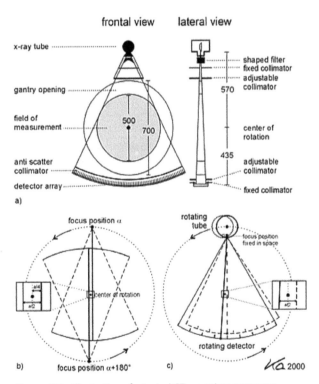

Figure 3.2. Illustration of a typical CT scanning geometry. (Reproduced, with permission, from Kalendar WA. *Computed Tomography: Fundamentals System Technology, Image Quality, and Applications*. 3rd ed. Erlangen, Germany: Publicis; 2011).

electrical signal into multiple parts; the more divisional parts the greater the accuracy. The parts are measured into bits, 1-bit divides the signal into two digital values. The ADC's dynamic range must be large to preserve the large dynamic range of the x-ray image. Converters with 16-bit resolution or greater are common in CT. These values determine the gray-scale resolution of the image. The final stage of DAS is transmission of the data to the computer. The output of the ADC data is routed to an image signal processor over high-speed optoelectronics by the use of lens and light diodes to facilitate data transmission for further signal processing and image reconstruction.

Steps of Data Acquisition

1. X-rays are produced
2. Detector measures the transmitted intensity
3. Intensities are amplified to increase their strength
4. Logarithmic amplifier converts the transmission measurements into attenuation and thickness data
5. Data are sent to the ADC to convert the analog information into discrete numbers (binary)
6. Digital data are transferred to the computer by means of optoelectronics

Data Acquisition and Sampling

As discussed above, the detectors need to possess certain characteristics in order to capture, absorb, and convert a transmitted intensity into a diagnostic image. This is only part of the process, having the ability to acquire enough samples on each detector is the next challenge. As the x-ray beam hits the patient, a certain number of photons pass directly through the patient to fall on the detectors. The detectors in turn, measure or samples the intensity of the photons hitting them. If not enough samples (photons) are obtained, an artifact can appear on the reconstructed image. This artifact is known as aliasing, which causes streaking; therefore, specific structures and spaces cannot be distinguished. To rectify the problem there needs to be an increase in the number of samples available for image reconstruction to improve the quality of the image. This is accomplished through:

Reduction of the slice thickness
- thinner slices aid in the reduction of the aliasing artifact related to under sampling

Closely packed detectors
- allow for more detectors available for data acquisition
  - ensure more samples per view
  - increase the total measurements taken

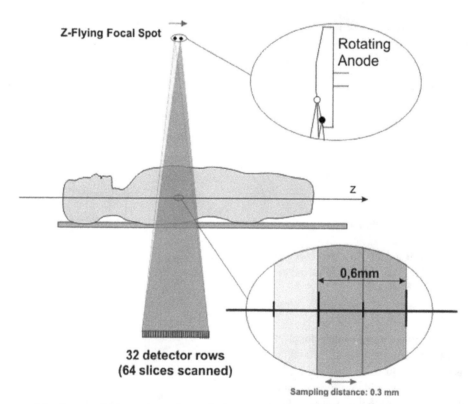

Figure 3.3. Diagram of the data acquisition and sampling in the z-direction utilizing the z-Sharp Technology. This technology doubles the efficiency of the sampling rate resulting in improved spatial resolution (Reproduced, with permission, from Kalendar WA. *Computed Tomography: Fundamentals System Technology, Image Quality, and Applications.* 3rd ed. Erlangen, Germany: Publicis; 2011).

Quarter shift detector
- older theory
- detectors are offset by a quarter detector
- central ray is offset by quarter of the sampling distance from the center of rotation
  - ray will again be shifted by a quarter in the opposite direction after 180-degrees
  - two measurements with the same ray are taken in opposite direction
    - sampling frequency is increased by a factor of two
      - this increases spatial resolution

Z-Sharp Technology (Fig. 3.3)
- Designed by Siemens Medical Solutions
- Z-flying focal spot
- magnetic field shapes and controls the beam within the tube
  - allows switching focus positions both in the fan and in the z-direction to provide overlapping sampling
- within microseconds double samples are obtained for each detector row at the same time per 360-degree rotation

Collimation/Beam Width

The purpose of collimation is to protect the patient by restricting the beam to the anatomy of interest. They are arranged to ensure a constant beam width at the detectors. Collimators affect patient dose and image quality by removing the scatter radiation, which improves axial resolution. CT scanner possesses two sets of collimators: prepatient collimation (at the x-ray tube) and postpatient (at the detectors).

Prepatient Collimation

The prepatient collimation is found between the x-ray tube and the patient, in order to define the dose profile according to the slice thickness. Collimation first begins at the tube housing, which provides a rough aperture dimension of the fan or cone beam. Within the gantry, there are two sets of collimators. The fixed collimator defines the maximum permissible beam and ensures proper alignment of the beam to hit the detector aperture. It is important to remember, as the number of detector rows increases, the x-ray beam becomes a cone and the detectors are angled to the center of rotation. The adjustable collimator, found as close to the gantry as possible, allows variable collimation for the desired total beam collimation and minimizes the amount of penumbra caused by the focal spot size.

Postpatient Collimation

The postpatient collimators are a fixed set located between each detector. The purpose of this collimation is to define slice thickness and minimize signal contribution from scatter radiation. This unnecessary signal input is called cross-talk. As CT vendors increased their detector rows greater than 64, scatter reduction became more imperative, since scatter radiation increases for large cone angles. Anti-scatter grids (ASG) were developed to rectify the scatter issue. These grids are placed in front of the detectors arranged in a 1D or 2D format system of thin lamellae made of strongly absorbing material.

Beam Width

Collimators close to the x-ray source determine the total x-ray beam width. Beam collimation width can be calculated by the produce of the number of detector rows and the detector aperture size. If a particular scanner utilized 16 detector rows with detector aperture of 1.2 mm, the total beam collimation would be expressed as 19.2 mm.

total beam collimation = number of rows × aperture size
total beam collimation = 16 × 1.2 mm
total beam collimation = 19.2 mm

Detector aperture size can also be calculated when the beam collimation and the number of detector rows are known. If the total beam collimation for a CT examination is 28.8 mm with 24 active detectors, the detector row collimation would be 1.2 mm.

detector aperture size = total beam collimation ÷ number of active detectors
detector row collimation = 28.8 mm ÷ 24
detector row collimation = 1.2 mm

The number of detector rows can also be calculated when the total beam width and the aperture detector size are known by the following equation:

number of detector rows = total beam collimation ÷ detector aperturesize

The total beam collimation for a CT examination chest is 20 mm with the detector aperture size of 0.5 mm, what is the number of active detector rows?

number of detector rows = 20 mm ÷ 0.5
number of detector rows = 40

Computer

The computer classification used in CT is a minicomputer-midrange. It is a multi-level computer with the ability to perform complex computations. The midrange computer deals efficiently with the convoluted mathematical input and produces output data at subsecond time intervals. These computers have networking capability that is connected to various terminals. The digital data processed by the computer can be sent to other scanners, picture archiving and communication systems (PACS), postprocessing workstation, CD burners, and laser printers. The important characteristics of the CT computer system are its large storage capacity and fast and efficient processing of various kinds of data.

Array Processor

An array processor is an extension of the computer's arithmetic logic unit capable of performing simultaneous computations or matrices of numbers. CT architectures were developed to accommodate fast image reconstruction and other image processing functions, such as image manipulations, networking data to other systems, and archiving image data. There are three types of processing architectures in CT, distributed processing, parallel processing, and pipelining processing.

Distributed processing
- information is processed by more than one computer connected by network system
- true distributed processing involves
  - separate computer for each task
  - combined work can contribute to larger goal

Parallel processing
- information is processed on one computer containing two or more CPUs
- tasks are distributed over available processors

Pipeline processing
- information is processed so that the output of one element is the input of the next one
- similar to an assembly line
- specialized in a particular type of operation
- process speeds execution time
  - this microprocessor does not wait for instructions

IMAGING PROCESSING

Reconstruction

The linear attenuation coefficients are given in projection values, termed the Radon transform; therefore, an inverse transformation needs to be carried out to determine these values in order to produce an image. The simplest form of reconstruction was the algebraic method of reconstruction performed by Hounsfield. This method used a linear system of equations to solve a problem. The mathematical steps were sequential since the first image matrices were 80×80, only 6,400 calculations needed to be performed. It took hours to perform these calculations, but an image

was produced revolutionizing the world of radiology. As technology increased in the computer world, new reconstruction methods were tried and improved. The three major CT reconstruction algorithms are back projection, filtered back project, and iterative.

Back Projection

Back projection, also known as summation method or linear superimposition method, is a simple procedure that does not require much understanding of mathematics. The process is performed in the spatial location domain by converting the data from the attenuation profile to a matrix. Let us take for instance one data point within the scanned object utilizing only four projections; the attenuation coefficient for each projection is determined by averaging the attenuation values for all projections that cross the data point, producing four interesting lines. This causes a major problem in clinical CT examinations because points outside the high density object receive some of the back projected intensity of the object resulting in an unsharp image. The type of artifact associated with back projection is known as the star pattern.

Filtered Back Projection

Filtered back projection is a type of reconstruction method known as the convolution method and was developed in order to eliminate the star pattern typical of the back projection method. This analytic method uses the Fourier transform to convert a signal in the spatial location domain to a signal in the spatial frequency domain. Once the waveform is divided into a series of sine and cosine functions of different frequencies and amplitudes, a mathematical filtering or convolution process is applied. The first advantage of the data being in the frequency domain is that it can be manipulated by changing the amplitudes of the frequency components in determining the properties of the reconstructed image in terms of spatial resolution and image noise. These convolution kernels vary from a soft or smooth image to an edge enhanced image. The other advantage is the frequency information can be used to measure image quality.

Reconstruction Algorithms/Convolution Filtering

High pass filtering
- algorithm that is intended to sharpen small objects in an image
- suppresses the low spatial frequencies in the image
- improves its overall detail
- practical applications
  - heads/skull fractures
  - extremities
  - spine
  - lung parenchyma

Low pass filtering
- process to smooth an image
- suppresses the high frequencies in the image
- smoothing is intended to reduce noise
  - which compromised image detail
- practical application
  - brain
  - volume 3D imaging
  - spine
  - extremities

Unsharp masking
- compromising algorithm
- processed low pass filtering algorithm is subtracted from the original raw data
  - produces an enhanced soft tissue image
- practical application
  - soft tissue structures
    - abdomen
    - mediastinum
    - muscle

Steps of CT Reconstruction

The progress of data from acquisition to image display

1. scan or measurement data
2. preprocessing
3. raw data
4. convolution filtering
5. filtered raw data
6. back projection
7. image data

Iterative Reconstruction

The iterative reconstruction method takes the attenuation coefficient intensities and projects them back onto the matrix with the assumption that all the intensities have the same value. This technique involves a series of corrections applied to the data to bring it into better agreement with the measured projections and then new corrections are applied until a satisfactory agreement is obtained. This algorithm was employed in the early development of CT, but was discontinued because it was difficult to get accurate ray sums because of quantum noise and patient motion, computer processing time, and to obtain an exact image, there needed to be more data sets then pixels. As computers became more sophisticated, iterative reconstruction algorithms were again introduced in the early 2000s. The purpose of using this process today is dose reduction. Individual manufacturers have their own noise reduction technique, such as ASIR (GE healthcare), IRIS, SAFIRE (Siemens), AIDR (Toshiba), and iDose (Phillips Healthcare), but they are all based on either the adaptive statistical iterative reconstruction or the

models photons and electric noise in the CT system Adaptive Statistical Iterative Reconstruction (ASIR).

Adaptive statistical iterative reconstruction is occasionally known as a hybrid IR algorithm because of its ability to blend with filtered back projection (FBP). The premise of this algorithm is to generate simulated data sets from estimation; then these estimated raw data sets are compared with the real measured data from the imaging system, followed by the comparison of the two data sets being projected back to the estimation step for future correction. This entire cycle continues until the difference between the estimated and measured data is within an acceptable range. The ASIR technique models photons and electric noise in the CT system.

Modeled Based Iterative Reconstruction

Modeled based iterative reconstruction has been shown to significantly improve image quality while reducing noise and artifacts in multislice CT scans in the initial research. This algorithm involves creating an accurate system model, a statistical noise model, and a prior model. The system model deals with the nature of the x-ray beam. The statistical noise model takes into account the size of an x-ray tube's focal spot and the 3D shape of detectors. The prior model is a regularization algorithm that corrects impractical conditions that could occur during reconstruction to speed up the process.

The advantage of both models is the reduction of image noise; thereby, allowing for the use of lower mAs. Using a low-dose protocol, a dose reduction of approximately 50% to 75% has been noted with improved low-contrast detectability.

Interpolation

With the introduction of spiral/helical CT scanning, additional algorithms were developed since different objects sections are measured at the start and end of any such segment. These data sets caused inconsistencies for image reconstruction due to translating the patient through the gantry, resulting in motion artifacts. The new preprocessing step is known as z-interpolation. The basic principle of z-interpolation is to estimate an unknown value of a function from two or more known values of the function about the location of the unknown value. The simplest approach to z-interpolation is linear interpolation between data measures for a given spiral position before and after the desired table position. The two types of z-interpolation used are 360- and 180-degree linear interpolation.

360-Degree Linear Interpolation

The 360-degree linear interpolation was most commonly used in the early days of spiral/helical CT. At every angular position of a 360-degree rotation, the planar slice is interpolated between two projection points in the data set that are closest to the chosen position along the z-axis. This interpolation generates 720-degrees of data resulting in a complete set of projections from the chosen z-position. The disadvantage of this method is that it degrades image quality by broadening the slice sensitivity profile, but provides the least image noise.

180-Degree Linear Interpolation

More advanced z-interpolations algorithms were developed due to the fact that x-ray attenuations are independent of direction. In other words, a ray between the tube and detectors is equal in both directions. This made it possible to compute a second spiral for the attenuation values along the ray between the tube and detectors in the opposite direction. By having both the projected spiral data and the virtual spiral data the planar slice is calculated from the 360-degree data set plus the fan angle of the x-ray beam. This algorithm became known as 180-degree linear interpolation (Fig. 3.4). This technique substantially narrowed the slice sensitivity profile because the distance between corresponding projections in the real and virtual spirals is less than between the corresponding projections in the real spiral alone. The data set generated by the virtual spiral is termed complementary data. The major advantages of 180-degree z-interpolation include: improved z-axis resolution, the generation of

thinner slices, and scanning at higher pitches. 180-degree z-linear interpolation results in higher noise than both conventional and 360-degree linear z-interpolation.

Types of Data

Measurement Data

Measurement data also known as scan data are the transmitted intensities hitting the detectors. This data undergo preprocessing to correct any errors that may have resulted from beam hardening, bad detectors, or scatter radiation. These corrections are made before the image reconstructed algorithm is applied.

Raw Data

Raw data are unprocessed computer data in the form of binary number. Once measurement data are preprocessed to correct for possible errors, they are sent to the ADC to convert the analog signal to discrete digital numbers where it becomes raw data. A protocol specific reconstruction algorithm is applied to the raw data to improve its quality. This data are processed immediately (known as prospective reconstruction) or can be stored in files in the image reconstruction system (IRS) for further use.

Image Data

Image data are the result of raw data being convoluted and processed by the computer. Once this process is completed

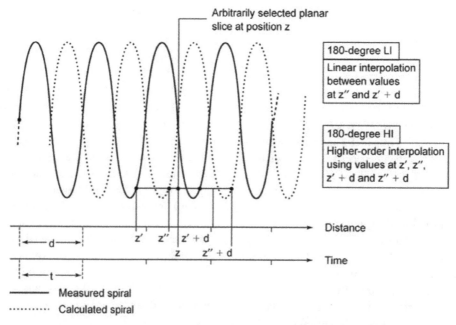

Figure 3.4. Illustration of how the 180° linear interpolation is used for image reconstruction. Note the data points are taken from the 180° with the complimentary data points used during the reconstruction process; therefore, two sets of images are generated, the spiral set and the virtual set. (Reproduced, with permission, from Seeram E, *Computed Tomography: Physical Principles, Clinical Applications, and Quality Control*. 3rd ed. St. Louis, MO: Saunders Elsevier; 2009).

a visible digital image appears on the scanner console. The only operation that can be performed on this data is reformation in the form of multiplanar or 3D manipulations. Image data can be copied to a CD and reviewed by means of a digital imaging and communication in medicine (DICOM) viewer or can be sent to a laser printer for hard copy viewing.

Prospective/Retrospective Reconstruction

Prospective Reconstruction

The image that is automatically reconstructed from the scan data is considered prospective data. Once the measurement data are corrected, they are sent to the ADC for digitization and raw data are produced when the convolution kernel is applied. The results of back projection to form a visible image viewed on the monitor can then be termed prospective reconstruction.

Retrospective Reconstruction

Retrospective reconstruction is the image reconstructed that occurs from the request of the technologist using raw data. As stated earlier, raw data are stored in the IRS and can be reprocessed to generate an entirely new set of images. Different slice thicknesses, slice increments, and convolution kernels can be changed to produce a new set of images. Retrospective reconstruction can only occur if the raw data are available.

Reconstruction Interval

Reconstruction interval or increment is the spacing between two adjacent slices. A contiguous interval is the one in which the thickness of the slice and the spacing between two slices are equal. When the reconstruction interval is half the thickness of the slice thickness, it is considered an overlapping interval. This type of interval is utilized to improve image quality. The last interval to discuss is gapping. A gapping interval occurs when there is considerable spacing between each slice. High-resolution CT chest images are an example of gapping when the slice thickness is 1 mm and the spacing between slices is 10 mm or greater.

POSTPROCESSING

Due to the nature of the CT scanner's geometry, scanning parameters are basically limited to transaxial imaging, except for direct coronals of the head or coronal and sagittal orientations of the extremities. The principle of postprocessing is to modify the reconstructed image data through the use of specialized software algorithms to create a desired image that is physically impossible or impractical to acquire or does not exist in a physical form

at all. The postprocessing techniques employed in CT are MPR, 3D techniques, and virtual reality techniques. It is important to remember that the postprocessing makes use of image reconstructed data as opposed to raw data.

Multi-Planar Reformation

MPR software reformats two-dimensional images at arbitrary planes defined by the operator, using the pixel data from a stack of transaxial images. Each pixel in the 512^2 matrix when used in conjunction with the slice thickness forms a voxel or volume of data representing the digital values of the scanned object. The MPR software extracts only those voxels from the data volume positioned one above the other with in the coronal or sagittal plane. An oblique or curved reformat is constructed in a similar way, but the image data need to be interpolated among adjacent voxels. When the size of the pixel and the slice thickness are equal, the reformatted image it is said to be isotropic, as opposed to an anisotropic reformatted image in which the pixel size and the slice thickness differ. Isotropic data produce the best image reformations, since very little data are lost during the postprocessing manipulations. It is important to remember that the image quality of the reformatted image is only as good as the image quality of the transaxial imaging. MPRs are a useful technique to follow pathological structures through multiple planes and when conditions require a second plane for diagnostic interpretation, as in the case or orbital imaging. Coronal reformats define the plane that passes through the body region from anterior to posterior, dividing the region into anterior and posterior sections. The clinical application for the use of coronal images may be in the evaluation of tumors of the liver, kidneys, or lower abdominal organs because coronals visualize specific structures in relationship to surrounding structures. The plane that passes through an anatomic region from left to right dividing the body into right and left sections is termed the sagittal reformat. Sagittal reformats are regularly used for extremity examinations to determine the extent of fractures and/or dislocations, bony fragments, or foreign bodies. These reformats are always performed in spinal examination to assess the spinal cord looking for fractures, misaligned spinal curves (kyphotic or lordoic), or bony fragments pressing on the spinal cord. For curved-planar reformats the operator defines the reformatted image on multiple reference images due to the fact that the structures of interest may leave and enter the reference image continually. This form of reformatted image is employed in CT angiography (CTA) and CT urography to straighten a blood vessel or ureter in the investigation of stenosis or blockage and to explore the pancreatic and bile duct.

3D Rendering (MIP, SSD, VR)

Three-dimensional rendering in CT is a process of generating an image from a 3D model (the patient) by means of computer processing and displaying it on the 2D computer screen. Computer graphics has played an integral role in the development and refinement of 3D imaging. This advanced visualization tool requires a hardware or software based approach to generate the images. The hardware based method uses stand-alone workstations to execute specialized algorithms, while the software based method utilized software coded algorithms to create the 3D images. The basic 3D rendering techniques are maximum intensity projection (MIP), minimum intensity projection (MinP), shaded surface display (SSD), and volume rendering (VR).

Maximum Intensity Projection

MIP is the simplest of the 3D rendering techniques, since it does not require high-tech computer hardware. This technique makes use of less than 10% of the data in the 3D volume. The images are generated by dividing the entire volume of interest into multiple thinner slabs and choosing a specific slice thickness for the resulting images (Fig. 3.5). The actual images are then reformatted displaying the maximum CT numbers. The clinical application of MIP is mainly used in CT angiography. CT angiography requires precise contrast enhanced vessels, otherwise the true extent of the artery may be excluded. Thin-slab MIP images can be pertinent in assessing pulmonary lesions and diffuse lung diseases. Superimposition is one of the main drawbacks of MIP imaging, since only the maximum Hounsfield unit (HU) is used in the image display. Another problem that can arise from this technique are image artifacts due to pulsating vessels and respiratory motion.

Minimum Intensity Projection

The process of generating MinP is similar to the maximum intensity technique except this technique makes use of only the minimum or lowest attenuation values to display the images. MinP is an essential tool in the evaluation of central tracheobronchial system, parenchymal density (in particular obstructive pulmonary disease and emphysema), and the intrahepatic bile ducts and the pancreatic duct. MinP is extremely limited in the detection of tumor associated changes.

Shaded Surface Display (SSD)

The principle behind Shaded Surface Display (SSD) is to realistically produce a 3D scene of the surface of a structure of interest from the acquired data set (Fig. 3.6). This

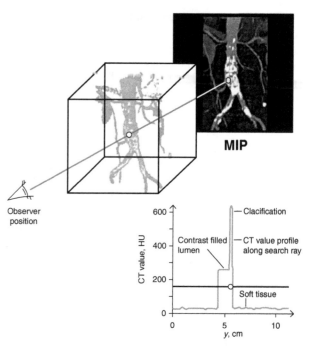

Figure 3.5. The illustration shows how the maximum intensity projection images are derived. The computer picks up all the intensities with an HU higher than the threshold projecting them to appear hyperdense and coming forward, while the lesser HU are projected back. As the image displays, the images are of high contrast. (Reproduced, with permission, from Kalendar WA. *Computed Tomography: Fundamentals System Technology, Image Quality, and Applications.* 3rd ed. Erlangen, Germany: Publicis; 2011).

process uses a segmentation technique that separates the object of interest from the background. The simplest way of generating these images is to define the object (skull, mandible, or an abdominal organ) and defining the range whose CT voxel attenuation threshold values do not exceed the threshold value of the volume of interest. Light illumination is the key element in this processing technique. Most hardware or software algorithms permit one virtual light source and vary the position of the source to display the details of the object. SSD is mainly used for the presence of findings as in the case of skeletal studies, since it can be rotated and viewed at any angle, but is rarely used for the diagnosis of complex anatomic or pathological situations. SSD is used less often today, but is well suited for interactive navigation through virtual endoscopy data sets.

Volume Rendering Technique (VRT)

Volume rendering, in the sense of the term, utilizes 100% of the volume data set making it a complex versatile procedure that produces images of higher image quality and

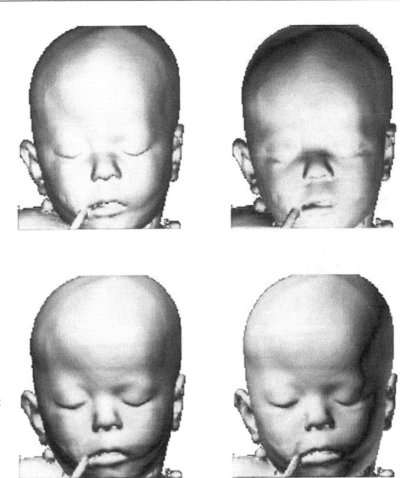

Figure 3.6. Image showing the effects of lighting on a surface rendered display image. Note the SSD image portrays contour and as the light shifts to different regions of the image, unique features of the reconstructed image appear. (Reproduced, with permission, from Seeram E, *Computed Tomography: Physical Principles, Clinical Applications, and Quality Control.* 3rd ed. St. Louis, MO: Saunders Elsevier; 2009).

provides more information than SSD or MIP techniques, because the entire data volume set is projected; therefore, it does not lose pertinent information (Fig. 3.7). Similar to SSD, VRT obtains its voxel data through a segmentation process by assigning different brightness levels or colors to the volume of interest. Opacity values (in range from 0% to 100%) are continuous and assigned to different tissues that make the 3D image. The three tissue types used for voxel classification are fat, soft tissue, and bone. Once segmentation or classification, another termed used for segmentation, has been established the rendering then takes place. The most common method of image projection is ray tracing. This process involves a mathematical ray that is sent from the observer's eye by means of the computer to pass through the actual 3D volume. The pixel intensities on the visual image are the average of all the intensities along the single ray for the entire volume of interest. This process is repeated for the entire 512^2 matrix. The major advantage of VRT is the elimination of superimposition of structures giving the viewer the opportunity

to observe both external and internal structures. Image noise may be a drawback causing irregularities of the object surfaces. Although MIPs are performed in CTA examinations, VRT is becoming the new standard for the display of the pulmonary vessels and the abdominal vessels in many institutions. The color coded VRT allows the radiologists to view the vessel lumen and calcified plaques in separate colors due to their attenuation values. It is also performed in skeletal fractures to demonstrate the position of fracture fragments as well as tendons, muscles, and the assessment of skin contours. VRT is superior to SSD due to the fact that it is less susceptible to partial volume effects and with pseudo defects in thin bone laminae and osteoporotic patients.

Quantitative Analysis

Calcium Scoring

The coronary artery calcium score is a measurement of the amount of calcium on the walls of the arteries that supply the heart muscle. The amount of hardening within

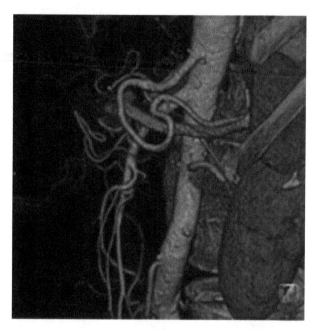

Figure 3.7. CT 3D volume rendered image of the aorta at the celiac axis. A 100% of the data is utilized to generate this image. The image can be rotated 360-degrees in order to delete superimposition. (Reproduced, with permission, from Kalendar WA. *Computed Tomography: Fundamentals System Technology, Image Quality, and Applications.* 3rd ed. Erlangen, Germany: Publicis; 2011).

an arterial wall is a disease termed atherosclerosis. An unenhanced CT scan of the heart is performed and the images are sent to a vendor specific workstation to calculate the Agatston score. This score is used to express the amount of calcium within the coronary arteries based on a slice by slice analysis. Once the images are loaded onto the workstation, a region-of-interest (ROI) is placed around a group of plaques located in each coronary artery and the program calculates the area on each section and multiplies it by a weighted factor depending on the maximum pixel number in the ROI. The sum of the individual scores generates the total calcium score. Calcifications are an early sign of coronary heart disease (CHD); therefore, a calcium score CT scan has the ability to show whether a patient is at risk for a heart attack or other heart problems before other signs and symptoms occur. The higher the Agatston score the more plaque present in the arteries and the greater the heart risk. If the score is more than 400, there is an increased likelihood of developing symptomatic heart disease (angina, heart attack, or even sudden death) in the next two to five years. If the score is more than 1,000, there is a 25% chance of having a heart attack within a year without medical intervention.

Ejection Fraction

With each heartbeat, the ventricles contract forcing blood out of their chambers, while during relaxation the ventricles refill with blood and the cycle continues usually 60 times per minute. With contraction, no matter how forceful, not all the blood leaves the ventricle; therefore, the percentage of blood leaving the ventricle is termed the ejection fraction. The ejection fraction is usually measured in the left ventricle, since it is the main pumping chamber of the heart. A cardiac CT angiogram is one method in which the ejection fraction is analyzed. A cardiac angiogram is performed according to the institutions protocol and the images are sent to a vendor specific workstation containing a software program with the ability to perform these measurements. Iodinated contrast media is required to differentiate the blood from the endocardial border. Two volumetric data sets at end diastole and end systole are reconstructed from each scan by means of retrospective electrocardiogram gating. The software package relies on the difference of the left ventricular cavity from the endocardium based on HU measurements. The reconstructed short-axis cine images of the heart are created and traced for ejection fraction calculations. As long as the contrast bolus timing is appropriate, there will be high contrast and spatial resolution resulting in a well-defined endocardial border. The workstation calculates the ejection fraction by measuring the ratio of blood ejected during systole (stroke volume) to blood in the ventricle at the end of diastole (end-diastolic volume). A left ventricle ejection fraction of 55 percent or higher is considered normal.

IMAGE DISPLAY

CT is in the classification of digital imaging processing. The analog intensities present at the detectors are converted by the analog-to-digital converter to become a digital image. The fundamental parameters of a digital image include matrix, pixels, voxels, and bit depth.

Pixel

A pixel is a 2D squared element that makes up the matrix (Fig. 3.8). Another name for a pixel is a picture element representing the tissue characteristic of the object. Each pixel in the CT image is related to the atomic number and mass density of the tissue and is assigned a brightness level for that particular area. When the field-of-view

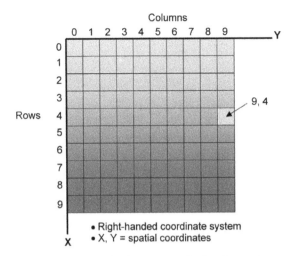

Figure 3.8. An example of a 9 × 9 matrix showing each square pixel. Each pixel is an exact location for an intensity generated by the detector. (Reproduced, with permission, from Seeram E, *Computed Tomography: Physical Principles, Clinical Applications, and Quality Control*. 3rd ed. St. Louis, MO: Saunders Elsevier; 2009).

(FOV) and the matrix size are known, the pixel size can be computed by the following mathematical equation:

$$\text{Pixel size} = \frac{\text{FOV}}{\text{Matrix}}$$

Once the individual pixel size is determined in the x-axis, the pixel area can be calculated by squaring the determined size:

$$\text{Pixel area}^2 = x\text{-axis} \times y\text{-axis}$$

Voxel

A voxel as opposed to a pixel in a digital image is a three-dimensional volume of tissue. A CT section has a fixed thickness; therefore, each pixel in the image matrix signifies a volume of tissue in the scanned z-axis. In most CT examinations, the slice thickness (z-axis) is 10 to 20 times larger than the x–y plane, giving the voxel the appearance of a matchstick. With the development of MDCT, this anisotropic shape can be replaced by isotropic voxels for larger body areas. The mathematical equation to find the voxel dimension is as follows:

$$\text{voxel volume}^3 = \text{pixel area}^2 \times \text{slice thickness}$$

This equation is imperative to remember when isotropic voxels are needed for 3D rendering reformations. In some cases the FOV or slice thickness may needed to be increased or decreased in order to produce these cubed shaped voxels.

Matrix

A matrix in the CT digital imaging world is defined as a two-dimensional array of numbers consisting of rows and columns in a square formation. In the CT scanning parameters, the matrix is always defined as 512. This means there are 512 pixels in the x-axis and 512 pixels in the y-direction. The size of the matrix has a significant relationship to image quality, especially spatial resolution. As the matrix size increases, the number of pixels increases; thus, improving the perception of details in the image. The matrix and the pixel size have the following relationship:

$$\text{Matrix} = \frac{\text{FOV}}{\text{Pixel size}}$$

The matrix size for a CT image is expressed as 512^2 denoting that within the entire matrix there are 262,144 pixels.

Image Magnification

Image magnification is a computer software program integrated into the CT system that allows the user to zoom an image on a computer monitor. In many cases, the purpose of magnifying a particular area of an image on the monitor is for distant and ROI measurements. Image data are used in the magnification process as opposed to raw data when a targeted reconstruction is desired. Image magnification does not change the original image quality of the reconstructed image, but degrades the display resolution.

Field-of-View (Scan vs. Display)

There may or may not be a difference between the SFOV reconstructed from the raw data and the DFOV that is shown on the viewing monitor. The SFOV is the area within the gantry from which the raw data are acquired located at the isocenter of the gantry. The SFOV is chosen by the technologist prior to the commencement of the examination depending on the body of interest. The protocol is chosen with the arc of the fan beam covering only the selected detectors in the x-direction. The allowable SFOVs are vendor specific ranging from 250 mm to usually a maximum of 500 mm. The main advantages of utilizing an SFOV with a narrower fan angle are:

Increased sampling rate
- improves spatial resolution
- used for examinations of the extremities, head, and in some institutions for cardiac imaging

Reduces radiation exposure to portions of the patient outside the SFOV

The DFOV determines how much of the collected raw data are used to create a reconstructed image. DFOVs that are too large make anatomic structures unnecessarily small; on the other hand, DFOVs too small may exclude important patient anatomy. It is important to select the optimal DFOV, since the reconstructed DFOV affects image quality by changing the size of the pixels. The smaller the pixel size the better the spatial resolution, since less ray averaging occurs. It is imperative to select the correct SFOV for the intended body part because the DFOV can be equal to the SFOV, but cannot be larger than the SFOV.

Windowing

Every pixel in the image matrix possesses a specific intensity and this intensity is assigned a gray scale value on the visible reconstructed image. The reconstructed image has a possibility of 4,096 shades of gray per pixel (2^{12}) ranging from $-1,024$ to $+3,072$ units. The human eye can process approximately 40 to 60 shades of gray; therefore, a process known as windowing is applied to visualize objects in the reconstructed image. Windowing is a computer visualization tool by which the image gray scale is manipulated with regard to the CT number of the structure of interest. Windowing contributes to the brightness and contrast of the displayed image. The two main components of windowing include window width and window level.

Window Width

Window width controls the contrast of the image by selecting a specific range of shades of gray from the Hounsfield scale displayed on the CT monitor (Fig. 3.9). The window width is chosen according to the attenuation values inherited in the anatomy of interest. Structures in close proximity to each other having small differences in their atomic numbers require a narrow width. A narrow window, using 80 to 300 shades of gray, increases the images contrast aiding in distinguishing gray matter from white matter in the brain and small density differences within the liver parenchyma. A wide window uses anywhere from 300 to 2,000 shades of gray decreasing image contrast. When the area of interest encompasses multiple attenuation values such as air, water, muscle, soft tissue, and bone within the same image, a window width of 300 to 500 highlights the individual structures. Images of the lung and bone require window widths from 1,000 to 2,000 shades of gray to accentuate the air spaces and bronchioles in the lungs and delineation between cortical bone, trabecular bone, and bone marrow. It is important to understand the effects window width has on image contrast (Fig. 3.10). As stated earlier, when the number of shades of gray decreases, image contrast increases giving the reconstructed image a black and white appearance. On the contrary, image contrast decreases as the width increases, since more shades of gray are available.

Window Level

Window level, center, or length controls the brightness of the image. The level is chosen according to the average attenuation value of the structure of interest and is found in the middle of the range of CT numbers used in the reconstructed image. The lung parenchyma is viewed with a window level from -500 to -800, since air has an attenuation value of $-1,000$. When the area of interest is bone, it is best to place the level at 500 to 800, since the attenuation of bone ranges from 250 to 1,000 HU. To include the attenuation of air, soft tissue, vessels, and bone as in the abdomen and mediastinum, a window level of 0 to 50 will suffice, since it encompasses all of the attenuation values. When the position of the window level changes, as in moving it to a higher

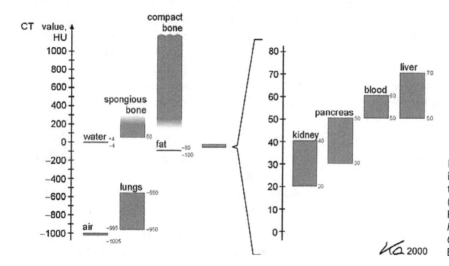

Figure 3.9. The Hounsfield scale showing the different values of different tissue types relative to the constant water. (Reproduced, with permission, from Kalendar WA. *Computed Tomography: Fundamentals System Technology, Image Quality, and Applications.* 3rd ed. Erlangen, Germany: Publicis; 2011).

HU value, the image will have a blacker appearance. The same is true for moving the level to a lower HU value, the image will now give the impression of being whiter (Fig. 3.11).

The combination of window width and window level plays an important role in optimizing the appearance of an image for precise interpretation; thus, the upper and lower limits of the gray scale can be calculated by the follow equations:

$$\text{Upper gray level value} = \text{WL} + \frac{\text{WW}}{2}$$

$$\text{Lower gray level value} = \text{WL} - \frac{\text{WW}}{2}$$

Note: CT numbers above the upper gray level will appear white, while CT numbers below the lower gray level value appear black.

Cine Mode

The development of multi-detectors CT scanning gave radiologist a large quantity of images (several hundred depending on the slice thickness utilized) to view per patient. To record these images, it took technologists an extensive amount of time, especially when multiple windows were needed for interpretation, let alone the cost of producing these films; therefore, approximately only a third of the images were actually documented. This process underutilized the MDCT scanners and in rare cases abnormalities were missed. When PACS workstations were introduced into facilities, radiologists not only had access to all image data, but had the ability to scroll through the images using the cine mode. With this mode, the observer has the capability of viewing images in the axial, coronal, or sagittal planes alone or using a combination of planes. The

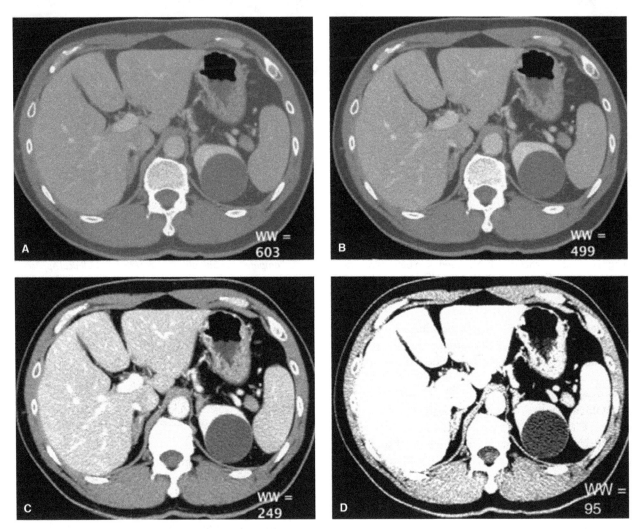

Figure 3.10. CT image of four different window widths with a constant window level. Notice how the image contrast changes as the shades of gray decrease (Reproduced, with permission, from Seeram E. *Computed Tomography: Physical Principles, Clinical Applications, and Quality Control.* 3rd ed. St. Louis, MO: Saunders Elsevier; 2009).

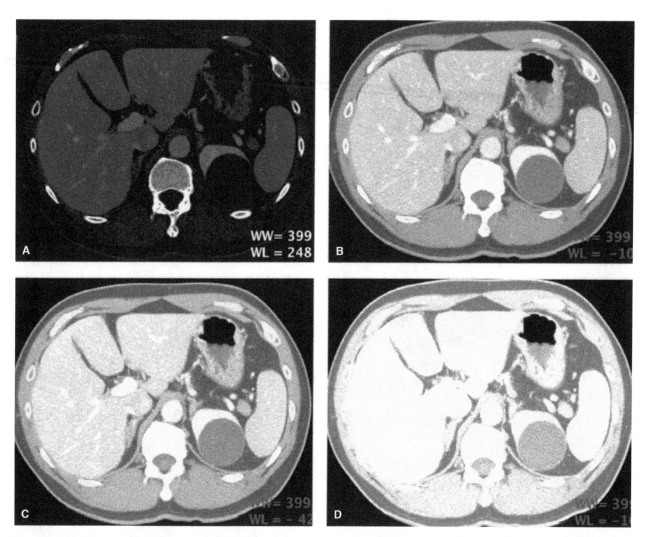

Figure 3.11. CT image of four different window levels with a constant window width. As the level descends down the HU scale, the image contrast also changes. (Reproduced, with permission, from Seeram E. *Computed Tomography: Physical Principles, Clinical Applications, and Quality Control.* 3rd ed. St. Louis, MO: Saunders Elsevier; 2009).

cine mode has several advantages including a more accurate evaluation of structures, it speeds up the interpretation time, and it increases the efficiency of the PACS system.

Region-of-Interest (ROI)

An ROI is a quantitative analytic measurement tool found on most CT scanners and PACS workstations. The ROI is a circular, oval, or rectangular geometric shaped area placed on an image that measures the pixel intensities in the area and records it as CT numbers or HU. The ROI readings, on many units, calculate the number of pixels within the region, the area of the region, the highest, lowest, and average (mean) pixel value in the region, and its standard deviation. This visualization tool affords the radiologist the proficiency to define the contents of a

lesion, the lesion's size in all three dimensions, and its shape. This recorded knowledge may save a patient an unnecessary invasive or noninvasive biopsy.

INFORMATICS

Hard/Electronic Copy

In the early days of CT imaging, images were recorded on hard copy film through the use of a multi-format camera. The analog intensities were transferred from the camera and onto film and transported into the radiology dark room using cassettes. This camera could record from 1 image per sheet up to 25 images per sheet. The multi-format camera was slow and labor-intensive to use in comparison to more modern imaging recording devices. As technology advanced the laser imaging recording systems became the gold standard. There were two types of lasers used for film imaging: the solid state laser diodes and gas lasers such as helium-neon. The 3M's solid state lasers performed better than the He-Ne gas lasers. The laser beam diameter is often in the order of 0.1 mm providing a broad gray-scale and excellent spatial resolution. A digital copy of the image on the viewing monitor was stored in the computer memory of the camera until a full sheet of images was complete; the film was then exposed and processed. The laser cameras were directly connected to a wet processor unit, but when dry processing became available, it increased workflow tremendously. Infra-red sensitive film was used in both systems. With the introduction of soft copy imaging, laser printing became an archaic process in fast paced CT facilities.

Soft copy recording is much faster and cheaper than hard copy films; therefore, patients now receive their images on a CD or DVD. For this form of recording, the CT scanner and/or the PACS units must be equipped with a CD or DVD burner. The digital imaging files are sent to the burner and transferred to the disk according to the DICOM standard. The disk is furnished with a DICOM viewer so that the images can be viewed on any computer. These disks are read-only-memory (ROM) so that the information on the CD or DVD cannot be erased.

DICOM was originally developed by the National Electrical Manufacturers Association (NEMA) and the American College of Radiology (ACR) for computerized axial tomography and magnetic resonance imaging images. In 1985, The ACR-NEMA committee was formed to explore ways of standardizing the interconnection of imaging devices and establishing a reasonable common ground for users and vendors. The original version specifies a hardware interface, a data dictionary, and a set of commands. The data dictionary is a comprehensive table of rules for the encoding of information associated with images; such as patient identification, date of birth, date of study, etc., with each vendor following the exact text format. In 1988, version 2.0 was published resulting in a messaging structure. In computer communications, a message is a stream of bits that represents information for transit from one device to another. The new standard is composed of two parts: a command segment and a data segment. Individual units of information, called data elements, are organized within the data dictionary into related groups. As with version 1.0, groups and elements are numbered with a pair of hexadecimal numbers designating a given group-element combination. The arrangement enabled a unique identification tag for that piece of

information. The length of every element and group is rounded to an even number to facilitate automatic error checking. An odd length detected at the receiving end is evidence of damage to the data set. When this occurs, the sending device is instructed to repeat the transmission. From the user's point of view, the element values are the most essential part of the message. This standard enables images to be transmitted from one vendor specific unit to a completely different vendor unit with no loss of information. The DICOM standard enables interoperability, which is considered important in reducing the cost of health care by eliminating the high cost of film and film storage, online PACS allowing small institutions to have images interpreted off-site so that the 24/7 radiologist coverage is not necessary and PACS workstations providing terabit archiving storage.

Archive

The term archive can be described as copying files to a long-term storage medium for backup and future retrieval. There are two approaches to secondary storage: sequential access/serial and direct access/random. Sequential access is referred to as reading or writing data records in sequential order, that is, one record after the other. A tape drive is an example of a sequential-access device because to get to, say point K on the tape, the drive needs to pass through points A through J. A magnetic tape is composed of a Mylar material coated with particles that magnetize the tape to record information. The tape looks like a movie reel and is positioned onto the tape drive and threaded, similar to threading a sewing machine, to pass by the read-write head on the drive and then moves onto a take-up real. The storage capacity of a tape reel ranged from 1,600 to 6,400 characters. Sequential-access files are faster to read and write if you always access records in the same order, but become very time consuming when a study in the middle of the tape needs retrieving. Sequential storage has become a thing of the past, since the tapes and tapes drives are too cumbersome for modern day technology. Direct or random access gives the operator the ability to read and write data in a random order. A disk drive is a random-access device, since the drive can access any point on the disk without passing through all intervening points. Magnetic or floppy disk was the first to be used. These disks are made of a flexible Mylar plastic encased in a plastic jacket coated with magnetic particles that allow data to be recorded and stored as binary code. The disks are composed of concentric tracks with 17 sectors per track allowing information to be written on these tracks where space is available. Each disk has a file directory indicating what sectors contain a particular patient's images. The common sizes for these disks are 3½ and 5¼ inch usually allowing for 4,000 bits of information per inch. As technology advanced, optical disk storage became available and engaged the use of a laser beam to read and write files. The laser beam is tightly focused to form a spot of light on the optical stylist, which then burns tiny pits onto the concentric tracks. There are three types of optical disks available:

- compact disc, read only memory (CD-ROM)
- write once, read many (WORM)
- erasable optical disk

A CD can hold megabits of information while a DVD holds kilobits of information. When PACS systems became the main stay of radiology departments, image storage is now being performed by the PACS workstation via a redundant array of independent disks (RAID) system. This hard disk system provides protection of data information. There are several levels of RAID organizations:

Data mirroring
- data copied to two hard disks
  - if one disk fails, the data are not lost, since they are saved on the other system
Data stripping
- data are distributed over several disks
  - one disk is used as a check disk
    - this disk identifies the placement of each file
  - if one disk fails
    - the check disk rebuilds the data

The storage of a RAID is in the form of terabits.

Picture Archiving and Communication Systems

PACS is an electronic system for archiving, transmitting, viewing, and manipulating images replacing hard-copy based means of managing medical images, such as film archiving. The universal format for PACS image storage and transfer is DICOM. Nonimage data, such as scanned documents, may be incorporated into PACS for reviewing using consumer industry standard formats like PDF once encapsulated in DICOM. PACS has the ability to deliver timely and efficient access to images, interpretations, and related data by placing the examination into a specific radiologist's workflow, such as neuro, chest, body, or muscular skeleton. PACS breaks down the physical and time barriers associated with traditional film-based image retrieval, distribution, and display. When images are transmitted to a PACS system they are encrypted and compressed during transportation for speed and security utilizing lossless compression. HIPPA requires PACS

images to be backed-up to eliminate image loss and sent to an off-site facility.

Networking

Networking involves the transmission of images and patient data from one location to another through the use of pathways. There are four network configurations used for transmission:

Bus topology
- only transmits data in one direction
- uses a common channel to connect all devices
- single cable (Ethernet) functions as a shared communication medium that devices, such as computers and printers, attach or tap into with an interface connector
- works best with a limited number of devices
Star topology
- consists of a host or file server
- computers, printers, or workstations are connected to the host
- transmission lines between them form a graph with the topology of a star
- server can handle very high utilization by one device without affecting others
Ring topology
- does not make use of a host or file server
- each device connects to exactly two other devices, forming a single continuous pathway in the form of a ring
- every device has access to the token and the opportunity to transmit
- point to point line configuration (device on either side) is quite easy to install and reconfigure
- adding or removing a device requires moving just two connections
- point to point line configuration makes it easy to identify and isolate faults

Area Networking

The three main types of area networks are local area networking (LAN), metropolitan area networking (MAN), and wide area networking (WAN). A LAN supplies networking capabilities to a group of computers in close proximity to each other as in an office building or home. A LAN networking system has the ability of being connected to other LANs. A MAN is a computer network larger than a LAN, covering an area of a few city blocks to the area of an entire city; hence, metropolitan, possibly including the surrounding areas. MAN links between LANs with wireless links using either microwave, radio, or infra-red laser transmission. Most companies rent or lease circuits from common carriers. A WAN is a network that covers a broad area, such as, telecommunications network that links across metropolitan, regional, national, or international boundaries using leased telecommunication lines. Recently with the spread of low cost of internet connectivity, many companies and organizations have turned to virtual private networking (VPN) to interconnect their networks, creating a WAN. Companies such as Citrix, Cisco, New Edge Networks, and Check Point offer solutions to create VPN networks.

IMAGE QUALITY

Image quality relates to how well the image represents the object scanned. The most important performance parameters that affect the quality of a CT image are as follows:

- high-contrast spatial resolution
- low-contrast resolution
- temporal resolution
- noise
- CT number
- uniformity
- artifacts

Spatial Resolution

The definition of high-contrast spatial resolution as stated by Seeram (2009), is the "system's ability to resolve, as separate forms, small objects that are very close together."

Measuring Spatial Resolution

There are two methods of quantifying spatial resolution: the direct measurement method and the indirect measurement method. In the days of single-slice CT scanning, the way of measuring spatial resolution was performed directly in terms of line pairs per centimeter or line pairs per millimeter using a line pair phantom. The line pair phantom is scanned, the observer reviews the reconstructed image counting the number of stripes visible. The metal strip and the space between the lines is a line pair, denoted as lp/cm. It is important to keep in mind that the unit of linear attenuation coefficient (μ) is per centimeter (cm^{-1}). Line pairs are counted to report the spatial resolution. As seen in the image below, the ability to resolve 21 lp/cm produces the best spatial resolution (Fig. 3.12). This form of measurement is fairly subjective due to the viewing window and the personal decision criteria.

The indirect measurement of spatial resolution is performed using a phantom with a 0.08 mm diameter tungsten wire submerged in water with the results being calculated from the point spread function that is subjected to the Fourier transformation to acquire the modulation transfer function (MTF). The MTF is a mathematical formula that measures the ratio of the accuracy of the image compared to the actual object scanned indicating its image fidelity. The MTF generates information concerning the entire frequency range in a quantitative and objective manner. Once the computations are completed, the results are displayed

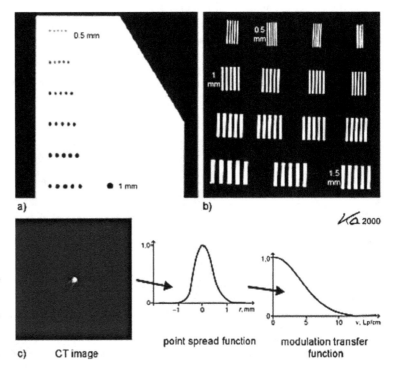

Figure 3.12. Images of different spatial resolution phantom test. (A) Hole pattern, (B) line pair/bar pattern, (C) wire phantom for MTF calculations using the point spread function. (Reproduced, with permission, from Kalendar WA. *Computed Tomography: Fundamentals System Technology, Image Quality, and Applications.* 3rd ed. Erlangen, Germany: Publicis; 2011).

on the scanner in lp/cm. It is not uncommon for modern CT scanner to have a limited resolution of 25 lp/cm.

With the introduction of volumetric CT scanning, cross-plane resolution has become an integral measurement tool that describes the slice sensitivity profile (SSP) of a series of scans (Fig. 3.13). The SSP is generated by the use of a ramp phantom or a delta phantom. The ramp phantom is the most straightforward using a thin strip of aluminum with a thickness of 0.1 mm. The aluminum stripe is placed at a shallow angle (usually a 23-degree angle) with respect to the x–y plane. Images are taken in the step-and-shoot fashion using a particular slice thickness (5–10 mm). The image is reconstructed and the wire measured. The measurement of the wire and the slice thickness should be equal. For spiral CT the ramp method does not suffice; therefore, an additional method termed the delta phantom is used. This method uses small thin plates or tiny spheres of high density and atomic number. The phantom is scanned in the spiral fashion along the z-axis. One revolution of the x-ray tube produces a slice sensitivity profile for that particular beam collimation. The slice sensitivity profile describes how thick a section is imaged and to what extent details within the section contribute to the signal. The effective section width is characterized by the full width of the profile at 50% of its maximum value (FWHM). The shape of the profile and the quality of the profile are not fully represented in the FWHM; therefore, the linear variable of a profile width of 10% of its maximum height has been established.

An image that is said to possess good spatial resolution allows the viewer the ability to distinguish peripheral borders of organs, vessels, and in some cases lesions from its surroundings. The factors affecting spatial resolution are:

Pixel size
Slice thickness
Sampling theorem

• pitch
Reconstruction algorithm
Focal spot size
Patient motion

Pixel Size

The pixel size as stated earlier is determined by the matrix size and the FOV. The information in a pixel is an average of all the intensities across the ray sum and is assigned one HU per pixel. When the object is smaller than the pixel, the densities within that pixel will be averaged with the density of other tissues contained in the pixel producing a less accurate HU for that pixel. For all intents and purposes large pixels will make it more likely multiple objects are contained within a pixel lending to an arbitrary HU. This comes into play when an ROI measurement of a lesion is taken to determine if the lesion is cystic, benign, or malignant. It is plan to see, smaller pixels are not prone to contain different densities, decreasing the possibility of volume averaging. To produce an image with the best spatial resolution, utilize the smallest DFOV possible without compromising anatomical structures.

Slice Thickness

Slice thickness accounts for the z-axis segmentation known as the voxel dimension. As with pixel size, slice thickness can contribute to volume averaging contributing to a less detailed or blurred image. Thin slice thicknesses are best used when looking for small details within the scanned object as in the case of HRCT images of the chest looking for granulomas or muscular skeleton imaging to determine fine fractures or loose bodies. Thin slices and small pixels may be counterintuitive, since they produce a noisier image degrading low-contrast detectability in the examination of the abdomen, pelvis, or brain tissue.

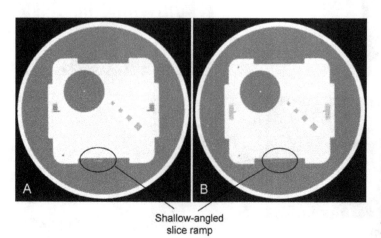

Shallow-angled
slice ramp

Figure 3.13. Image of a CT phantom demonstrating a shallow angled ramp slice for the measurement of SSP. Image A measured a 5 mm slice, while image B used a 10-mm collimation. Both phantoms were scanned using the step-and-shoot method. (Reproduced, with permission, from Seeram E. *Computed Tomography: Physical Principles, Clinical Applications, and Quality Control.* 3rd ed. St. Louis, MO: Saunders Elsevier; 2009).

Sampling Theorem

The sampling theorem is based on the Nyquist theorem stating that the sampling rate must be at least twice the highest analog frequency component. For a true replication of an object, the pixel dimension must be half the size of the intended object. Sampling is imperative in order to reproduce an image with almost the exact characteristics as the object. CT accomplishes sampling in several ways; detector sampling (as discussed above), digitization accomplished through the use of the ADC, and pitch. To increase the number of data samples, manufacturers have designed scanners that double sample the detectors by means of the quarter-shift technology and the z-Sharp sampling. When the analog signal produced at the detectors is converted into digital information by the ADC, the ADC samples the analog signal at various times to measure its strength. It is safe to say that the more samples produced the higher the chance the image will represent the object. The most important characteristics of the ADC are its speed and accuracy, for which they are inversely proportional to each other. The faster the ADC is at converting the signal into digital format, the less accurate the delineation of the object scanned. Pitch is the one factor of sampling controlled by the technologists. Pitch in its simplest terms is the ratio of the table feed per 360-degree rotation and the total beam collimation. It can be expressed with the following equations:

$$\text{Pitch} = \frac{\text{table speed}\left(\dfrac{\text{mm}}{\text{sec}}\right) \times \text{gantry rotation time (sec)}}{\text{total bean collimation}}$$

$$\text{Pitch} = \frac{\text{table feed (mm)}}{\text{total beam collimation}}$$

Note: table feed = table speed (mm/sec) × gantry rotation time (sec)

When the table speed moves at the same distance as the total beam collimation, it is said to have a pitch of 1:1, as the table speed moves at a distance larger than the beam width, the pitch increases degrading spatial resolution. In viewing pitch in the sampling perspective, lower pitch factors ($\leq$0.5) produce more samples, since the table movement is slower and the patient is being sampled or exposed to the radiation beam at a slower pace. The major disadvantage of these low pitch factors is the extra amount of radiation dose the patient receives. In choosing pitch, the technologist must justify if the outcome outweighs the risk.

Reconstruction Algorithm

High pass algorithms (bone or detail algorithms) accentuate the difference between neighboring pixels optimizing spatial resolution, but have a negative effect on noise. Low pass algorithms (standard or smooth algorithms) reduce the difference between adjacent pixels, producing a smooth image appearance thus reducing the appearance of image noise, but at the cost of degrading spatial resolution.

Focal Spot Size

The focal spot size, the scanner geometry, the detector aperture size and spacing, and the movement of the focus are important geometric factors affecting resolution specifically spatial. As long as the CT scanner is installed so that the optical focal spot is similar to a quadratic shape at the center of the detector array, the focal spot size does not need to be small. CT utilizes such a restricted beam width, the focal spot size of the CT scanner is appropriate for sequencing the aliasing artifact, increasing spatial resolution.

Patient Motion

Movement of the object during data acquisition results in inconsistencies of the measured projection. The inconsistencies not only cause unsharpness (degrading spatial resolution), but also cause streak artifacts in the reconstructed CT image.

Contrast Resolution

Contrast resolution can be described as the ability to distinguish one soft tissue from another with similar densities as their background. The term low contrast detectability (LCD) is used to describe contrast resolution in CT. CT has the capability to image tissues that vary only slightly in density and atomic number, thus detecting density difference from 0.25% to 0.5%. When the difference between the object and background is small LCD improves. The factors affecting LCD include:

Noise
Photon flux
* patient size
Slice thickness
Sensitivity of the detectors
Reconstruction algorithms
Image display/recording

Noise

Noise plays an important role in LCD and can be defined as the undesirable fluctuation of pixel values in an image of a homogeneous material. The noise value can be measured by means of the standard deviation (σ) indicating the amount of variance among pixel values in a desired ROI. Noise can be distinguished on an image as a grainy mottled appearance. There are several types of noise that can appear on an image, such as quantum mottle, computational noise, and electronic noise. Of the three types, quantum mottle can be controlled by the operator. Quantum mottle occurs when there are an insufficient number of photons reaching the detectors and measured. It is inversely related to the number of photons detected to produce an image. As the number of photons reaching the detectors and recorded increases the noise in the image decreases. Number of photons detected per pixel is referred to as signal-to-noise ratio (SNR). SNR compares the level of desired signal to the level of the background noise as denoted in the following equation:

$$SNR = \frac{\text{mean HU of the ROI}}{\text{background HU of the ROI}}$$

Computational noise is due to mathematical errors made by the computer when calculating the linear attenuation coefficient of an object during image reconstruction. Electronic noise is due to physical inherited limitations of the CT system. This type of noise is predisposed by the electronics in the detector photodiode, data acquisition system, and minimally by scatter radiation.

Photon Flux

Photon flux is primarily dependent on the combination of kVp, mAs, and beam filtration. These factors affect both quantity and quality of photons reaching the detectors with mAs directly influencing the number of x-ray photons needed to produce a CT image. The effect of increasing the mAs to produce more photons increases dose. Dose increases linearly with mAs per scan. By doubling the mAs the SNR increases by 40% which in turn improves contrast resolution, but at the cost of increased radiation dose. mAs are directly proportional to radiation dose. Since CT utilizes high kVp in the range of 100 to 140, kVp incurs a slight effect on noise. Increasing kVp results in a higher photon flux; thus increasing the number of photons and decreasing the noise. For all intense purposes, this may seem ideal, but the visibility of low contrast objects may be compromised. These low contrast objects depend on low energy photons which are rather less for the higher tube currents. Increasing kVp without reducing mAs also increases dose. Beam filtration is somewhat stable in CT, but it is imperative to choose the correct bow tie filter when scanning to shape the beam properly. Patient size affects the attenuation of the beam, thus the photon flux at the detectors. Utilizing one technique for all patients may be detrimental, since larger patients attenuate more x-ray photons, leaving fewer to reach the detectors. This results in a reduction of the SNR, increased noise consequently degrading contrast resolution.

Slice Thickness

Slice thickness is represented by the volume of tissue within the voxel. Increase in slice thickness increases the depth of the voxel allowing more x-ray photons to hit the detectors, which in turn decreases noise. As with the increase of kVp, an increase of slice thickness can obscure the visibility of small objects by increasing the partial volume effect. Slice thickness should be chosen according to the area of interest.

Detector Sensitivity

Detectors must be capable of discriminating among small differences in x-ray attenuation required to measure small differences in soft tissue contrast, in the order of at least 1%. The preventative maintenance program established by the manufacturer requires the detectors be checked for their capture, absorption, and conversion properties. If the detectors are not efficient enough, more photons will be needed to be produced to result in a signal.

Reconstruction Algorithms

Reconstruction algorithms possess a dramatic effect on contrast resolution. Low pass algorithms (standard or smooth) are used for image smoothing. They enhance the perceptibility of low-contrast lesions, such as metastatic disease, brain, and abdomen imaging all of which demonstrate subtle differences in subject contrast. These algorithms suppress the high frequencies, thus smoothening the image reducing noise and improving contrast resolution.

Image Display

The size and resolution of the monitor and viewing distance also affect contrast resolution. As the viewing distance increases for large screens, the ease of detecting low-contrast images improves. Computers that have a large spectrum of windowing/leveling manipulation techniques tend to have improved low-contrast resolution. It is important to remember that the contrast resolution on the image is only as good as the inherited resolution.

Temporal Resolution

Temporal resolution refers to the precision of a measurement with respect to time. Often there is a trade-off between temporal resolution and spatial resolution. Fast acquisitions result in less samples (profiles) taken thus degrading spatial resolution. In previous years, temporal resolution did not play a significant role in CT imaging, but with the introduction of cardiac imaging, temporal resolution has become a hot topic. One method to improve temporal resolution to reduce or eliminate motion is by increasing scan speed. Even though modern MDCT scanners have the capability of producing scan speeds as low as 33 milliseconds, it is not sufficient enough to completely freeze the motion of the beating heart; therefore, manufacturers developed specific cardiac reconstruction algorithms. These specific algorithms are known as the 180-degree multi-cardio delta (MCD) and the 180-degree multi-cardio interpolation (MCI). The MCD makes use of the projected data of 180-degrees plus the fan angle and the effective scan time is roughly 55% of the rotation time having the effective scan time approximately 165 ms. The slice sensitivity profile is defined exactly with the pitch chosen to correspond to the heart frequency. If the heart cycle is shorter than the effective scan time, degradation can occur. This procedure allows for a substantial reduction of the motion artifact and a 40% increase in temporal resolution. The MCI algorithm utilizes the patient's ECG to reconstruct the data only during the selected heart phase. This technique allows for a significant reduction in the effective scan time (<100 ms). A disadvantage of this method is that the slice sensitivity profile is not exact and the heart motion path has to stay constant to avoid motion unsharpness.

Quality Assurance

The terms "quality assurance" and "quality control" are often used interchangeably and should not be confused even though, both refer to ways of ensuring the quality of a CT scanner. The terms, however, have different meanings. Quality assurance (QA) is any systematic process of checking the CT scanner performance to verify whether the scanner is meeting specified requirements and operating at a tolerable level. Quality control (QC) on the other hand reviews the results of the quality assurance testing and makes corrections to improve the scanner's performance. Quality assurance programs are developed by the individual institutions with guidelines from regulatory agencies, medical physicist, manufacturing engineers, radiologist, and in some cases CT technologists. These programs were first established to guarantee high image quality by providing the radiologist the maximum information for correct interpretation and foster good quality patient care. A reputable QA program will define scanner problems before it effects image quality and the resolutions can be performed in a timely manner resulting in reduced scanner downtime.

There are three basic tenets of a good quality assurance program:

1. The program must be performed on a regular periodic basis—some tests are performed on a daily basis, monthly, semiannually, or yearly.
2. Prompt interpretation of the measurements—guidelines are established at time of instillation and upgrades are added to aid the technologist or medical physicist in the acceptable limits of the machine.
3. Results must be documented in a consistent format—this gives the observer the opportunity to see subtle changes.

CT Number

The end result of the CT measurement is the CT number, calculated from the linear attenuation coefficient of the object, by scaling with the respective coefficient for pure water and given in HU. A CT number can be determined by the following equation:

$$\text{CT number} = \frac{\mu(\text{tissue}) - \mu(\text{water})}{\mu(\text{water})} \times 1,000$$

Using the scaling factor of water it is safe to say that the accuracy of all CT numbers depends on the CT number for water in a homogeneous material; therefore, CT number is an important QA test. The test is performed using either a commercial 20 cm water phantom or a 1 gallon plastic container filled with water. All QA testing must be performed using a standard patient protocol. The phantom is scanned with an ROI encompassing an area of 2 to 3 cm^2 positioned in the center of the phantom. The expected result for the average CT number of water should be 0 with a tolerance of $+/-3$. This test should be performed on a daily basis. A cause for this test failure could be a miscalibration. If performing a recalibration does not rectify the problem, service should be notified.

Noise (Standard Deviation)

The noise test also requires the use of a 20 cm water phantom. As with the CT number test, an ROI area of 2–3 cm^2 is placed in the center of the phantom. The results of the test depend on the type of algorithm used (higher with sharp algorithms and lower for smooth algorithms) but should stay steady from day to day. If the measurement increases, it indicates more variation in the pixel to pixel CT numbers and poorer low contrast detectability. The cause of this failure may be due to low x-ray output or an increase in electronic noise, and it must be reported to the service engineer.

Cross Field Uniformity

The terms uniformity or homogeneity can be interchanged with their simplest meanings being the same; therefore, the goal of uniformity is to maintain a constant CT value for water, over the entire cross-section of a homogeneous water phantom (Fig. 3.14). This test is performed using a 20 cm or a 32 cm water phantom. An ROI with the area measurement of 2 to 3 cm² is placed in the center of the phantom, one at the 12 o'clock position, one at the 3 o'clock position, one at the 6 o'clock position, and one at the 9 o'clock position. It is important to place the peripheral ROIs approximately one ROI diameter away from the edge. The measurements of each ROI should not deviate more than 4 to 5 HU of each other. If the results demonstrate a high number in the center of the phantom the image reveals cupping, whereas a low value in the center relative to the edges reveals capping. The cause of cupping or capping is the result of beam hardening. This test should be performed monthly or biannually depending on the institution.

Linearity

Linearity refers to the relationship of the CT number of the reconstructed object to the measured linear attenuation coefficient. Linearity is measured using a Catphan phantom with distinctive materials representing bone, contrast, fat, water, and air. The linear attenuation coefficient values of each material are plotted against its respective CT number. A line graph demonstrating a straight line indicates an acceptable linearity QA test.

High Contrast Spatial Resolution

The QA test for high contrast spatial resolution was discussed earlier in this chapter. For the direct and indirect measurement a scanner possessing the best spatial resolution will resolve the largest number of lp/cm. The baseline is established at time of instillation and checked biannually and compared. When the scanner falls below the set

specification, the cause may be from an enlarged focal spot, mechanical wear of the gantry due to motion, or misalignments of the electromechanical components along with vibrations or detector failures.

Contrast Resolution (LCD)

A contrast resolution phantom contains a strip of polystyrene inserted in the phantom. The strip has a series of holes with decreasing diameters drilled in the plastic and the phantom is filled with water and an additional material such as methanol or sucrose to bring the fluid's CT number close to the plastic. The observer will review the reconstructed image looking for the smallest holes visible comparing the finding to the original specifications. This test should be performed biannually. Some causes of the failure are due to a decreased x-ray output, tungsten coating build-up, and electronic noise. Once a failure is discovered, a service engineer must be notified.

This is a brief review of some of the QA testing performed by a technologist. Many institutions have dedicated QA technologists so that the consistency is maintained. More advanced testings are performed by the medical physicist such as dose, signal-to-noise ratio (SNR) and contrast-to-noise ratio (CNR).

ARTIFACT RECOGNITION AND REDUCTION

CT artifacts seriously degrade the quality of a CT image, since they are described as inconsistencies between the reconstructed CT numbers in the image and the true attenuation coefficients of the object. Artifacts can affect the image to the point of undiagnostic use; therefore, it is

a)

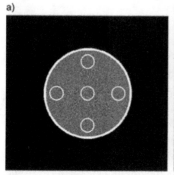

b)

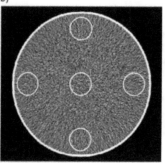

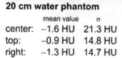

20 cm water phantom		
	mean value	σ
center:	−1.6 HU	21.3 HU
top:	−0.9 HU	14.8 HU
right:	−1.3 HU	14.7 HU
bottom:	−0.9 HU	14.6 HU
left:	−1.3 HU	14.9 HU

32 cm water phantom		
	mean value	σ
Center:	−3.0 HU	68.5 HU
top:	−1.6 HU	34.8 HU
right:	−0.9 HU	34.2 HU
bottom:	−0.9 HU	35.1 HU
left:	−0.1 HU	35.3 HU

Figure 3.14. CT water phantom used to measure homogeneity. Image A is the typical 20 cm head phantom, while image B is the 32 cm body phantom. The ROIs contained within the images should have a near 0 measurement and the difference between the central ROI and the peripheral ROI's should not exceed 5 HU. (Reproduced, with permission, from Kalendar WA. *Computed Tomography: Fundamentals System Technology, Image Quality, and Applications.* 3rd ed. Erlangen, Germany: Publicis; 2011).

imperative for technologists to understand why artifacts occur and how they can be prevented or suppressed. The three main sources of CT artifacts are:

- Physics-based
- Patient-based
- Scanner-based

Artifacts in this section will be described according to their definition, cause, appearance, and rectification.

Physics Based

Beam Hardening Artifact

Definition

As a beam passes through an object, the laws of physics interaction with matter state that the mean energy increases because the lower energy photons are absorbed more than the higher-energy photons producing a more penetrating beam of radiation. The degree to which beam hardening occurs depends on the composition of the tissue, more for bone and less on fat. There are two types of beam hardening artifacts seen on CT images: cupping and streaks and dark bands.

Cause

Cupping

- the cupping artifact occurs when the beam becomes harder through the center of the object
- the attenuation coefficient decreases towards the edges of the object
- the beam
  - becomes more energetic when it reaches the detectors resulting in the attenuation profile being different from the ideal profile that would be obtained without beam hardening

Streaks and Dark Bands

- the rotating tube causes
  - the beam to be hardened more at certain angle positions than other, especially when translating through areas of high attenuation objects to low attenuation object, exiting at high attenuation objects
  - detectors are unable to calibrate the erroneous data

Appearance

Cupping

- periphery of the image is lighter
- center of the image is darker
  - homogeneous water phantom—the CT number in the center of the image are higher than the CT number at the peripheral of the image

Streaks and dark bands

- dark streaks can be found between two high attenuation objects, such as metal, bone, iodinated contrast, or barium

- bright streaks are seen adjacent to the dark streaks
- these artifacts are a particular problem in the posterior cranial fossa, and with metal implants

Rectification

Filtration

- adding 0.1 to 0.4 mm of AL to the inherited filtration

Beam hardening correction software

- that assumes an average amount of beam hardening, given the measured attenuation
  - higher atomic number materials such as metal cause a higher than average amount of beam hardening, and will thus not be fully corrected
- iterative reconstruction using uncorrected projection data
  - metal and bone are then detected using an HU cutoff
  - the data are projected forward to determine how much bone and metal are present in each detector measurement
  - this information is then used to perform a custom beam hardening correction for each detector element
- dual energy
  - reduces beam hardening effects by scanning at two different energies
  - the information can be used to derive virtual monochromatic images
    - does not suffer from beam hardening effects

Partial Volume Averaging Artifact

Definition

- Partial volume averaging arises when tissues of widely different absorption are encompassed on the same CT voxel producing a beam attenuation proportional to the average value of these tissues

Cause

Object is partially lying within an individual slice

- more than one tissue type is contained within a particular voxel

Generating skewed linear attenuation coefficient value (Fig. 3.15)

- producing inconsistencies among the tissue values

Appearance

- Streak-shaped dark and light bands
- Shading

Rectification

Best avoided by utilizing

- thin acquisition section widths
  - necessary when imaging parts of the anatomy that rapidly change in the z-axis

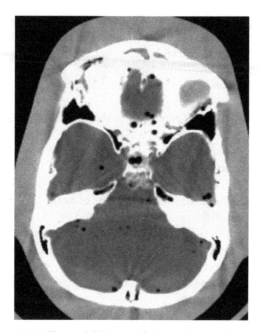

Figure 3.15. The axial CT image of a brain phantom. The image was acquired using a 7 mm slice width to observe the streaking effect between the temporal bones. (Reproduced, with permission, from Seeram E. *Computed Tomography: Physical Principles, Clinical Applications, and Quality Control.* 3rd ed. St. Louis, MO: Saunders Elsevier; 2009).

Edge Gradient Artifact

Definition

- CT system is not able to resolve two small objects with very different densities of high frequency or high contrast. Instead of imaging these two small structures as separate entities, the CT system sees them as one structure.

Cause

System's inability to process high spatial frequency signal required for sharp edges

Common sites

- dense bone and surrounding tissue
- bowel loops with contrast
- blood vessels with IV contrast
- areas around biopsy needles

Appearance

- Edges or borders of these high frequencies are blurred to a certain degree
- Streaks

Rectification

Using a bone, sharp, high frequency algorithm during reconstruction

- mathematically enhances the edges of structures by diminishing structural blurring
- this algorithm produces an increase in image noise

Thinner slices

Low HU-value oral contrast

- VoLumen or water

Patient Based Artifacts

Motion

Definition

- Motion refers to any movement or change in position or time. There are two types of motions: voluntary and involuntary. Voluntary motion is actual physical movement of the patient during data acquisition. Involuntary motion is an action done without or against one's will.

Cause

Voluntary

- movement of the patient
- respiratory

Involuntary

- cardiac
- bowel

Appearance

Blurring

Double images

Streaks

- occur between high contrast edges and the x-ray tube position when the motion occurs

Rectification

Avoidance by the technologists

- positioning aids may be sufficient for most patients
- immobilization by the means of sedation
  - pediatric patients
  - incoherent patients
- utilizing short scan times
- utilizing faster scanners with more detector rows
  - allows greater volume per revolution
- inspiration techniques
- sensitivity of the image to motion depends on the orientation of the motion
  - preferably to start and end position of the tube that is aligned with the primary direction of the motion
  - vertically at 0 or 180-degrees

Manufactures solutions

- software correction
- body scan mode
  - automatically applies reduced weighting to the beginning and end views to suppress their contribution to the final image

- may lead to an increase in noise in the vertical direction of the resultant image depending on the shape of the patient
- specialized motion correction is available on some scanners
  - one technique is the correction of fluid interface
- cardiac gating
  - rapid motion of the heart leads to severe artifact in images of the heart and artifacts that can mimic disease in associated structures
    - dissected aorta
    - small coronary arteries
  - techniques developed to produce images by using data from a fraction of the cardiac cycle (least cardiac motion)
  - achieved by a combination of ECG tracing with specialized methods of image reconstruction

Metallic Artifacts

Definition

- Inconsistencies of the projected data on the reconstructed image due to the high density of the metal

Causes

Presence of high density objects (usually made of metal)

- dental fillings
- metal prosthetic devices
- surgical clips

Primary reason that streaks occur from metal objects

- the objects exceed the maximum attenuation value that a CT system can image
  - 1,000 HU
    - coincides with the attenuation value of cortical bone
- metal has a higher attenuation value greater than cortical bone
- the computer can only assign the highest value it knows
  - metallic type objects exceed the dynamic range of the detectors in the detector array
  - resulting in the metallic object being unable to be faithfully imaged

Appearance

- Streaks

Rectification

Avoidance by the technologist

- removal of all metal objects
  - jewelry
  - bridges

- nonremoval objects, such as dental fillings, prosthetic devices, and surgical clips
  - angulation of the gantry to exclude these items
- increase the technical parameters
  - especially kVp
    - help with penetration
- utilizing thinner slice widths

Manufactures solutions

- interpolation techniques to substitute the over range values in attenuation profile
  - metal objects are usually considered opaque and data corresponding to the rays through the metal objects are defined as missing data
  - inaccurate metal data are replaced with forward projected values
  - instead of trying to look through the metal to see soft tissue
    - the technique looks around the metal
  - use of this metal artifact reduction method is sometimes limited
    - loss of detail around the metal–tissue interface
      - especially when structures within a few millimeters of metal are blurred out

Out of Field Artifact

Definition

- Any portion of the patient lying outside the SFOV, giving the computer incomplete information relating to this portion

Cause

Patients arms at their side

IV tubing containing contrast medium lying within the gantry

Exceptionally large patients—exceeding the selected SFOV

- extra tissues are blocking detectors and attenuating the photons

Blocking the reference channels at the sides of the detector array

- interferes with data normalization

Appearance

- Streak artifact occurs throughout the entire image
- Bright rim at the edge of the field of reconstruction

Rectification

- Position patient with arms above the head
- Make sure nothing is touching the gantry aperture

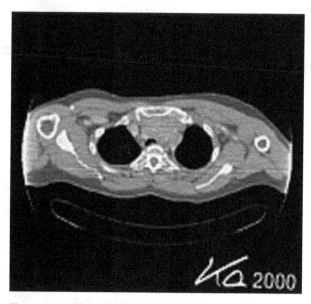

Figure 3.16. CT axial image depicting an out-of-field artifact. The streaking on either side of the shoulder lends the observer to believe the subject was larger than the SFOV. (Reproduced, with permission, from Kalendar WA. *Computed Tomography: Fundamentals System Technology, Image Quality, and Applications.* 3rd ed. Erlangen, Germany: Publicis; 2011).

- Make sure the SFOV is larger than the object being scanned (Fig. 3.16)
- Some manufacturers monitor the reference data channels for inconsistencies and avoid using data that appear suspicious

Scanner Based Artifacts

Ring Artifacts

Definition
- An artifact that emerges as a circular structure centered on the position of the axis of rotation within the image impairing the diagnostic quality of the image

Causes
One detector out of calibration
- third generation scanner
  - detector will give a consistently erroneous reading at each angular position

Single slice scanner solid-state detectors
- more susceptible when central detectors are affected

Rectification
Recalibrating the detector is sufficient to fix this artifact
- although occasionally the detector itself needs to be replaced

Software corrections
- that characterizes and corrects detector variation

Tube Arcing Artifact

Definition
- Tungsten vapor from anode and cathode intercepts the projectile electrons intended for collisions with the target

Cause
Arcing causes a momentary loss of x-ray output
- contaminates the signal at the detectors affecting proper image reconstruction

Degradation of the vacuum within the tube
- resulting in increased gas pressure

Appearance
There is no specific pattern for this artifact
Depending on the degree of arcing
- a single streak to multiple streaks can appear
- usually not noticed on transaxial image
  - reformatted images (sagittal and coronal)
  - hypodense rippling effect across the entire image

Cone Beam Artifact

Definition
- An artifact that arises due to the beam geometry representing a cone rather than fan angle

Cause
Incomplete or insufficient projection samples due to the cone beam geometry in MDCT scanners
As the number of sections per rotation increases
- wider collimation is required
  - with detector rows 16 channels or greater
- x-ray beam becomes cone-shaped

Appearance
Leads to a shading artifact around the off-axis objects
- it is more pronounced for the outer detector rows than for the inner ones

Rectification
Specialized 3D reconstruction algorithms
When high image resolution is imperative and the speed of the scan acquisition is not as important
- protocols may be designed so that only the center rows of the detector array are used

Artifacts come in the appearance of streaks, shading, rings, and dark bands, which severely diminish the quality of an image. Modern CT manufacturers have implemented special software corrections to combat a number of artifacts, but it is still the responsibility of the technologist to be able to recognize and minimize artifacts.

Review Questions

Multiple Choice: Select the one single best answer.

1. Which of the following is **not** considered a degradation of the reconstruction image due to an artifact?

   (A) degrading the image quality
   (B) segmenting the voxel data
   (C) affecting the perceptibility of detail
   (D) leading to misdiagnosis

2. What are the two principal demands placed on an x-ray tube for CT imaging?

   (A) heat dissipation and bean filtration
   (B) high x-ray intensity and heat dissipation
   (C) high x-ray intensity and rotation speed
   (D) line focus principle and rotating anode

3. Which of the following photon interactions produce a photon that is deflected from its original site of interaction?

   (A) characteristic radiation
   (B) Compton interaction
   (C) Photoelectric interaction
   (D) deterministic effect

4. In the early days of CT scanning, reconstruction algorithms were very antiquated. What type of reconstruction algorithm was performed by Hounsfield during his first experiments?

   (A) back projection
   (B) filtered back projection
   (C) algebraic reconstruction
   (D) iterative reconstruction

5. What is defined as the z-axis segmentation?

   (A) voxel
   (B) pixel
   (C) matrix
   (D) FOV

6. A digital image is composed of multiple pixels. What is considered a characteristic of a pixel?

   (A) cube-shaped volume of tissue
   (B) unit of linear attenuation
   (C) two-dimensional square of data
   (D) unit of x-ray exposure in air

7. What is considered an electronic system for archiving, transmitting, viewing, and manipulating images in the radiology department?

   (A) DICOM
   (B) PACS
   (C) HIS
   (D) RIS

8. What is one of the advantages to using high kVp during CT imaging?

   (A) reduction of imaging time
   (B) reduction of reconstruction time
   (C) reduction of radiation intensity at the image receptor
   (D) reduction of radiation dose

9. A CTA study was performed on a patient suspected of having an abdominal aneurysm. The 3D technologist requested the voxels to be isotropic to eliminate loss of detail. Which of the following constitutes an isotropic voxel?

   (A) one in which all sides are equal
   (B) one in which the slice thickness is larger than the pixel area
   (C) one in which the image needs to be reconstructed on a smaller matrix
   (D) one in which the pixel size is smaller than the slice thickness

10. If one wants to increase the contrast resolution of an image, which of the following would be the best factor to change?

    (A) increase of mAs
    (B) increase of kVp
    (C) increase of beam filtration
    (D) decrease of kV

11. A matrix can be described by which of the following characteristics?

    (A) aperture size used during data acquisition
    (B) relationship between the field-of-view and the pixel size
    (C) relationship between the field-of-view and the reconstruction algorithm
    (D) volume of tissue

12. Slip rings are employed in helical CT to conduct high voltage power to what components in the gantry?

    (A) x-ray tube and couch
    (B) x-ray tube and detector acquisition system
    (C) cooling and detector acquisition system
    (D) generator and the cooling system

13. Which of the following key performance parameters of image quality are considered indirectly proportional to each other?

    (A) spatial resolution and noise
    (B) contrast resolution and linearity
    (C) temporal resolution and contrast resolution
    (D) spatial resolution and temporal resolution

14. Which of the following is the best way of reducing the partial volume averaging artifact?

    (A) faster slice acquisitions
    (B) iterative reconstruction
    (C) thinner slice acquisitions
    (D) increased tube output

15. What is a useful characteristic of a gas-filled detector for CT imaging?

    (A) no afterglow
    (B) high detector efficiency
    (C) direct digitization
    (D) DAS not required

16. If the μ for soft tissue is 0.215 and the μ for water is 0.206, what is the correlated HU for soft tissue?

    (A) 43 HU
    (B) 2,000 HU
    (C) −43 HU
    (D) 1,000 HU

17. What occurs when the interspace distance between detectors is reduced?

    (A) detector response time is reduced
    (B) patient dose is increased
    (C) signal acquisition time is increased
    (D) total detector efficiency is increased

18. Which of the following reconstruction algorithms is known as the convolution method?

    (A) back projection
    (B) filtered back projection
    (C) algebraic reconstruction
    (D) iterative reconstruction

19. A CT examination of the abdomen was performed on a patient complaining of left upper abdominal pain. Upon reviewing the image, a blurring occurred at the air/fluid level of the stomach. What was the possible cause of this artifact?

    (A) beam hardening
    (B) edge gradient
    (C) motion
    (D) cone beam

20. What is the name given to the algorithm that compares an assumption with the measured values, makes corrections, and repeats the cycle?

(A) analytical reconstruction

(B) back projection

(C) iterative reconstruction

(D) Fourier reconstruction

21. What is the DFOV for a particular image having a pixel size of 0.625 mm and the matrix size of 10,242?

(A) 320 mm

(B) 320 cm

(C) 640 mm^2

(D) 640 mm

22. Of the following, what organization was responsible for the development of the DICOM standard?

(A) ACRIN

(B) ASRT-ARRT

(C) ACR-NEMA

(D) NASA

23. How is it possible to increase the energy of a CT examination?

(A) raising the mAs

(B) lowering the kVp

(C) changing the scanned field of view

(D) raising the kVp

24. Which of the following is considered the area within the gantry from which the raw data are acquired located at the isocenter of the gantry?

(A) Display field of view (DFOV)

(B) reconstruction algorithm

(C) Scan field of view (SFOV)

(D) detector cell size

25. A CT examination was performed on a patient presenting with lung cancer. The radiologist wants to determine if the disease metastasized to the patient's thoracic spine. Which of the following convolution filters would you use to retrospectively reconstruct the image for this appropriate interpretation?

(A) bone

(B) smooth

(C) standard

(D) ultra-smooth

26. What type of artifact is found in the pelvis running across the two femoral heads, especially when a prosthesis is present?

(A) edge gradient

(B) aliasing

(C) cone beam

(D) beam hardening

27. What is considered a computer visualization tool responsible for controlling the brightness and contrast of an image on the computer monitor?

(A) 3D volume rendering

(B) multiplanar reformation

(C) region of interest measurements

(D) windowing

28. Which of the following is an important component of the ADC?

(A) converts continuous signal into discrete numbers

(B) second step in image digitization

(C) converts digital signal into analog signal

(D) assigns an integer to the brightness value that was sampled

29. Which of the following reconstruction algorithms models photons and electric noise in the CT system?

(A) filtered back projection reconstruction

(B) adaptive statistical iterative reconstruction

(C) modeled based iterative reconstruction

(D) algebraic reconstruction

30. Which of the following is **not** a tenet of a good quality assurance program?

(A) documentation

(B) prompt interpretation

(C) radiologist is responsible for all testing

(D) performed on a regular basis

31. What technical factor determines the quantity of photons reaching the detectors?

    (A) kVp
    (B) mAs
    (C) pitch
    (D) filters

32. What is the most straightforward technical way to reduce or eliminate the motion of an object?

    (A) increasing scan speed
    (B) removing metal objects
    (C) gantry angulation
    (D) decreasing slice thickness

33. What generation CT scanner utilized a translate–translate scanning geometry principle with 5–30 detector linear array assembly?

    (A) first generation
    (B) second generation
    (C) third generation
    (D) fourth generation

34. One of the new z-interpolation process is 180° linear interpolation. Which of the following is **not** an advantage of 180° linear interpolation?

    (A) scanning at pitches >2
    (B) narrower slice sensitivity profile
    (C) improved z-axis resolution
    (D) reduced noise

35. Which of the following is **not** an advantage of cine viewing?

    (A) more accurate evaluation of structures
    (B) calculates the mean pixel values in an area
    (C) speeds up the interpretation time
    (D) increases the efficiency of the PACS system

36. Which of the following is the appropriate type of gas utilized in gas ionization detectors?

    (A) helium
    (B) argon
    (C) xenon
    (D) neon

37. Which of the following forms of data is required to be preprocessed?

    (A) raw data
    (B) image data
    (C) measurement data
    (D) retrospective data

38. Anti-scatter grids (ASG) have been incorporated in MDCT scanners. What is the purpose of these grids?

    (A) prevent cross-talk
    (B) define slice thickness
    (C) rectify the scatter issue with an increased cone beam
    (D) define the maximum permissible beam

39. Which of the following allows the technologist to alter the displayed picture contrast?

    (A) increasing kVp
    (B) decreasing mAs
    (C) window controls
    (D) retrospective reconstruction

40. A CT phantom was scanned with the results stating the CT numbers of the uniform phantom were identical throughout the phantom. What QA test was performed?

    (A) spatial resolution
    (B) low contrast resolution
    (C) linearity
    (D) cross field uniformity (homogeneity)

41. CT scanners utilize a multitude of complex computations; therefore, they employ a midrange computer. Which of the following is **not** a characteristic of a midrange computer?

    (A) networking capability
    (B) dealing efficiently with the convoluted mathematical input
    (C) fast and efficient processing
    (D) small storage capability

42. Which of the following is a characteristic of a homogeneous radiation beam?

    (A) all photons have the same energy
    (B) the quantity and quality of the beam changes as it passes through an absorber
    (C) all photons have different energies
    (D) known as a polychromatic beam

43. A CTA of the heart requires 128 detector row channels and each detector element is 0.6 mm, what is the total beam collimation?

    (A) 213.3 mm
    (B) 76.8 cm
    (C) 213.3 cm
    (D) 76.8 mm

44. The QA test for standard deviation employs a water filled 20-cm phantom with an ROI placed in the center of the images, what is the general purpose of this QA test?

    (A) spatial resolution
    (B) noise
    (C) contrast resolution
    (D) temporal resolution

45. A particular CT examination requires the slice thickness to be 5 mm and the spacing between each slice to be 5 mm, what type of reconstruction interval is this considered?

    (A) overlapping interval
    (B) prospective interval
    (C) contiguous interval
    (D) gapping interval

46. Which of the following types of CT computer architecture requires a high structured environment that allows hardware and software to communicate, share resources, and exchange information freely?

    (A) parallel processing
    (B) serial processing
    (C) multiprocessing
    (D) distributed processing

47. Which of the following QA test requires the use of a Catphan phantom with inserts representing specific body densities?

    (A) spatial resolution
    (B) linearity
    (C) noise
    (D) CT number

48. The attenuation of a beam of radiation depends on several factors. Which of the following factors does **not** influence attenuation?

    (A) the atomic number of the material
    (B) the electrons per gram of tissue
    (C) the energy of the radiation beam
    (D) the acquisition geometry

49. What classification of image manipulation stacks the image data to generate a new series of images in a plane or orientation different from the perspective image?

    (A) prospective reconstruction
    (B) multiplanar reformation
    (C) object-based analysis
    (D) scene-based analysis

50. Of the following, what is considered an image display technique used to optimize image viewing by means of gray scale manipulations?

    (A) windowing
    (B) cine mode
    (C) image magnification
    (D) multiplanar reformation

51. A CT examination of the hip was performed with a table speed of 40 mm at a 0.5 second gantry rotation time using a 32 detector row and a 0.625 detector aperture, what is the pitch?

    (A) 0.3:1
    (B) 0.5:1
    (C) 1:1
    (D) 1.2:1

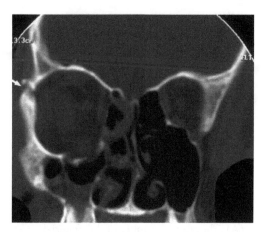

Figure Q3.1. Reproduced, with permission, from Grey ML, Ailinani JM, *CT and MRI Pathology: A Pocket Atlas*. 3rd ed. New York, NY: McGraw-Hill; 2012.

52. Figure Q3.1 demonstrates a fracture of the lateral wall of the right orbit. Which of the following window levels was most likely used to display the image?

    (A) −700 HU
    (B) 0 HU
    (C) +150 HU
    (D) + 600 HU

53. Various 3D rendering techniques are used today to enhance diagnostic interpretation. Which of the follow techniques is best utilized for the evaluation of the central tracheobronchial system?

    (A) maximum intensity projection
    (B) volume rendering
    (C) surface rendering
    (D) minimum intensity projection

54. What is the range of CT numbers if the window width is 450 and the window level is 50?

    (A) −275 to 175
    (B) 275 to −175
    (C) 500 to −400
    (D) −500 to 400

Answers and Explanations

1. **(B)** CT artifacts seriously degrade the quality of a CT image, since they are described as inconsistencies between the reconstructed CT numbers in the image and the true attenuation coefficients of the object. Artifacts can affect the image to the point of undiagnostic use; therefore, it is imperative for technologists to understand why artifacts occur and how they can be prevented or suppressed. *(Kalendar, 3rd ed., pp. 130–131)*

2. **(B)** With the introduction of spiral/helical CT scanning new technical advancements are needed to be made in order to deal with the continually rotating tube for longer periods of time. The construction of a larger anode (200 mm) allows for the use of higher tube currents. The heat capacity with these disks is also increased with an improvement in heat dissipation. *(Seeram, 3rd ed,. pp. 115–116)*

3. **(B)** Compton interaction occurs between moderate energy x-rays (above 75 keV) and outer shell electrons resulting in the ionization of the target atom. A portion of the energy is absorbed and a photon is produced with reduced energy. When that photon ejects from the site of interaction, it is deflected from that of the original photon. Due to its change in direction, this form of interaction is termed a scattering process. Since CT filters the x-ray photons as they leave the x-ray tube, short energy wavelengths are produced making the beam harder and a higher chance of the photon to penetrate the body to produce a signal at the detectors. *(Sprawls, Radiation Interaction with Matter, online)*

4. **(C)** The simplest form of reconstruction was the algebraic method of reconstruction performed by Hounsfield. This method used a linear system of equations to solve a problem. The mathematical steps were sequential since the first image matrices were 80 × 80, only 6,400 calculations needed to be performed. *(Seeram, 3rd ed., p. 5)*

5. **(A)** A voxel is synonymous with volume element for a 2D CT image in the z-axis direction. The voxel is expressed by the width of the sides of the pixels (area) and the width of the slice. *(Kalendar, 3rd ed., p. 386)*

6. **(C)** A pixel is a two-dimensional picture element that represents the smallest discrete block in a digital image display field. Multiple pixels compose the image matrix with each pixel representing a brightness level in the reconstructed image based on the atomic number and mass density of the tissue. *(Seeram, 3rd ed., p. 64)*

7. **(B)** Picture Archiving and Communication System (PACS) is one of the two key elements that form the radiology department's information infrastructure. The term PACS encompasses a broad range of technologies necessary for the storage, retrieval, distribution, manipulation, and display of images. *(Seeram, 3rd ed., p. 51)*

8. **(D)** One of the advantages of utilizing a high-frequency generator is the ability to use high kVp to minimize the photoelectric absorption which in

turn reduces radiation dose. Higher kVp means that the photons have higher energies and can penetrate thicker object. The radiation dose is proportional to the square of the kVp. *(Seeram, 3rd ed., p. 114, 231)*

9. **(A)** The term isotropic is described as uniformity in all orientations. For a CT image this means the x, y, and z planes must have the same dimensions. *(Prokop, p. 4)*

10. **(A)** Photon flux is primarily dependent on the combination of kVp, mAs, and beam filtration with mAs being the most straightforward technical factor to change when contrast resolution is required. mAs is directly proportional to the number of photons produced and the patient dose received. *(Seeram, 3rd ed., pp. 196–198)*

11. **(B)** As long as the FOV and the pixel size are known, the matrix size can be calculated

$$\text{Matrix} = \frac{\text{FOV}}{\text{pixel size}}$$

(Seeram, 3rd ed., p. 64)

12. **(B)** The purpose of slip-ring technology was to first eliminate the cable needed to transmit voltage from the generator to the gantry. The slip-ring assembly consists of a series of conductive rings for providing continuous high-voltage power to the generator, x-ray tube, collimators, and detector acquisition system. *(Seeram, 3rd ed., p. 112)*

13. **(D)** Temporal resolution refers to the precision of a measurement with respect to time. Often there is a trade-off between temporal resolution and spatial resolution. Fast acquisitions result in less samples (profiles) taken thus degrading spatial resolution. *(Seeram, 3rd ed., p. 198)*

14. **(C)** The best method to reduce the partial volume averaging artifact is to reduce the width of the slice. In the case of an image producing too much noise, several slices can be summed producing an image with less noise and without the scan-induced artifact. *(Kalendar, 3rd ed., p. 132)*

15. **(A)** Gas ionization detectors do not produce after-glow, since they do not employ scintillation

material. The detectors use gas (xenon) ionization chambers which convert x-ray energy directly into electrical energy. The disadvantage of these detectors is their low QDE and they can produce detector pile-up. *(Seeram, 3rd ed., pp. 122–125)*

16. **(A)**

$$\text{CT number} = \frac{\mu(\text{tissue}) - \mu(\text{water})}{\mu(\text{water})} \times 1,000$$

$$\text{CT number} = \frac{0.215 - 0.206}{0.206} \times 1,000$$

$$\text{CT number} = 0.43 \times 1,000$$

$$\text{CT number for soft tissue} = 43 \, \text{HU}$$

(Kalendar, 3rd ed., p. 354)

17. **(D)** When there are gaps between detectors, there is a possibility a photon will not hit the intended detector; thus, causing no signal. When the detectors are firmly packed together, this phenomenon is less likely to occur resulting in an increased total detector efficiency. *(Seeram, 3rd ed., pp. 122–123)*

18. **(B)** The filtered back projection of reconstruction uses a method similar to back projection, since it averages the attenuation values for all projections that cross the data point, but performs the process in the spatial frequency domain. In using the frequency data, a mathematical kernel is applied to manipulate the amplitudes to reconstruct the image with either a sharp or soft appearance. *(Kalendar, 3rd ed., p. 30)*

19. **(B)** Edge gradient artifacts occur because of the CT system's inability to process high spatial frequency signal required for sharp edges. When two densities of different atomic number are scanned in the same plane, such as barium and air in the stomach, the system sees them as one structure, resulting in a blurring at the borders or edges of the high frequency object. *(Hale, 2013)*

20. **(C)** The iterative reconstruction method takes the attenuation coefficient intensities and back projects them onto the matrix with the assumption that all the intensities have the same value. This technique involves a series of corrections applied to the data to bring it into better agreement with the measured

projections and then new corrections are applied until a satisfactory agreement is obtained. *(Seeram, 3rd ed., p. 141)*

21. **(D)** The DFOV is the product of the pixel size and the matrix size

    DFOV = pixel size × matrix size

    DFOV = 0.625 mm × 1024

    DFOV = 640 mm

    (Seeram, 3rd ed., p. 64)

22. **(C)** Digital Imaging and Communication in Medicine (DICOM) was originally developed by the National Electrical Manufacturers Association (NEMA) and the American College of Radiology (ACR) for computerized axial tomography and magnetic resonance imaging images. In 1985, The ACR-NEMA committee was formed to explore ways of standardizing the interconnection of imaging devices and establishing a reasonable common ground for users and vendors to transmit digital data files. *(DICOM PS3.1)*

23. **(D)** kVp is a qualitative measure of the x-ray beam; therefore, an increase in kVp produces an increase in photon energy. The typical ranges of kVp in CT are 100 to 140 kVp. *(Mayer-Smith, 2104)*

24. **(C)** The SFOV is the region or volume for which complete data sets can be acquired. The size depends on the fan angle. The object to be scanned must be within the SFOV to avoid artifacts due to data inconsistencies. *(Kalendar, 3rd ed., p. 121)*

25. **(A)** In order to visualize small bony details or lesions in the spine a high-pass convolution kernel is needed for image reconstruction. This kernel is intended to sharpen small objects in an image by suppressing the low spatial frequencies in the image, improving the overall detail of the image. *(Seeram, 3rd ed., pp. 75–76)*

26. **(D)** Beam hardening occurs due to the laws of physics interaction with mater. As a beam passes through an object, the mean energy increases, because the lower energy photons are absorbed more than the higher energy photons producing a more penetrating beam of radiation. The degree to which beam hardening occurs depends on the

composition of the tissue, more for bone and less on fat. These artifacts are a particular problem in the posterior cranial fossa, with metal implants, and between dense bone and soft tissues. *(Boas, 2012)*

27. **(D)** Windowing is a computer visualization tool by which the image gray scale is manipulated with regard to the CT number of the structure of interest. The two main components of windowing include window width (controls contrast) and window level (controls the brightness levels). *(Seeram, 3rd ed., pp. 169–170)*

28. **(A)** The transmitted data produce a signal at the detectors, which is in analog form. In order for the computer to process this information, it must be converted into discrete or binary numbers. This process is performed by the ADC. *(Seeram, 3rd ed., pp. 128–129)*

29. **(B)** Adaptive statistical iterative reconstruction is a hybrid algorithm that blends with filtered back projection (FBP). It estimates raw data sets and compares the sets to the measured data sets from the CT system. This process is repeated until an acceptable range has been reached. The ASIR technique models photons and electric noise in the CT system to suppress noise, reduce dose, by lowering mAs, and improve low-contrast detectability. *(Honours, 2014)*

30. **(C)** A good quality assurance program requires the testing to be performed on a regular basis designated by the quality control team, the measurements should be interpreted upon completion of the test to assure the scanner is working according to its standards, and good documentation is required so that measurement can be compared from test to test. *(Seeram, 3rd ed., pp. 408–481)*

31. **(B)** Quantity refers the number of photons. Tube current in CT is calculated by the product of the true mA and the rotation time. In MDCT the term effective mAs is utilized, which denoted the mAs per slice. This relationship is given by the following equation: Effective mAs = true mAs/pitch. *(Mayer-Smith, Seeram, 3rd ed., p. 230)*

32. **(A)** Faster scanners reduce motion artifact because the patient has less time to move during the acquisition. This can be accomplished with

faster gantry rotation or more x-ray sources. More detector rows allow a greater volume to be imaged in a single gantry rotation, thus increasing the distance between step-off artifacts from motion on coronal or sagittal reformats. *(Boas, 2012)*

33. **(B)** The second generations scanner employed a translate–translate scanning principle in which the tube and detectors would translate across the patients, translate back, and then rotate the assemble 10-degrees. When there are 5 to 30 detectors incorporated in the scanner, it increases its performance by 5 to 30 times compared to the first generation scanners. *(Prokop, p. 3; Seeram 3rd ed., p. 105)*

34. **(D)** The major advantages of 180-degree z-interpolation include: improved z-axis resolution, the generation of thinner slices, and scanning at higher pitches. These advantages are accomplished, since two data sets (spiral and virtual) are generated in opposite direction of each other. *(Prokop p. 12)*

35. **(B)** Cine viewing is an image display tool that allows the user to interpret a large amount of data sets. This tool became imperative with the inception of MDCT. Its main advantages are that it provides a more accurate evaluation of structures, speeds up the interpretation time, and increases the efficiency of the PACS system. *(Prokop, p. 48)*

36. **(C)** Gas ionization detectors are filled with the noble or inert gas, xenon at high pressure (pressurized to about 30 atmospheres to increase the number of gas molecules available). This is done to achieve high x-ray absorption. *(Kalendar, 3rd ed., p. 368)*

37. **(C)** Measurement data undergo preprocessing to correct any errors that may have resulted from beam hardening, bad detectors, motion artifacts, or interpolation artifacts. These corrections are made before the image reconstructed algorithm is applied. *(Seeram, 3rd ed., p. 144)*

38. **(C)** Anti-scatter grids (ASG) were developed to rectify the scatter issue notably seen in detector system having 64 or more detectors. The x-ray beam becomes a cone lending to an increase of penumbra. These grids are placed in front of the detectors arranged in a 1D or 2D format system of thin lamellae made of strongly absorbing material. *(Kalendar, 3rd ed., p. 51)*

39. **(C)** Window width controls the contrast of the image by selecting a specific range of shades of gray from the Hounsfield scale displayed on the CT monitor. The window width is chosen according to the attenuation values inherited in the anatomy of interest. It is important to understand the effects window width has on image contrast. As the number of shades of gray decreases, image contrast increases giving the reconstructed image a black and white appearance. On the contrary, image contrast decreases as the width increases, since more shades of gray are available. *(Seeram, 3rd ed., pp. 170–177)*

40. **(D)** The terms uniformity or homogeneity can be interchanged with their simplest meanings are the same; therefore, the goal of uniformity is to maintain a constant CT value for water, over the entire cross-section of a homogeneous water phantom. The measurements of each ROI should not deviate more than 4 to 5 HU of each other. *(Kalendar, 3rd ed., p. 112)*

41. **(D)** A midrange computer was known in the past as a minicomputer. This computer is smaller than a mainframe computer, but larger than a microcomputer (personal computer). The midrange computer deals efficiently with the convoluted mathematical input and produces output data at subsecond time intervals. Its major characteristics are its large storage capacity and fast and efficient processing of various kinds of data. *(Seeram, 3rd ed., p. 33)*

42. **(A)** In a homogenous beam (gamma ray), all the photons have the same energy. This type of beam is also known as a monochromic or monoenergetic beam. The homogeneous beams like the gamma rays that Hounsfield used for his first CT device satisfied the requirements of the Lambert–Beer law for image reconstruction. *(Seeram, 3rd ed., pp. 90–91)*

43. **(D)** total beam collimation = number of rows $\times$ aperture size

    total beam collimation = 128×0.6

    total beam collimation = 76.8

(Seeram, 3rd ed., p. 272)

44. **(B)** The noise value can be measured by means of the standard deviation (ǒ) indicating the amount of variance among pixel values in a desired ROI. Noise can be distinguished on an image as a grainy mottled appearance. The noise test requires the use of a 20 cm water phantom. The results of the test depend on the type of algorithm used (higher with sharp algorithms and lower for smooth algorithms) but should stay steady from day to day. If the measurement increases, it indicates more variation in the pixel to pixel CT numbers and poorer low contrast detectability. *(Seeram, 3rd ed., pp. 482–483)*

45. **(C)** A contiguous interval is one in which the thickness of the slice and the spacing between two slices are equal. *(Seeram, 3rd ed., pp. 260–262)*

46. **(D)** The distributed processing system processes information by more than one computers connected by a network system. It is characterized by having each computer perform a particular task and the combined work contributes to a larger goal. *(Seeram, 3rd ed., p. 34)*

47. **(B)** Linearity refers to the relationship of the CT number of the reconstructed object to the measured linear attenuation coefficient. Linearity is measured using a Catphan phantom with distinctive materials representing bone, contrast, fat, water, and air. The linear attenuation coefficient values of each material are plotted against its respective CT number. A line graph demonstrating a straight line indicates an acceptable linearity QA. test *(Seeram, 3rd ed., p. 202; Kalendar, 3rd ed., pp. 113–114)*

48. **(D)** The problem in CT is to determine the attenuation of the tissues and use this information to reconstruct an image of the slice of tissue. Attenuation is the reduction of the intensity of a beam of radiation as it passes through an object, some photons are absorbed, but others are scattered. The attenuation of the beam is dependent on the electrons per gram of tissue, the atomic number of the tissue, tissue density, and the radiation energy used. *(Seeram, 3rd ed., p. 89)*

49. **(B)** The principle of multiplanar reformation is to reconstruct a new series of images at arbitrary or even curved planes defined by the operator, using the pixel data from a stack of transaxial images. With the introduction of MDCT, coronal and sagittal reformats became a common postprocessing technique. *(Kalendar, 3rd ed., pp. 48–50)*

50. **(A)** Windowing is a computer visualization tool by which the image gray scale is manipulated with regard to the CT number of the structure of interest (Fig. E3.2). Windowing contributes to the brightness and contrast of the image. The two main components of windowing include window width and window level. *(Seeram, 3rd ed., p. 171)*

51. **(C)**

$$\text{pitch} = \frac{\text{table speed}\left(\dfrac{\text{mm}}{\text{sec}}\right) \times \text{gantry rotation}(\text{sec})}{\text{total beam collimation}}$$

$$\text{pitch} = \frac{40\,\text{mm} \times 0.5\,\text{sec}}{32 \times 0.625}$$

$$\text{pitch} = \frac{20\,\text{mm/sec}}{20\,\text{mm}}$$

$$\text{pitch} = 1 : 1$$

(Kalendar, 3rd ed., p. 89)

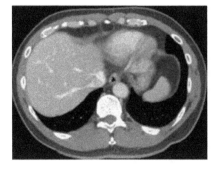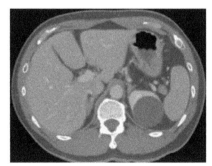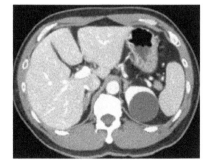

Figure E3.2. The CT axial image above demonstrate three distinct windowing techniques. (A) 450WW and 50WL enhances organs with regards to bone, air, and contrast. (B) 2000WW and 600WL, improves the bone detail of the ribs and spine. (C) 150WW and 50WL increases image contrast enhancing the liver parenchymal Reproduced, with permission, from Seeram E. *Computed Tomography: Physical Principles, Clinical Applications, and Quality Control.* 3rd ed. St. Louis, MO: Saunders Elsevier; 2009.

52. **(D)** Figure Q3.1 demonstrates a bone window which enhances the bony details of the fracture. Window level, center, or length controls the brightness of the image. The level is chosen according to the average attenuation value of the structure of interest and is found in the middle of the range of CT numbers used in the reconstructed image. When the area of interest is bone, it is best to place the level at 500 to 800, since the attenuation of bone ranges from 250 to 1,000 HU. *(Kalendar, 3rd ed., p. 32)*

53. **(D)** Minimum intensity projection (MinP) technique uses the minimum or lowest attenuation values to display the images. This protocol aids in diagnosing abnormalities of the central tracheobronchial system and for localizing extrabronchial air collections and in demonstrating strictures, concentric stenosis, and dilations. *(Prokop, p. 60)*

54. **(A)** The equation for calculating CT window range is:

$$WL + \frac{WW}{2} \qquad\qquad WL - \frac{WW}{2}$$
$$50 + \frac{450}{2} \qquad\qquad 50 - \frac{450}{2}$$
$$50 + 225 \qquad\qquad 50 - 225$$
$$275 \qquad\qquad -175$$

(Seeram, 3rd ed., p 172)

Subspecialty List

33. Physics and Instrumentation — Radiation Interaction with Matter — Acquisition (Geometry)

34. Physics and Instrumentation — Image Processing — Interpolation

35. Physics and Instrumentation — Image Display — Cine

36. Physics and Instrumentation — CT System Principles, Operations, and Components — Detector Configuration

37. Physics and Instrumentation — Image Processing — Raw data vs image data

38. Physics and Instrumentation — CT System Principles, Operations, and Components — Collimation/ Beam Width

39. Physics and Instrumentation — Image Display — Windowing

40. Physics and Instrumentation — Image Quality — Uniformity

41. Physics and Instrumentation — CT System Principles, Operations, and Components — Computer and Array Processor

42. Physics and Instrumentation — Radiation Interaction with Matter — Physical Principles (Attenuation)

43. Physics and Instrumentation — CT System Principles, Operations, and Components — Collimation/ Beam Width

44. Physics and Instrumentation — Image Quality — Standard Deviation

45. Physics and Instrumentation — Image Processing — Reconstruction Interval

46. Physics and Instrumentation — CT System Principles, Operations, and Components — Computer and Array Processor

47. Physics and Instrumentation — Image Quality — Linearity

48. Physics and Instrumentation — Radiation Interaction with Matter — Physical Principles (Attenuation)

49. Physics and Instrumentation — Image Processing — Multiplanar Reformation

50. Physics and Instrumentation — Image Display — Windowing

51. Physics and Instrumentation — Image Quality — Spatial Resolution

52. Physics and Instrumentation — Image Display — Windowing

53. Physics and Instrumentation—Image Reconstruction—3D Reformation

54. Physics and Instrumentation — Image Display — Windowing

CHAPTER 4

Practice Test 1
Questions

1. What is the purpose of performing an unenhanced CT scan of the liver?

   (A) to demonstrate hepatocellular carcinoma
   (B) to demonstrate hepatomas
   (C) to demonstrate cirrhosis
   (D) to demonstrate fatty infiltrates

2. Which dural fold lines the longitudinal fissure?

   (A) falx cerebelli
   (B) tentorium cerebelli
   (C) falx cerebri
   (D) infundibulum

3. In patients with liver dysfunction or who are in cardiac failure and who have normal renal function, metformin should be discontinued at the time of an examination or procedure using intravenous iodinated contrast media and withheld for how many hours post injection?

   (A) 12 hours
   (B) 24 hours
   (C) 48 hours
   (D) should not receive iodinated contrast media

4. What arterial branch of the aorta arises at L1 and is posterior to the neck of the pancreas?

   (A) celiac artery
   (B) SMA
   (C) iliac artery
   (D) phrenic artery

5. The floor of the third ventricle is formed by what organ of the brain?

   (A) thalamus
   (B) caudate nucleus
   (C) midbrain
   (D) hypothalamus

6. Which of the following is a potential complication from the use of barium sulfate as an oral contrast agent?

   (A) leakage
   (B) extravasation
   (C) colitis
   (D) pancreatitis

7. A set of ROIs is recorded on a CT image of the abdomen, one placed within the liver and one placed within the spleen; this is often used to document which of the following conditions?

   (A) splenomegaly
   (B) fatty infiltrate of the liver
   (C) sickle cell disease
   (D) lymphoma

8. What CT imaging plane is the most common entity for identifying pars defects?

   (A) transaxial
   (B) sagittal
   (C) coronal
   (D) 3D-shaded surface rendering

9. What is the purpose of the slip-ring technology employed in modern CT scanners?

   (A) capacity for continuous acquisition protocols
   (B) decrease temporal resolution
   (C) increase tube loading
   (D) employ single data acquisition protocols

10. How should lead shielding (if being utilized) be placed on the patient during a CT examination of the brain?

    (A) under the patient's body region not being examined
    (B) under and over the patient's body region not being examined
    (C) over the patient's body region
    (D) no need to use shielding for a CT examination

11. The approach to patients about to undergo a contrast-enhanced examination has three general goals. Which of the following is **not** part of this methodology?

    (A) to assure that the administration of contrast is appropriate for the patient and the indication
    (B) to be unconcerned about the patient's medical history
    (C) to minimize the likelihood of a contrast reaction
    (D) to be fully prepared to treat a reaction should one occur

12. The thalamus and hypothalamus are a part of which section of the brain?

    (A) cerebrum
    (B) diencephalon
    (C) midbrain
    (D) cerebellum

13. Name an advantage of utilizing the Fourier transform for image reconstruction:

    (A) manipulation of data in the spatial frequency domain
    (B) manipulation of data in the spatial location domain
    (C) calculating the intensities along the ray sum
    (D) calculating the CT number of the given intensities

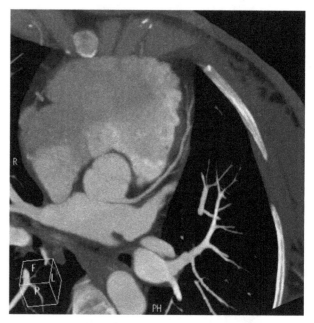

Figure Q4.1 Reproduced, with permission, from Grey ML, Ailinani JM. *CT and MRI Pathology: A Pocket Atlas.* 2nd ed. New York, NY: McGraw-Hill; 2012.

14. Figure Q4.1 above demonstrates which of the following 3D techniques?

    (A) volume rendered (VRT)
    (B) maximum intensity projection (MIP)
    (C) minimum intensity projection (MinIP)
    (D) multiplanar reformation (MPR)

15. Heating is a process which lowers the viscosity of a contrast agent; at what temperature should an LOCM be at the time of injection?

    (A) 98.6°F
    (B) 72°F
    (C) 32°F
    (D) 102°F

16. A particular CT image has a matrix size of 512^2 and a field-of-view (FOV) of 360 mm, what is the pixel area?

    (A) 0.7 mm
    (B) 4.9 mm^2
    (C) 0.7 cm^2
    (D) 0.49 mm^2

17. Peritoneal ligaments serve to connect organs with another organ or to the abdominal wall; what is the function of the hepatorenal ligament?

    (A) connects the stomach to the liver
    (B) connects the liver to the kidney
    (C) connects the gall bladder to the hepatic flexure
    (D) connects the stomach to the diaphragm

18. Which of the following scientist theory states the sampling rate must be at least twice the highest analog frequency component?

    (A) Hounsfield
    (B) Cormack
    (C) Nyquist
    (D) Radon

19. Name the space between the dura mater and arachnoid meningeal layers:

    (A) epidural space
    (B) subdural space
    (C) prearachnoid space
    (D) subarachnoid space

20. Which of the following medication is not an essential drug found on the emergency cart?

    (A) Solu-Medrol
    (B) Nitrostat
    (C) Ambien
    (D) Vasopressin

21. Which of the following refers to the ability of the CT detector to capture, absorb, and convert x-ray photons into electrical energy?

    (A) efficiency
    (B) stability
    (C) response time
    (D) dynamic range

22. The primary vendors of CT systems (GE, Siemens, Toshiba, and Philips) all have systems available which will reduce radiation dose. Which of the following is a commonplace technique that optimizes the dose to the patient while maintaining constant image quality?

    (A) subsecond scanning
    (B) hybrid detector array
    (C) dual energy scanning
    (D) automatic tube current modulation

23. Which of the following pathological infections cause damage to the heart valves and valve leakage?

    (A) pneumonia
    (B) pulmonary embolism
    (C) tuberculosis
    (D) carditis

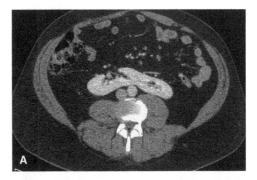

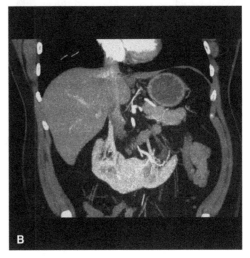

Figure Q4.2 Reproduced, with permission, from Grey ML, Ailinani JM. *CT and MRI Pathology: A Pocket Atlas.* 2nd ed. New York, NY: McGraw-Hill; 2012.

24. What pathological condition is demonstrated in Figure Q4.2?

    (A) pyelonephritis
    (B) vascular injury
    (C) renal cyst
    (D) horseshoe kidney

25. Patients at risk for stroke or heart attack may be prescribed anticoagulant medications. When performing an invasive procedure, it is imperative to check the patient's INR results. Which of the following INR ratios is appropriate for a patient on anticoagulant medication?

    (A) 1.0–2.0
    (B) 1.5–1.7
    (C) 2.0–3.0
    (D) 3.5–5.0

26. Which of the following organs is a triangular-shaped gland consisting of lymphoid tissue and is located in the superior portion of the mediastinum inferior to the manubrium?

    (A) thalamus gland
    (B) thymus gland
    (C) submandibular gland
    (D) thyroid gland

27. What structure in the brain produces cerebrospinal fluid from the blood?

    (A) pia mater of the brain
    (B) capillaries on the surface of the brain
    (C) choroid plexuses of the ventricles
    (D) subarachnoid space

28. Which of the following is **not** an advantage of today's iterative reconstruction algorithm?

    (A) reduces noise
    (B) improves image quality
    (C) reduction in mAs
    (D) increase in kVp

29. Extravasation can be defined as an accidental administration of intravenous contrast media into the extravascular space/tissue around the infusion site by an indirect or direct leakage. Once an extravasation or infiltration is noted, steps should be taken to make the patient comfortable. Which of the following is **not** a step in remedying the situation?

    (A) remove the needle
    (B) withdraw the fluid from the subcutaneous tissue
    (C) apply pressure on the injection site
    (D) administer either a moist hot or cold compress

30. Which of the following pathological conditions is characterized by a heterogeneous response to pulmonary injury?

    (A) pulmonary embolism
    (B) pulmonary thrombosis
    (C) hepatopulmonary syndrome
    (D) adult respiratory distress syndrome (ARDS)

31. Which of the following detector array systems consist of several solid-state small detectors of the same dimension that are arranged in rows of identical thickness?

    (A) hybrid array
    (B) adaptive array
    (C) matrix array
    (D) variable array

32. What ligament extends from the anterior part of the tibial spine and attaches to the posterior part of the medial surface of the lateral femoral condyle?

    (A) posterior cruciate ligament
    (B) anterior cruciate ligament
    (C) lateral collateral ligament
    (D) medial collateral ligament

33. What is the mathematical calculation to determine the voxel dimension of a digital image?

    (A) $voxel\,volume = \dfrac{FOV}{matrix}$
    (B) $voxel\,volume = pixel\,size \times slice\,thickness$
    (C) $voxel\,volume = pixel\,area \times slice\,thickness$
    (D) $voxel\,volume = \dfrac{pixel\,area}{slice\,thickness}$

34. Which of the following refers to a method by which the patient is systematically scanned by the x-ray tube and detectors to collect enough information for image reconstruction?

(A) beam geometry

(B) data acquisition

(C) sampling

(D) projection reconstruction

35. A CT examination of the abdomen/pelvis typically results in an effective dose in which of the following ranges?

(A) 3 to 10 mGy

(B) 10 to 15 mR

(C) 3 to 10 mSv

(D) 3 to 8 Gy

36. What is the pitch having a table feed of 15.36, a gantry rotation of 0.3 seconds, and a detector collimation of 128 × 0.3 mm?

(A) 0.4:1

(B) 0.12:1

(C) 1:1

(D) 1.2:1

37. When a drug is injected directly into a vein, it is termed an intravenous injection. Which of the following is **not** a common anatomical site for the injection of contrast media for a CT examination of the chest?

(A) cephalic vein

(B) basilic vein

(C) basilar vein

(D) median cubital vein

38. The liver is divided into lobes according to their surface anatomy; which lobe is located in the anterior inferior surface?

(A) caudate

(B) left lobe

(C) quadrate

(D) right lobe

39. What CT artifact occurs when the object being scanned is outside the scan-field-of-view (SFOV)?

(A) out of field

(B) partial volume averaging

(C) cone beam

(D) motion

40. A fracture of the anterior arch categorized by bursting of the ring of the C1 vertebrae is a characteristic of which of the following spinal fractures?

(A) hangman's fracture

(B) traumatic type 4 spondylolisthesis

(C) Jefferson's fracture

(D) metastatic disease of the cervical

41. Which of the following conditions may put a patient at risk following the administration of IV contrast media?

(A) muscular dystrophy

(B) myasthenia gravis

(C) pregnancy

(D) HIV/AIDS

42. What pathological condition results from blood collection between the dura mater and the arachnoid mater?

(A) epidural hematoma

(B) subdural hematoma

(C) subarachnoid hematoma

(D) sinusitis

43. Which of the following is an attribute of the adjustable pre-patient collimators?

(A) prevent afterglow

(B) allows variable collimation for the desired total beam collimation

(C) maximizes the amount of penumbra caused by the focal spot size

(D) as close to the focal spot as possible

44. What is the most common malignant abdominal tumor in children ages 1 to 5?

    (A) renal lymphoma
    (B) polycystic kidney disease
    (C) angiomyolipoma
    (D) nephroblastoma

45. Which of the following preprocessing techniques broadens the slice sensitivity of the reconstructed data?

    (A) 360-degree *z*-interpolation
    (B) high-pass convolution filtering
    (C) 180-degree *z*-interpolation
    (D) low-pass convolution filtering

46. Which of the following laboratory test is of clinical use when there is a suspicion of deep venous thrombosis (DVT) or pulmonary embolism?

    (A) D-dimer
    (B) PTT
    (C) INR
    (D) AST

47. Which of the following cerebral lobes is located deep within the Sylvian fissure?

    (A) parietal lobe
    (B) temporal lobe
    (C) occipital lobe
    (D) insula

48. Which of the following are recommended by the Center for Devices and Radiological Health as a CT dose descriptor?

    (A) ionization chamber measurements
    (B) $CTDI_{volume}$
    (C) dose profile
    (D) projection profile

49. Which of the following pathological conditions is a major risk factor for stroke and can lead to brain damage?

    (A) salivary stone obstruction
    (B) goiter
    (C) carotid artery stenosis
    (D) jugular vein thrombosis

50. Which of the following angiocatheter gauge is the optimal IV access most commonly used in children?

    (A) 20 gauge
    (B) 24 gauge
    (C) 18 gauge
    (D) 22 gauge

51. A CT examination of the internal auditory canal possesses a DFOV of 10 cm and a pixel size of 0.195 mm; what is the matrix size?

    (A) 512^2
    (B) 320^3
    (C) 256^2
    (D) 192^2

52. Which chamber of the heart comprises the largest portion of the anterior surface of the chest and receives deoxygenated blood from the right atrium and forces it into the pulmonary trunk for transportation to the lungs?

    (A) right ventricle
    (B) right atrium
    (C) left atrium
    (D) left ventricle

53. Which of the following statements is **true** concerning the celiac trunk?

    (A) it is superior to the renal arteries on the abdominal aorta
    (B) it is the only unpaired visceral branch of the aorta
    (C) it divides into the gastric, splenic, and mesenteric arteries
    (D) it branches from the aorta at the level of L2/L3 vertebral level

54. What type of artifacts can arise from insufficient projection sampling or from insufficient view sampling?

    (A) aliasing
    (B) motion
    (C) beam-hardening
    (D) interpolation

55. Premedication is given to patients who are at risk for an adverse event when given an iodinated contrast media. Which of the following medications is used in emergency situations for these patients?

    (A) Naproxen
    (B) Digitalis
    (C) Solu-Cortef
    (D) Gastrografin

56. What refers to the retention of excess gas in all or part of the lungs during any phase of expiration?

    (A) pulmonary fibrosis
    (B) pleural edema
    (C) pleural effusion
    (D) air trapping

57. Contrast resolution is superior with CT examinations principally because of what feature?

    (A) collimation
    (B) low kVp
    (C) high-pass convolution kernel
    (D) postprocessing

58. What structure may appear as a calcified midline structure on CT scans?

    (A) clivus
    (B) falx cerebri
    (C) pineal gland
    (D) dipole

59. Which of the following is recognized as the number one aseptic priority?

    (A) sterilization of the CT table
    (B) not shaking hands with the patient
    (C) handwashing
    (D) changing linen after each patient interaction

60. Which of the following is a characteristic of raw data?

    (A) known as scan data
    (B) undergoes corrections for errors that occurred
    (C) can be sent to a laser printer for hard-copy viewing
    (D) is the unprocessed computer data in the form of binary numbers

61. Which of the following traumatic pathological processes within the abdominal cavity presents with attenuation values within 20 HU of the aorta and is a life-threatening situation?

    (A) cyst
    (B) abscess
    (C) ascites
    (D) hemorrhage

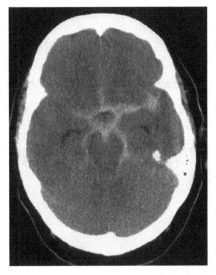

Figure Q4.3 Reproduced, with permission, from Grey ML, Ailinani JM. *CT and MRI Pathology: A Pocket Atlas.* 2nd ed. New York, NY: McGraw-Hill; 2012.

62. What pathological condition is demonstrated in Figure Q4.3?

    (A) epidural hematoma
    (B) subdural hematoma
    (C) subarachnoid hematoma
    (D) metastatic lesion

63. Computed tomography systems typically report two pieces of information related to radiation dose about each scan, which of the following represents these dose measurements?

    (A) MSAD and $CTDI_{100}$
    (B) $CTDI_{100}$ and $CTDI_W$
    (C) DLP and $CTDI_{100}$
    (D) $CTDI_{volume}$ and DLP

64. Specialized in-dwelling catheters are used to monitor critically ill patients and those who need long-term care. Which of the following catheters are used to measure cardiac output?

    (A) Port-A-Cath
    (B) PICC
    (C) Hickman
    (D) Swan-Ganz

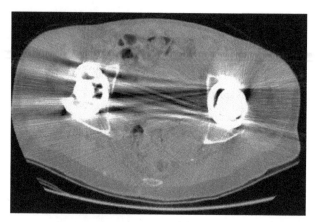

Figure Q4.5 Reproduced, with permission, from Seeram E. *Computed Tomography: Physical Principles, Clinical Applications, and Quality Control.* 3rd ed. St. Louis, MO: Saunders Elsevier; 2009.

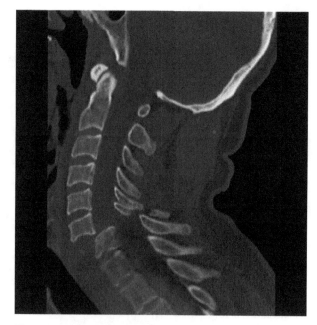

Figure Q4.4 Reproduced, with permission, from Grey ML, Ailinani JM, *CT and MRI Pathology: A Pocket Atlas.* 2nd ed. New York, NY: McGraw-Hill; 2012.

65. The CT sagittal image in Figure Q4.4 demonstrates a greater than 75% slipping of C6 over C7. Which of the following pathological conditions does this represent?

    (A) traumatic type 4 spondylolisthesis
    (B) traumatic type 2 spondylolisthesis
    (C) spondylolysis
    (D) traumatic type 1 spondylolisthesis

66. The artifact depicted in Figure Q4.5 arises due to which of the following reasons?

    (A) patient involuntary motion
    (B) inconstancies of the projected data on the reconstructed image due to the high density of the metal
    (C) object is partially lying within an individual slice
    (D) insufficient projection sampling

67. Which of the following is located in the retroperitoneal space?

    (A) spleen
    (B) liver
    (C) ileum
    (D) abdominal aorta

68. Which of the following is a characteristic of a heterogeneous beam?

    (A) all photons have the same energy
    (B) attenuation causes the quality or mean energy of the photons to be altered by the absorber
    (C) it is considered a monochromatic beam
    (D) attenuation causes the number of photons to remain the same, while the mean energy increases

69. A particular CT image possesses a pixel size of 0.68 mm; what is the DFOV that was used during reconstruction?

    (A) 750 mm
    (B) 348 mm
    (C) 237 mm
    (D) 512 mm

70. Anaphylactic shock is a life-threatening condition that can result in respiratory or cardiac arrest. Which of the following would **not** be a sign or symptom of an anaphylactic reaction?

    (A) itching of palms hands and sole of the feet
    (B) cool, clammy skin
    (C) dysphagia
    (D) erythema

71. A 64-slice CT scanner has a total beam collimation of 38.8 mm for a CT examination of the abdomen and pelvis. What is the size of each detector aperture?

    (A) 0.3
    (B) 0.6
    (C) 1.2
    (D) 2.4

72. Which of the following diseases occurs when a small segment of the talus bone begins to separate from its surrounding region due to a lack of blood supply?

    (A) osteochondral dissecans
    (B) LisFranc fracture
    (C) osteonecrosis
    (D) osteosarcoma

73. Temporal resolution can be improved by employing what technical factor?

    (A) increase kVp
    (B) decrease mA
    (C) increase gantry rotation time
    (D) decrease slice thickness

74. Which of the following pathological conditions of the kidneys will demonstrate a hyperdense structure within the renal pelvis or renal parenchyma?

    (A) renal cell carcinoma
    (B) renal stone
    (C) polycystic kidney disease
    (D) horseshoe kidney

75. Which of the following contrast media listed below does **not** increase the osmolality of the blood serum?

    (A) Ioxaglate meglumine
    (B) Diatrizoate meglumine
    (C) Ioversol
    (D) Iothalamate meglumine

76. What is defined as the spacing between each reconstructed image?

    (A) reconstruction algorithm
    (B) reconstruction interval
    (C) prospective data
    (D) retrospective reconstruction

77. Which of the following pathological diseases requires the CT technologist to perform an HRCT scan with the patient in the prone position?

    (A) cystic fibrosis
    (B) asbestosis
    (C) pleural effusion
    (D) pulmonary embolism

78. Which of the following requirements was recently added as a requirement by the U.S. Food and Drug Administration to avoid radiation injuries?

    (A) dose check
    (B) dose limits
    (C) dose optimization
    (D) dose justification

79. In relationship to the vertebral column, where is the pancreas located?

    (A) fifth and eighth thoracic vertebrae
    (B) ninth and eleventh thoracic vertebrae
    (C) twelfth thoracic and second lumbar vertebrae
    (D) second and fourth lumbar vertebrae

80. The typical flow rate for a CTA of the chest requires 5 cc/s utilizing 100 cc of nonionic contrast media for a total duration time of 20 seconds. The patient habitus is larger than normal; so the radiologist asks for the amount of contrast to be increased to 125 cc. What will the duration time be for this examination?

    (A) 25 seconds
    (B) 28 seconds
    (C) 30 seconds
    (D) 32 seconds

81. When images are transmitted to a PACS system or other devices, they are encrypted and compressed during transportation for speed and security. What type of compression is required by Health Insurance Portability and Accountability Act (HIPAA) for the transmission of medical data?

    (A) lossy
    (B) irreversible
    (C) truncated
    (D) lossless

82. Which of the following pathological conditions is caused by a deficiency in hormone synthesis?

    (A) salivary gland abscess
    (B) goiter
    (C) thymus CA
    (D) carotid stenosis

83. Which of the following is the cause of the aliasing artifact?

    (A) increase in the photon energy as it passes through matter
    (B) x-ray absorption
    (C) gas ionization detectors
    (D) limited number of samples

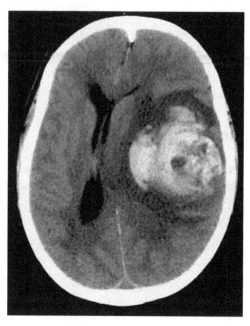

Figure Q4.6 Reproduced, with permission, from Seeram E. *Computed Tomography: Physical Principles, Clinical Applications, and Quality Control.* 3rd ed. St. Louis, MO: Saunders Elsevier; 2009.

84. What pathological condition is demonstrated in Figure Q4.6?

    (A) brain infarct
    (B) cerebral hematoma
    (C) epidural hematoma
    (D) acoustic neuroma

85. A patient arrives in the CT department with a closed chest tube inserted in the posterior inferior chest wall. In what position should the drainage system be placed when moving this patient from the stretcher to the CT table?

    (A) below the level of the patient's chest to avoid reverse flow
    (B) the unit should be placed between the patient's legs to avoid spillage of the fluid
    (C) the unit should be placed on an IV pole as to not dislodge the tube
    (D) patients with chest tubes should not be transported

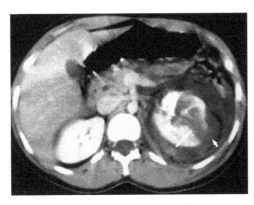

Figure Q4.7 Reproduced, with permission, from Grey ML, Ailinani JM. *CT and MRI Pathology: A Pocket Atlas.* 2nd ed. New York, NY: McGraw-Hill; 2012.

86. What pathological condition is demonstrated in the Figure Q4.7?

(A) renal cell carcinoma

(B) pyelonephritis

(C) kidney laceration

(D) angiomyolipoma

87. What is the range of CT numbers if the window width is 2,000 and the window level is 700?

(A) −1,700 to 300

(B) 1,700 to −300

(C) 2,300 to 1,650

(D) −2,300 to 1,650

88. Which artery appears as a T-shaped structure on cross-sectional images?

(A) pulmonary trunk

(B) right common carotid artery

(C) splenic artery

(D) bifurcation of the iliac arteries

89. Which of the following is a newer CT-derived value in milligrays (mGy) that incorporates patient size as a modifying correction factor to better estimate patient dose?

(A) CTDI$_W$

(B) SSDE

(C) MSAD

(D) DLP

90. A CT water phantom was scanned and the linear attenuation coefficient of a particular pixel on the image measured 0.0004; what does this coefficient represent in terms of structures?

(A) water

(B) air

(C) fat

(D) calcium

91. What would the delivered volume amount of contrast media be for a flow rate of 3 cc/s and a duration time of 40 seconds?

(A) 75 cc

(B) 85 cc

(C) 100 cc

(D) 120 cc

92. What 3D technique is said to be a realistically looking 3D view of the contour of the structure of interest within the acquired volume data set?

(A) minimum intensity projection

(B) shaded surface display

(C) volume-rendered technique

(D) multiplanar reformations

93. What ligament of the female pelvis passes laterally from the cervix and upper vagina to the fascia overlying the obturator internus muscle?

(A) broad ligament

(B) cardinal ligament

(C) round ligament

(D) uterosacral ligament

94. Which of the following QA test requires the operator to place 5 ROIs within a homogeneous water phantom?

(A) contrast resolution

(B) uniformity

(C) linearity

(D) bed index

95. What is the arch-shaped structure that makes up the inferior margin of the septum pellucidum?

    (A) fornix
    (B) foramen of Monroe
    (C) interventricular foramen
    (D) cerebral aqueduct

96. What refers to the general structure of a computer and includes both the elements of hardware and software?

    (A) midrange
    (B) architecture
    (C) control unit
    (D) arithmetic logic unit

97. Which of the following oxygen administration system is designed to deliver the volume of oxygen that meets the patient's specific needs?

    (A) nonrebreathing mask
    (B) nasal cannula
    (C) oxygen tent
    (D) Venturi mask

98. At what vertebral level does the adult spinal cord end?

    (A) T12
    (B) L1
    (C) L2
    (D) S2

99. The MTF can be used to estimate spatial resolution at which of the following frequencies?

    (A) at high spatial frequencies
    (B) at low spatial frequencies
    (C) at all spatial frequencies
    (D) by converting an LSF to an ERF

100. CT is the imaging choice for the diagnosis of blunt abdominal/pelvic trauma. Which of the following can be a cause of a ruptured bladder?

    (A) blow to the lower abdomen when the bladder is extended and/or a pelvic fracture
    (B) aneurysm in the internal iliac artery
    (C) thrombosis of the renal artery
    (D) blow to the lower abdomen when the rectum contains feces

101. Following the injection of an iodinated contrast media, the technologist noticed the patient's eyes and face are swollen, but claims he/she is feeling fine. Which of the following type of contrast reaction is this patient experiencing?

    (A) mild
    (B) moderate
    (C) severe
    (D) CIN

102. A CT image was produced with a 1.0-mm detector aperture size and was displayed using a 512^2 matrix and a 10-cm DFOV. What is the voxel dimension for this image?

    (A) $0.19 \text{ mm} \times 0.19 \text{ mm} \times 1.0 \text{ mm}$
    (B) $1.9 \text{ mm} \times 1.9 \text{ mm} \times 1.0 \text{ mm}$
    (C) $5.1 \text{ mm} \times 5.1 \text{ mm} \times 1.0 \text{ mm}$
    (D) $0.19 \text{ mm} \times 0.19 \text{ mm} \times 1.0 \text{ cm}$

103. An ER patient presents with sudden chest pain, shortness of breath (SOB), and left leg swelling. The patient states he/she had just returned from an 8-hour plane ride. Which of the following is the possible diagnosis the ER physician suspects?

    (A) pulmonary embolism
    (B) cystic fibrosis
    (C) pulmonary fibrosis
    (D) sarcoidosis

104. The Image Wisely and Image Gently campaigns provide information to radiologists, patients, and referring physicians about imaging examinations and appropriate tests for pediatric and adult populations, respectively. Which of the following is **not** a caveat of their efforts?

   (A) do not image for uncomplicated headache
   (B) do not image if cancer is expected in children
   (C) do not image for pulmonary embolism without a moderate-to-high pretest probability
   (D) do not perform CT for appendicitis in children until ultrasound has been considered

105. All CT generation scanners have their advantages and disadvantages. Which of the following is a disadvantage of the third-generation scanner?

   (A) allows for better x-ray beam collimation
   (B) increased scatter radiation
   (C) produce only tomographic sections of the brain
   (D) highly sensitive to detector performance which results in the appearance of ring artifact

106. In order to produce good image quality, the detectors must obtain enough sample to produce the reconstructed image. Which of the following is **not** a way of providing adequate samples?

   (A) closely packed detectors
   (B) quarter-shift detector system
   (C) increasing pitch
   (D) z-Sharp technology

107. Which of the following contrast agents is a dimer that consist of a molecule with two benzene rings each with three iodine atoms and **does not** dissociate in water?

   (A) Visipaque
   (B) Isovue
   (C) Optiray
   (D) Conray

108. Which of the following is illustrated by #12 in Figure Q4.8?

   (A) pedicle
   (B) transverse foramen
   (C) ventral rami
   (D) intervertebral foramen

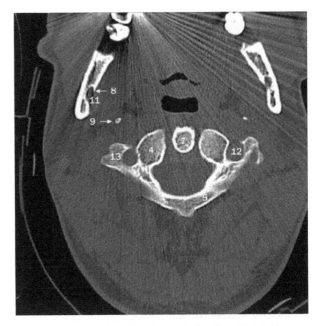

Figure Q4.8 Reproduced, with permission, from Weir J, Abrahams PH, Spratt JD, et al. *Imaging Atlas of Human Anatomy.* 4th ed. St. Louis, MO: Mosby Elsevier; 2011.

Refer to Figure Q4.8 to answer Questions 108–110.

109. The structure labeled #7 in Figure Q4.8 is

   (A) lateral mass of the atlas
   (B) occipital bone
   (C) odontoid process
   (D) transverse ligament attachment

110. Which of the following demonstrates the posterior arch of C1 in Figure Q4.8?

   (A) 13
   (B) 4
   (C) 12
   (D) 5

111. Which of the following reconstruction algorithms improves the appearance of contrast resolution?

   (A) high-pass convolution kernel
   (B) bone kernel
   (C) ultra-high kernel
   (D) smooth kernel

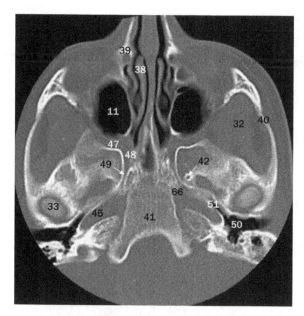

Figure Q4.9 Reproduced, with permission, from Weir J, Abrahams PH, Spratt JD, et al. *Imaging Atlas of Human Anatomy.* 4th ed. St. Louis, MO: Mosby Elsevier; 2011.

Refer to Figure Q4.9 to answer Questions 112–114.

112. In Figure Q4.9, #33 represents which anatomical structure?

(A) mandibular condyle
(B) mastoid atrium
(C) internal auditory canal
(D) foramen rotundum

113. Which of the following is illustrated by #41 in Figure Q4.9?

(A) occipital condyle
(B) mastoid process
(C) temporal bone
(D) clivus

114. Which of the following is demonstrated by #50 in Figure Q4.9?

(A) mastoid air cells
(B) middle ear
(C) semicircular canal
(D) internal auditory canal

115. Which of the following vessels does not drain directly into the IVC?

(A) right suprarenal vein
(B) left renal vein
(C) right phrenic vein
(D) left gonadal vein

116. In what CT scanner does cone beam artifacts occur?

(A) first generation
(B) third generation with single detector
(C) fourth generation with ≥16 detector channels
(D) third generation with ≥16 detector channels

117. What type of data have been convoluted and back projected into the image matrix?

(A) raw data
(B) scan data
(C) image data
(D) prospective data

118. The American College of Radiology has set values for maximum doses for CT examinations that range from 20 mSV for abdomen to 75 mSV for the head. Technologists have the responsibility to make sure they are adhering to the principles of radiation safety. Which of the following cardinal principles of radiation protection lessens the skin dose to the patient?

(A) ALARA
(B) time
(C) shielding
(D) distance

119. A CT examination of the brain was performed using a 300-mm SFOV and a 250-mm DFOV. The radiologist requested the images be reconstructed with a DFOV of 350-mm. What is needed to perform this new reconstruction?

(A) raw data targeting the images outside the SFOV
(B) image data targeting the images outside the SFOV
(C) measurement data to preprocess the data to include more detector information
(D) images are not able to be reconstructed to size larger than 300 mm

120. What muscle group is located on the anterolateral portion of the neck and originates from the transverse process of the cervical spine with its insertion point on the first and second ribs?

(A) scalene muscle

(B) trapezius muscle

(C) rhomboid muscle

(D) supraspinatus muscle

121. If all other parameters are held constant, doubling the pitch will have what effect on patient exposure?

(A) halve

(B) double

(C) quadruple

(D) remain the same

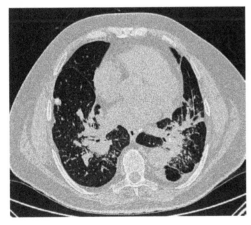

Figure Q4.10 Reproduced, with permission, from Grey ML, Ailinani JM. *CT and MRI Pathology: A Pocket Atlas.* 2nd ed. New York, NY: McGraw-Hill; 2012.

122. Figure Q4.10 demonstrates increasing opacification involving the mid-lung with marginal lung nodules and atelectasis. Which of the following diseases does this represent?

(A) pulmonary embolism

(B) pulmonary stenosis

(C) pulmonary thrombosis

(D) sarcoidosis

123. The voxel volume of an isotropic digital image is 0.125 mm³, and the slice thickness is 0.5 mm; what is the pixel area?

(A) 0.5 cm

(B) 0.25 mm²

(C) 0.5 mm²

(D) 0.25 cm

124. What organ of the female pelvis is a muscular tube that connects the uterine cavity with the exterior?

(A) fornix

(B) rectouterine pouch

(C) cervix

(D) vagina

125. Which of the following statements is **not true** concerning the preprocedural phase of patient education?

(A) two unique identifier are used to confirm patient identification

(B) an explanation of how the contrast media will be filtered through the body

(C) obtaining a proper medical history

(D) providing the patient with the proper instructions on the procedure

126. What is the term used for the group of detector electronics positioned between the detector array and the computer?

(A) hybrid detector arrays

(B) data acquisition system

(C) optoelectronic data transmissions

(D) analog-to-digital converter

127. The CT attenuation of extravasated blood (hemorrhage) depends on a number of factors. Which of the following factors **does not** apply?

(A) age of hemorrhage

(B) location of hemorrhage

(C) presence of clots

(D) amount of hemorrhage extravasation

128. Which of the following equations represents SNR?

(A) $SNR = mean\,ROI \times background\,ROI$

(B) $SNR = \dfrac{(mean\,ROI) - (background\,ROI)}{standard\,deviation}$

(C) $SNR = \dfrac{background\,ROI}{mean\,ROI}$

(D) $SNR = \dfrac{mean\,ROI}{background\,ROI}$

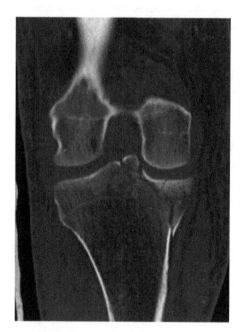

Figure Q4.11 Reproduced, with permission, from Grey ML, Ailinani JM. *CT and MRI Pathology: A Pocket Atlas*. 2nd ed. New York, NY: McGraw-Hill; 2012.

129. The image in Figure Q4.11 depicts, which of the following pathological conditions?

(A) bone contusion
(B) lateral collateral ligament tear
(C) tibial plateau fracture
(D) baker cyst

130. Which of the following CT examinations can be successfully performed with noisier images, and thus lower doses to the patients?

(A) brain
(B) soft tissue
(C) liver
(D) lungs

131. Which of the following types of data can be retrieved for later use?

(A) raw data
(B) image data
(C) measurement data
(D) convoluted data

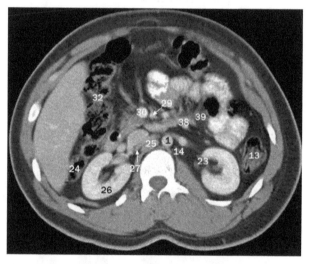

Figure Q4.12 Reproduced, with permission, from Weir J, Abrahams PH, Spratt JD, et al. *Imaging Atlas of Human Anatomy*. 4th ed. St. Louis, MO: Mosby Elsevier; 2011.

Refer to figure Q4.12 to answer Questions 132–134.

132. What number in Figure Q4.12 illustrates the superior mesenteric artery?

(A) 30
(B) 29
(C) 25
(D) 38

133. Which of the following is demonstrated by #24 in Figure Q4.12?

(A) right hepatic flexure
(B) gall bladder
(C) transverse colon
(D) ileum

134. Which of the following is illustrated by #23 in Figure Q4.12?

(A) left renal artery

(B) left renal vein

(C) left renal pelvis

(D) cyst in the left kidney

135. Which of the following pathological processes is characterized by a volume loss of a portion of a lung?

(A) asthma

(B) emphysema

(C) atelectasis

(D) pulmonary fibrosis

136. Which of the following artifacts give the appearance of a bright rim at the edge of the field of reconstruction?

(A) metal

(B) motion

(C) out of field

(D) beam hardening

137. CT enteroclysis involves combining which of the following techniques?

(A) barium enema and CT enterography

(B) barium swallow and CT angiography

(C) small-bowel enteroclysis and CT enterography

(D) small-bowel enteroclysis and virtual colonoscopy

138. What type of CT computer architecture employs one computer with two or more CPUs to process its data?

(A) parallel processing

(B) sequential processing

(C) pipeline processing

(D) distributed processing

139. What organ of the body is situated between the fundus of the stomach and the diaphragm?

(A) splenic flexure of the colon

(B) spleen

(C) pancreas

(D) gall bladder

140. The bronchus intermedius supplies air into which of the lung lobes?

(A) left middle lobe

(B) left lower lobe

(C) right upper lobe

(D) right middle lobe

141. The dimension of a voxel may be decreased by which of the following methods?

(A) decreasing the slice width

(B) decreasing the pixel size

(C) increasing the section width

(D) increasing the DFOV

142. What is the narrow inferior-third section of the uterus called?

(A) body

(B) fundus

(C) cornua

(D) cervix

143. When a CT x-ray beam experiences beam hardening, what happens to the mean photon energy of the beam?

(A) decreases

(B) increases

(C) is unaffected

(D) beam hardening and beam energy are not related

144. IV contrast reactions develop in all different forms. The term urticaria is used to describe which of the following types of reactions?

(A) bronchospasms

(B) hives

(C) feeling of warmth

(D) dizziness

145. Islet cell tumor is a collective term applied to tumors arising from endocrine cells in which organ of the body?

    (A) thyroid
    (B) pancreas
    (C) uterus
    (D) thymus

146. Which of the following postprocessing techniques extracts only those voxels from the data volume positioned one above the other within the coronal or sagittal plane?

    (A) prospective reconstruction
    (B) multiplanar reformation
    (C) object-based analysis
    (D) scene-based analysis

147. Which of the following glands are depicted as high-attenuation structures on CT images?

    (A) thyroid gland
    (B) parotid gland
    (C) submandibular gland
    (D) sublingual gland

148. What pathological process is the leading cause of work-related disabilities with a treatment regimen of nonsteroidal anti-inflammatory drugs used for pain?

    (A) avascular necrosis
    (B) osteoporosis
    (C) osteoarthritis
    (D) unicameral

149. If an MDCT scanner is equipped with 64 detectors and each detector possess a detector aperture size of 0.3 mm, what is the total beam collimation?

    (A) 10.5 mm
    (B) 15.2 mm
    (C) 19.2 mm
    (D) 38.8 mm

150. CT has the sensitivity for the detection of small tumors and is significantly useful for staging with the use of thin sections. In the TNM staging of pancreatic tumors, what does T2 represent?

    (A) carcinoma in situ
    (B) infiltration of the stomach, spleen, colon, and/or large vessels
    (C) tumor limited to pancreas but >2 cm
    (D) multiple regional lymph node metastases

151. What is the purpose of the intercostal muscles?

    (A) assist in forced expiration
    (B) push the abdominal viscera inferiorly
    (C) fixes the intercostal spaces rigid
    (D) act to elevate and protract the scapula

152. Which of the following liver tumors display an intense almost inhomogeneous enhancement during the arterial phase?

    (A) hypovascular lesions
    (B) hypervascular lesions
    (C) metastatic lesions
    (D) primary lesions

153. Which of the following artifacts occurs because of inconstancies of the projected data on the reconstructed image due to the high-density structure(s)?

    (A) cone beam
    (B) tube arcing
    (C) partial volume
    (D) metal

154. What heart valve prevents blood from flowing back into the left atrium from the left ventricle?

    (A) tricuspid valve
    (B) bicuspid valve
    (C) semilunar valve
    (D) chordae tendineae

155. Networking or connectivity became an essential aspect when radiology departments were urged to become filmless. Which of the following area networks covers an area of a few city blocks to the area of an entire city?

   (A) Local area network (LAN)
   (B) Wide area network (WAN)
   (C) Metropolitan area network (MAN)
   (D) World wide web (WWW)

156. Which ventricle forms the apex of the heart and has the function of pumping blood into the aorta?

   (A) right atrium
   (B) left atrium
   (C) right ventricle
   (D) left ventricle

157. Which of the following allows the technologist to alter the displayed picture contrast?

   (A) increasing kVp
   (B) decreasing mas
   (C) window width
   (D) retrospective reconstruction

158. Which ligament of the uterus extends out like a fan from the lateral wall of the cervix and vagina with the function of suspending the uterus above the bladder?

   (A) round ligament
   (B) broad ligament
   (C) cardinal ligament
   (D) uterosacral ligament

159. The beam collimation for this particular MDCT scanner is 12 mm and each detector aperture size is 0.5 mm, how many detector rows does this scanner possess?

   (A) 8
   (B) 12
   (C) 24
   (D) 64

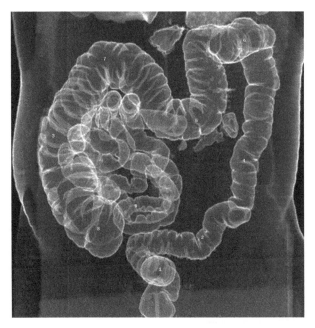

Figure Q4.13 Reproduced, with permission, from Weir J, Abrahams PH, Spratt JD, et al. *Imaging Atlas of Human Anatomy.* 4th ed. St. Louis, MO: Mosby Elsevier; 2011.

Refer to figure Q4.13 to answer Questions 160–162.

160. In Figure Q4.13 above, which of the following is illustrated by #6?

   (A) splenic flexure
   (B) transverse colon
   (C) descending colon
   (D) sigmoid colon

161. The structure labeled #9 in Figure Q4.13 is the

   (A) descending colon
   (B) ascending colon
   (C) terminal ileum
   (D) transverse colon

162. What 3D-rendering technique is illustrated in Figure Q4.13?

   (A) volume rendering (VRT)
   (B) surface-shaded display (SSD)
   (C) multiplanar reformation (MPR)
   (D) BE view

163. A female patient arrived in the ER complaining of right-sided back pain. A CT of the abdomen and pelvis was ordered and performed. During the interpretation of the images, the radiologist noticed a radiopaque density on her second lumbar spine and requested the images be retrospectively reconstructed in a bone reconstruction algorithm. Which of the following types of data can be used to perform this bone reconstruction?

    (A) scan data
    (B) raw data
    (C) measurement data
    (D) image data

164. Name the pathological condition that occurs as an interruption in the blood flow within the bone:

    (A) avascular necrosis
    (B) osteoporosis
    (C) osteoarthritis
    (D) unicameral

165. Name the detector array system consisting of thin detectors at the center and thicker detectors on either side of the central detectors:

    (A) hybrid array
    (B) adaptive array
    (C) nonuniform array
    (D) uniform array

Answers and Explanations

1. **(D)** Under normal circumstances, the spleen is approximately 10 HU lower than the liver. Fatty infiltrates may be focal or diffuse within the liver. Imaging characteristics of the liver on a computed tomography (CT) image demonstrate hypodense attenuation in appearance, as compared to that of the spleen, on an unenhanced series. *(Webb, p. 214)*

2. **(C)** The longitudinal fissure is a long, deep furrow dividing the cerebrum into two hemispheres. Located within this fissure is the falx cerebri. *(Kelley, 3rd ed., pp. 102–103)*

3. **(C)** Patients on the drug metformin for the treatment of type II diabetes have been placed into one of three categories by the American College of Radiology. Category I—patients with normal renal function and no known comorbidities: metformin does not need to be discontinued and post renal function test are not necessary. Category II—patients with multiple comorbidities who apparently have normal renal function: metformin should be discontinued at the time of an examination or procedure using intravenous (IV) iodinated contrast media and must be withheld for 48 hours post injection. Category III—patients with known renal dysfunction: metformin should be suspended at the time of contrast injection, and cautious follow-up of renal function should be performed until safe reinstitution of metformin can be assured. It is important to follow your institution's policies for the management of patients taking metformin. *(The American College of Radiology Manual. p. 44)*

4. **(B)** The SMA branches approximately 1 cm below the celiac trunk at approximately the level of L1. *(Madden, 3rd ed., p. 327)*

5. **(D)** The hypothalamus is formed by the floor and part of the lateral wall of the third ventricle. It is a relatively small organ, but controls many bodily functions related to maintaining homeostasis or stability within the body. *(Madden, 3rd ed., p. 17)*

6. **(A)** The most serious complication resulting from the use of barium in the gastrointestinal tract is leakage into the mediastinum or peritoneal cavity. The possible complications of a barium leak depend on the site at which it occurs. Esophageal leakage may cause mediastinitis. Stomach, duodenal, and small intestinal leakage may result in peritonitis. Escape of barium from the colon, where the bacterial count is highest, carries high mortality related to leakage of stool. No permanent harmful effects with the use of a water-soluble contrast media in the mediastinum, pleural cavity, or peritoneal cavity have been shown to occur. *(The American College of Radiology Manual, p. 57)*

7. **(B)** Normal liver attenuation is approximately 10 HU higher than the splenic parenchyma; therefore, if the liver measures a lower attenuation on an unenhanced CT scan, this most likely indicates a fatty infiltrate. The most common causes of fatty infiltrates in the United States is alcoholism. *(Grey, p. 260)*

8. **(B)** CT imaging utilizing sagittal reformations is the most common entity for identifying pars

defects. A pars defect is due to spondylolysis. This defect is usually a fracture of the vertebral arch between the superior and inferior facet joints (specifically, the pars interarticulares), occurring on one or both sides. *(Webb, p. 379)*

9. **(A)** The major advantage of slip-ring technology is for continuous rotation of the x-ray tube in order to produce a volume of data. It allows for faster scanning times with the elimination of interscan delays, and the ability of acquiring data in one breath-hold, eliminating motion. *(Seeram, 3rd ed., p. 113)*

10. **(B)** Shielding in CT is intended to protect not only the patient's sensitive organs (gonadal, breast, eyes, and thyroid), but also personnel and the general public. Through the public hype of radiation exposure in CT, patients are concerned about exposure. Due to the thin collimation, most exposure to the gonadal region is derived from internal scatter, except for direct exposure; therefore, there is no need for such a concern. When shielding patients the under and over method should be employed, due to the nature of the x-ray beam rotating around the patient. *(Seeram, 3rd ed., pp. 242–243)*

11. **(B)** The main goal of providing a safe environment for patients undergoing contrast-enhanced studies depends on obtaining an appropriate and adequate history for each patient, preparing the patient appropriately for the examination, having equipment available to treat reactions, and ensuring that an experienced staff is available to treat even the most severe reactions readily at hand. *(The American College of Radiology Manual, p. 5)*

12. **(B)** The thalamus and hypothalamus are located in the diencephalon. The thalamus is made up of a pair of large oval gray masses interconnected with most areas of the brain. It makes up a large portion of the walls of the third ventricle and is the relay station to and from the cerebral cortex for all sensory stimuli, except for the olfactory nerves. The hypothalamus is situated below the thalamus posterior to the optic chiasm forming the floor of the third ventricle. *(Kelley, 3rd ed., p. 113)*

13. **(A)** The first advantage of the data being in the frequency domain is that it can be manipulated by changing the amplitudes of the frequency components to determine the properties of the reconstructed image in terms of spatial resolution and image noise. *(Seeram, 3rd ed., pp. 142–143)*

14. **(B)** The 3D technique performed on the CT cardiac study is a maximum intensity projection (MIP). The CT procedure for coronary studies utilizes a rapid bolus of IV contrast with an injection delay to gain complete enhancement of the coronary arteries. The algorithm for rendering MIPs is such that it only brings forward tissues with the highest intensity being displayed. The MIP image in figure 4.1 validates a near complete occlusion of the right coronary artery. *(Grey, 2nd ed., p. 165; Seeram, 3rd ed., pp. 352–354)*

15. **(A)** Viscosity is determined by the number of particles and the attractions among the particles. The contrast media used in CT injections possess high viscosity. The process of making the injection tolerable is to reduce the friction, allowing the fluid to flow more freely. This is accomplished by heating the agent to body temperature. *(Adler, 5th ed., p. 296)*

16. **(D)** The formula for calculating pixel size is as follows:

$$pixel\,size = \frac{FOV}{matrix}$$
$$= \frac{360\,mm}{512}$$
$$= 0.7\,mm$$
$$pixel\,area = length \times width$$
$$= 0.7\,mm \times 0.7\,mm$$
$$= 0.49\,mm^2$$

(Seeram, 3rd ed., p. 64)

17. **(B)** The hepatorenal ligament is a peritoneal ligament that is not a ligament in its true sense, but a region of the mesentery connecting the liver to the kidney. *(Kelley, 3rd ed., p. 406)*

18. **(C)** The Nyquist theorem or sampling theorem states that the sampling rate must be at least twice the highest analog frequency component. For the analog-to-digital conversion (ADC) to result in a faithful reproduction of the signal, samples of the

analog waveform must be taken frequently. The number of samples per second is called the sampling rate or sampling frequency. *(Seeram, 3rd ed., p. 193)*

19. **(B)** The subdural space is an artificial space created by the separation of the arachnoid mater from the dura mater as a result of trauma, pathologic process, or the absence of cerebrospinal fluid (CSF). *(Kelley, 3rd ed., p. 90)*

20. **(C)** An emergency cart or crash cart is equipped with specific essential items and medications for use when a patient's condition worsens. Solu-Medrol sterile powder is an anti-inflammatory glucocorticoid, which contains methylprednisolone sodium succinate as its active ingredient. This medication is used to reduce symptoms such as swelling and allergic reactions. Solu-Medrol is used when a similar drug cannot be taken by mouth or when a very fast response is needed. Nitrostat is a vasodilator that relaxes the walls of blood vessels and increases circulation. Vasopressin is a vasoconstrictor, which causes contraction of muscle cells in the walls of blood vessels, narrowing their internal diameter in order to raise blood pressure. Ambien is a sedative used to treat insomnia; therefore, it would not be a drug found in the emergency cart. *(Ehrlich, 8th ed., pp. 294–297)*

21. **(A)** The purpose of the detectors is to capture the radiation beam from the patient and convert it into electrical signals, thus converting this information into binary-coded information. Its efficiency can be defined as its ability to capture, absorb, and convert x-ray photons to electrical signals. *(Seeram, 3rd ed., pp. 122–123)*

22. **(D)** Automatic tube current modulation dynamically changes the mA or mAs of the x-ray tube as the examination progresses. The x-ray tube current changes as a function of the changes along the z-axis of the patient (longitudinal tube current modulation) or as a function of changes in attenuation through the patient as the tube travels around the patient (angular tube current modulation). The ultimate method of patient dose reductions would be a combination of longitudinal and angular tube current modulation. *(Hale, 2013)*

23. **(D)** Carditis is an inflammation of the heart tissue leading to valvular disease. This infection may damage or destroy the heart valves. In severe cases,

the damaged valves may need to be replaced. *(Kelley, 3rd ed., p. 331)*

24. **(D)** A horseshoe kidney is a common renal fusion anomaly in which two functioning kidneys on each side of the midline are connected by an isthmus of functioning renal parenchyma. The isthmus crosses midline between the aorta and the inferior vena cava. *(Prokop, p. 651; Grey, 2nd ed., p. 288)*

25. **(C)** The therapeutic range of international normalized ratio (INR) for patients on medications such as warfarin or heparin is between 2.0 and 3.0. An increase in INR may be contraindicated for invasive procedures and contrast media examinations. *(Ehrlich, 8th ed., p. 223)*

26. **(B)** The thymus gland is a lymphatic organ responsible for the development of cellular immunity. It is located in the superior portion of the mediastinum. In newborns, this gland is usually larger than the heart, but gradually decreases in size with age. *(Kelley, 3rd ed., p. 323)*

27. **(C)** The choroid plexus produces CSF from the blood to fill the ventricles. The plexus lines the lateral ventricles, roof of the third ventricle, and inferior medullary velum of the fourth ventricle. *(Kelley, 3rd ed., p. 99)*

28. **(D)** The advantage of both the adaptive statistical iterative reconstruction and the model-based iterative reconstruction is the reduction of image noise; thereby, improving image quality and allowing the use of lower mAs and kVP. Using a low-dose protocol, a dose reduction of approximately 50% to 75% has been reported, with improved low-contrast detectability. *(Honours, 2014)*

29. **(B)** The first step when an extravasation occurs is to remove the needle and apply pressure to the injection site. There is much controversy whether moist heat or cold compresses should be applied. Heat has been found to improve absorption of the extravasation as well as in improving blood flow, particularly distal to the site. Many radiologists prefer to use cold compresses and have reported that it may be helpful for relieving pain at the injection site. The most commonly reported severe injuries after extravasation of low osmolar contrast media (LOCM) are compartment syndromes,

defined as a condition in which a muscle swells but is constricted by the connective tissue around it, which cuts off blood supply to the muscle. Less common injuries involve skin ulceration and tissue necrosis. Close clinical follow-up for several hours is essential for all patients in whom extravasations occur. *(Adler, 5th ed., p. 283; The American College of Radiology Manual, p. 17)*

30. **(D)** Adult respiratory distress syndrome (ARDS) is the result of pulmonary injury that can be divided into three phases. Stage I (within the first 24 hours) presents with vasodilation, interstitial and alveolar edema, and capillary stasis with thrombosis leading to interstitial thickening. Stage II demonstrates alveolar shadowing due to hemorrhage and fibrin deposition occurring within 2 to 7 days. Stage III is the chronic fibrotic stage resulting in interstitial fibrosis, lung distortion. In many cases, mediastinal emphysema and pneumothorax is frequently seen. CT is the superior modality in finding this pathology. *(Prokop, pp. 368–369)*

31. **(C)** Matrix detectors consist of multiple detector rows of identical width. Depending on the total beam collimation all or only a specific number of detectors will be exposed. Several combinations can exist. For instance, a 16-row detector array with aperture size of 1.25 can produce the following effects:

    (1) 16 × 1.25 mm, beam collimation of 20 mm
    (2) 4 × 1.25 mm, beam collimation of 5 mm
    (3) 4 × 2.5 mm, beam collimation of 10 mm
    (4) 4 × 3.75 mm, beam collimation of 15 mm

    (Prokop, p. 21; Seeram, 3rd ed., p. 287)

32. **(B)** The anterior cruciate is a round ligament extending from the anterior part of the tibial spine and attaching to the posterior part of the medial surface of the lateral femoral condyle. Its purpose is to prevent hyperextension and anterior displacement of the tibia. *(Kelley, 3rd ed., p. 695)*

33. **(C)** When the pixel size and slice thickness are known, the voxel volume can be equated by multiplying the pixel area and slice thickness. *(Sprawls, Computed Tomography Image Formation, 2014)*

34. **(B)** Data acquisition refers to a technique by which the patient is systematically scanned by the x-ray tube and detectors to collect enough information to produce a CT image path. The mechanisms that encompass the data acquisition schema are the beam geometry, which denotes the size, shape, and the motion of the x-ray beam, and the physical components that shape and define the beam, measure its transmission through the patient, and convert the data into digital data for computer input. The data acquisition geometries have changed dramatically through the modernization of technology. *(Seeram, 3rd ed., pp. 88–89)*

35. **(C)** Effective dose is used to quantify the risk from partial body exposure to that from an equivalent whole-body dose. The Sievert (Sv) is the unit of effective dose. The typical CT examination of the abdomen and pelvis yields an effective dose from 3 to 10 mSv. *(Seeram, 3rd ed., p. 220)*

36. **(A)** The formula for calculating the pitch is as follows:

$$pitch = \frac{table\ feed}{total\ beam\ collimation}$$
$$= \frac{15.36}{128 \times 0.3\ mm}$$
$$= \frac{15.36}{38.4}$$
$$= 0.4 : 1$$

(Kalendar, 3rd ed., p. 89)

37. **(C)** The most common anatomical sites used for the administration of contrast media include the: cephalic vein, located on the lateral side of the arm, the basilic vein, situated on the medial side of the arm, and the median cubital vein, connecting the cephalic and basilic veins located in the cubital fossa. Since power injectors are utilized as an administration method in CT, the veins in the hand should only be used if the vein is sturdy enough to withstand the needle gauge and flow rate required for the examination. *(Adler, 5th ed., p. 283)*

38. **(C)** The quadrate lobe can be found on the anterior inferior surface of the left lobe of the liver between the gall bladder and the ligamentum teres. *(Kelley, 3rd ed., p. 413)*

39. **(A)** The out-of-field artifact is the result of any portion of the patient or an object lying outside the

scan-field-of-view (SFOV), giving the computer incomplete information relating to this portion. The main causes of this artifact are patients' arms at their side, IV tubing containing contrast media lying within the gantry, or exceptionally large patients exceeding the selected SFOV. *(Kalendar, 3rd ed., p. 132).*

40. **(C)** A C1 fracture is usually the cause of direct pressure on the top of the head. This can be due to a swimming- or diving-related accident. It is known as Jefferson's fracture that occurs as two fractures in the anterior arch and two in the posterior arch of the C1 vertebra. *(Grey, 2nd ed., p. 122)*

41. **(C)** Diagnostic iodinated contrast media have been shown to cross the human placenta and enter the fetus when given in usual clinical doses. There is insufficient evidence to conclude that low osmolar contrast media are without any risk with respect to the fetus; therefore, the ACR recommends that all imaging facilities have policies and procedures in place to identify pregnant patients prior to the performance of any examination involving administration of iodinated contrast media. If a patient is known to be pregnant, the potential added risks of contrast media should be considered and discussed with the patient and her referring physician before proceeding with the study. Nonemergent CT examinations should be withheld until the patient is no longer pregnant. *(The American College of Radiology Manual, p. 94)*

42. **(B)** Subdural hematoma is a form of "traumatic brain injury." Blood collects between the dura mater (the outer protective covering of the brain) and the arachnoid (the middle layer of the meninges (the middle layer of the meninges). CT imaging is the preferred radiological modality, since it is fast and noninvasive. *(Grey, 2nd ed., pp. 86–87)*

43. **(B)** The adjustable collimator, found as close to the gantry as possible, allows variable collimation for the desired total beam collimation and minimizes the amount of penumbra caused by the focal spot size. *(Kalendar, 3rd ed., p. 51)*

44. **(D)** Nephroblastoma or Wilms' tumor develops from immature renal parenchyma found in children from the ages of 1 to 5 years. It has been found that 15% of cases are bilateral. The tumor appears as a large heterogeneous mass causing renal deformity. *(Prokop, p. 669)*

45. **(A)** At every angular position of a 360-degree rotation, the planar slice is interpolated between two projection points in the data set that are closest to the chosen position along the z-axis. This interpolation generates 720 degrees of data resulting in a complete set of projections from the chosen z-position. The disadvantage of this method is that it degrades image quality by broadening the slice sensitivity profile, but provides the least image noise. *(Prokop, p. 11)*

46. **(A)** D-dimer measurement is an important step in the diagnostic strategy of clinically suspected acute pulmonary embolism (PE). The D-dimer blood test measures one of the breakdown products of a blood clot. If this test is normal, then the likelihood of a PE is very low. The standard diagnostic approach of patients with clinically suspected acute PE and a positive plasma D-dimer measurement requires further imaging studies such as compression ultrasonography, computed tomography pulmonary angiography (CTPA), or ventilation–perfusion lung scan. It should be noted that the clinical usefulness of the D-dimer measurement is limited in elderly patients. *(Righini, 2014)*

47. **(D)** The insula, commonly called the inner lobe, is located deep within the Sylvian or lateral fissure. It may also be referred to as the Island of Reil. The function of this lobe is not totally understood, but its stimulation produces visceral sensations and autonomic responses. *(Madden, 3rd ed., pp. 17–18)*

48. **(B)** Volume CT dose index ($CTDI_{volume}$) is internationally recognized and is arguably the most important measure of the radiation output from the CT scanner. The milligray is the unit of $CTDI_{volume}$, a measured quantity used only with CT. It is measured by using a pencil ionization chamber placed in a standard circular plastic (polymethyl methacrylate) phantom. The $CTDI_{volume}$ reported by the scanner is an estimate of the average radiation dose within a volume of tissue only if the tissue is the same size and attenuation as the plastic phantom. Thus, $CTDI_{volume}$ is one of the key radiation descriptors in CT and is useful for comparing different scanner outputs from different imaging protocols

and for comparing the same examination type on different CT machines. *(Mayer-Smith, 2014)*

49. **(C)** Carotid artery stenosis is a major risk factor for stroke and can lead to brain damage. It is caused by a narrowing of the carotid artery(ies) caused by buildup of plaque inside the artery wall that reduces oxygen-rich blood flow to the brain. *(Prokop, p. 892)*

50. **(B)** A research study conducted by Indrajit et al. showed that a 24-gauge angiocatheter placed in a peripheral location can be safely power injected using a maximum flow rate of approximately 1.5 mL/s and a maximum pressure of 150 pounds per square inch (PSI). When access is thought to be tenuous, however, a hand injection of contrast media should be strongly considered to minimize risk of vessel injury and extravasation. *(Indrajit, 2015)*

51. **(A)** The equation to determine matrix size is as follows:

$$matrix\ size = \frac{FOV}{pixel\ size}$$

The first step in completing this problem is to employ a dimensional analysis by converting the FOV of 10 cm to 100 mm, in order to ensure that the solutions to problems yield the proper units; then, proceed with the equation

$$matrix\ size = \frac{100\ mm}{0.195\ mm}$$
$$= 512^2$$

(Seeram, 3rd ed., p. 64)

52. **(A)** The right ventricle receives deoxygenated blood from the right atrium and forces it into the pulmonary trunk for transportation to the lungs. On CT images, it is the most anterior of the heart chambers. *(Kelley, 3rd ed., pp. 336–337)*

53. **(A)** The celiac trunk is a very short vessel that lies on the anterior wall of the abdominal aorta just after the aorta passes through the diaphragm and superior to the renal arteries. The trunk divides into the left gastric artery, the common hepatic artery, and the splenic artery at approximately the level of the first lumbar vertebra. *(Kelley, 3rd ed., p. 474)*

54. **(A)** An aliasing artifact occurs when insufficient samples are obtained for image reconstruction. There are several ways of rectifying this artifact: acquiring the largest possible number of projections per rotation, quarter-detector shift, and the z-Sharp technology. These corrections are model specific. *(Seeram, 3rd ed., p. 213)*

55. **(C)** Several premedication regimens have been proposed to reduce the frequency and/or severity of reactions to contrast media, with hydrocortisone sodium succinate (Solu-Cortef) 200 mg intravenously recommended for emergency patients having a necessity of receiving iodinated contrast media. This medication must be administered every 4 hours (q4h) until contrast study commences along with diphenhydramine 50 mg IV administered 1 hour prior to the contrast injection. IV steroids have not been shown to be effective when administered less than 4 to 6 hours prior to contrast injection. *(The American College of Radiology Manual, p. 9)*

56. **(D)** Air trapping is evaluated using inspiration and expiration chest series. On inspiration, air fills the lungs and the CT number is very low. As the patient expels air, the CT number becomes higher; this attenuation of the voxels is predominantly the result of interstitial tissue. Patients with disease will fail to show an increase in attenuation. *(Prokop, p. 301)*

57. **(A)** Contrast resolution is superior because of the finite collimation available in CT scanners. Collimators affect patient dose and image quality by removing scatter radiation, which improves axial resolution. CT scanners are equipped with two types of collimations: pre-patient, which defines the beam width and the dose profile according to the detector configuration, and the pre-detectors, located between the patient and the detector array. These collimators improve the slice sensitivity profile by giving it a more rectangular shape. An additional set of collimators at the detector array decreases the effective detector element width (some manufacturers, 0.625–1.2 mm) thus increasing the conceivable geometric resolution. *(Kalendar, 3rd ed., p. 51)*

58. **(C)** The pineal gland is an endocrine structure (attached to the roof of the third ventricle), which secretes the hormone melatonin. This hormone aids

the regulation of the day–night cycles and is responsible for reproductive functions. On cross-sectional image, the pineal gland may be calcified. *(Madden, 3rd ed., p. 15)*

59. **(C)** Aseptic technique is a set of specific practices and procedures performed under carefully controlled conditions with the goal of minimizing pathogens in any clinical setting. Handwashing is considered a way of preventing fatal infections spreading from individual to individual. An essential role in all healthcare facilities should be to cleanse hands before and after each patient interaction. *(Adler, 5th ed., p. 217)*

60. **(D)** Raw data is unprocessed computer data in the form of binary numbers. A protocol-specific reconstruction algorithm is applied to the raw data to improve its quality. These data are processed immediately and stored in files in the image reconstruction system (IRS) for further use, if needed. *(Seeram, 3rd ed., p. 144)*

61. **(D)** Abdominal trauma from a sharp or blunt force most often results in intra-abdominal hemorrhage. On CT images, the active bleeding appears as a hyperdensity flowing from the area of injury to depressions in the abdomen and/or pelvis. The discovery of this pathology is an indication of a life-threatening hemorrhage that needs immediate surgical intervention. *(Webb, p. 194; Prokop, p. 605)*

62. **(C)** Subarachnoid hemorrhage is a collection of blood in the space between the arachnoid mater and pia mater. On CT images, a hyperdensity appears within the subarachnoid space, especially in the basal cisterns and into the pathways of the CSF. *(Grey, 2nd ed., pp. 84–85)*

63. **(D)** The two dose measurements reported on each CT scan are the CTDI$_{volume}$ and the dose length product (DLP). These dose measurements represent an approximation of the absorbed dose a patient will receive. The formal definition of CTDI$_{volume}$ only takes into account the radiation emitted over the length of a 100-mm scan. The actual dose averaged over the full volume of the scan will increase with scan length. The DLP parameter attempts to take into account the different lengths along the patient. It is defined as the

average CTDI$_{volume}$ for the scan multiplied by the length of the scan in cm. This unit is represented by the following equation mGy*cm (representing the radiation intensity, CTDI$_{volume}$ and the extension, the scan length. *(Mayer-Smith, 2014)*

64. **(D)** The Swan-Ganz catheter consists of several lumina and a balloon at its tip to keep it in place. The main purpose of this catheter is to measure cardiac output and right heart pressure with an indirect purpose of measuring left heart pressure and lung pressure. If the catheter is equipped with a fiberoptic infrared sensor, it has the means of measuring the balance between oxygen supply and oxygen demand. *(Ehrlich, 8th ed., pp. 409–410)*

65. **(A)** This sagittal CT-reformatted image using the bone/detail algorithm demonstrates a traumatic type 4 spondylolisthesis. Spondylolisthesis occurs in 60% of patients with spondylolysis. Ninety percent of this pathological condition occurs at the L5–S1 interspace, whereas cervical spondylolisthesis is rare in the cervical spine, having a 1% incidence rate. *(Grey, 2nd ed., p. 100)*

66. **(B)** Metal artifacts occur when the object(s) being imaged exceed the maximum attenuation value that a CT system can image. They appear as streaks on the reconstructed image, which can severely degrade the quality of the image. Metal artifacts are particularly pronounced with high atomic number metals such as iron or platinum, and less pronounced with low atomic number metals such as titanium. *(Boas, 2012; Seeram, 3rd ed., p. 207)*

67. **(D)** Retroperitoneum consists of structures posterior to the peritoneum. The retroperitoneal space is located between the diaphragm and the pelvic brim and is divided into the anterior pararenal, perirenal, and posterior pararenal compartments by the anterior and posterior renal fascia. It houses organs such as the kidneys, ureters, adrenal glands, and pancreas, most of the duodenum, ascending and descending colon, aorta, inferior vena cava, and uterus. The abdominal aorta or descending aorta lies on either side of the vertebral column. *(Madden, 3rd ed., p. 326)*

68. **(B)** The attenuation of a heterogeneous beam of photons (e.g., x-ray tube), as the quantity or number of photons is reduced by an absorber (tissue),

and equal thickness of absorber now reduces a smaller percentage of photons as the photons pass through the absorber. In this case, the quality or mean energy of the photons is altered by the absorber (tissue). The lower-energy photons are absorbed, so the mean photon energy increases, thus increasing the penetration power of the beam. This is known as "beam hardening." *(Seeram, 3rd ed., pp. 89–91)*

69. **(B)** The DFOV can be calculated by the product of the pixel size and the matrix size. When the matrix size is not indicated, it is assumed the matrix for CT images is 512. The equation is as follows:

$$DFOV = pixel\,size \times matrix\,size$$
$$= 0.68\,mm \times 512$$
$$= 348\,mm$$

(Seeram, 3rd ed., p. 193)

70. **(A)** Anaphylaxis is rapid in onset and is believed to be caused by the release of histamine from certain cells of the lungs, stomach, and lining of the blood vessels. These reactions are so severe that death can occur. A technologist should be familiar with signs of anaphylaxis that include tingling, itching of the palms of the hands and soles of the feet, difficulty swallowing, throat construction, and expiratory wheezing which may progress into laryngeal and bronchial edema. *(The American College of Radiology Manual, p. 102; Ehrlrich, 8th ed., p. 319)*

71. **(B)** The formula for calculating detector aperture is as follows:

$$detector\,aperture\,size = \frac{total\,beam\,collimation}{number\,of\,active\,detectors}$$
$$= \frac{38.8}{64}$$
$$= 0.6\,mm$$

72. **(A)** Osteochondral dissecans is the result of the isolated loss of blood flow to a portion of the talus bone. Usually, this occurs in conjunction with a history of chronic stress. It is sometimes also known as an osteochondral fracture of the talus or chip fracture of the articular surface or a chondral fracture of the talus. *(Prokop, p. 973)*

73. **(C)** One method to improve temporal resolution is to reduce or eliminate motion by increasing scan speed. In previous years, temporal resolution did not play a significant role in CT imaging, but with the introduction of cardiac imaging, temporal resolution has become a key parameter. Specific reconstruction algorithms, such as the 180-degree multi-cardio delta (MCD) and the 180-degree multi-cardio interpolation (MCI) have increased the effectiveness of temporal resolution by utilizing the 180-degree projected data and the fan angle along with employing the patient's ECG cycle. *(Kalendar, 3rd ed., p. 100; Seeram, 3rd ed., pp. 198–200)*

74. **(B)** Renal stone appears as a hyperdense structure on CT imaging due to its calcium or uric acid composition. *(Grey, 2nd ed., p. 298)*

75. **(C)** The iodine concentration of Ioversol is maintained without increasing the number of particles in solution; therefore, it does not increase the osmolality of the blood serum and does not change the osmotic pressure in the bloodstream. The advantage of a lower-osmolality media is that they are more water soluble (hydrophilic) and are less likely to be reactive with cells that can trigger allergic events. *(Adler, 5th ed., pp. 295–296)*

76. **(B)** Reconstruction interval is a unique parameter of spiral/helical CT. It can also be referred to as reconstruction increment or reconstruction spacing. There are three distinct types of reconstruction intervals: contiguous, overlapping, and gapping. The overlapping interval improves image quality and decreases partial volume averaging. *(Seeram, 3rd ed., pp. 260–262)*

77. **(B)** If asbestosis is suspected, a low-dose series of the chest is performed with the patient in the prone position. This allows the radiologist to compare the images in the supine and prone position looking for fibrotic and pleural thickening changes with positional change. *(Prokop, pp. 347–348)*

78. **(A)** Dose check was recently added as a requirement by the U.S. Food and Drug Administration to avoid radiation injuries. Dose check is a software upgrade that allows CT operators to set a maximum $CTDI_{volume}$ value for each specific

protocol and to alert the operator when any change in scan parameters are chosen that can lead to values higher than the limit. *(Mayer-Smith, 2014)*

79. **(C)** The pancreas is a long narrow retroperitoneal organ that lies posterior to the stomach and extends transversely at an oblique angle between the duodenum and the splenic hilum. The head is nestled in the second portion of the duodenum at approximately the level of L2/L3, whereas the tail extends into the splenic hilum at approximately T12. *(Kelley, 3rd ed., p. 437)*

80. **(A)** The equation to determine duration time when the amount of contrast and the flow rate are known is as follows:

$$duration\ time = \frac{volume}{flow\ rate}$$
$$= \frac{125\,cc}{\dfrac{5\,cc}{sec}}$$
$$= 25\,seconds$$

(Prokop, pp. 97–98)

81. **(D)** The term data compress describes the reduction of redundant data bits within an image. The recurring data are reduced or eliminated by an encryption code with a program that uses a particular type of compression algorithm. The two types of compression are lossy or irreversible and lossless or reversible compression. Lossless or reversible compression does not cause any data loss in the compression-decompression process; therefore, the decompressed file is identical in every way to the original file. CT utilizes the lossless compression algorithm termed discrete wavelet transform (DVT), which is required by HIPPA (Health Insurance Portability and Accountability Act). *(Seeram, 3rd ed., pp. 51: 77–78)*

82. **(B)** Goiters may be related to an increase in the thyroid-stimulating hormone (TSH) due to a deficiency in normal hormone synthesis. *(Grey, 2nd ed., p. 148)*

83. **(D)** Image quality depends on the number of projections to reconstruct an image. If an inadequate number of samples are obtained during data acquisition, the aliasing artifact may occur, thus triggering misregistration by the computer of information relating to sharp edges and small objects. *(Seeram, 3rd ed., p. 213; Kalendar, 3rd ed., p. 350)*

84. **(B)** The hyperdensity seen in the image lends the radiologist to interpret this case as a cerebral hematoma. The large hematoma is causing a large midline brain shift. *(Seeram, 3rd ed., p. 397)*

85. **(A)** A chest tube placed in the inferior chest wall drains fluid that collects in the base of the pleural space. Closed chest drainage systems must always be kept below the level of the patient's chest to avoid reverse flow. Any disturbance of the chest tube may result in reversing the intended treatment and possibly cause a collapsed lung. *(Ehrlich, 8th ed., pp. 408–409)*

86. **(C)** This enhanced CT image shows low-density areas of the parenchyma of the left kidney consistent with a deep laceration and hematoma. The hematoma is depicted by its hypodense appearance. *(Grey, 2nd ed., p. 291)*

87. **(B)** The equation for calculating CT window range is:

$$WL + \frac{WW}{2} \qquad WL - \frac{WW}{2}$$
$$700 + \frac{2{,}000}{2} \qquad 700 - \frac{2{,}000}{2}$$
$$700 + 1{,}000 \qquad 700 - 1{,}000$$
$$1{,}700 \qquad\qquad -300$$

The window range for the above WW and WL is 1,700 to −300. *(Seeram, 3rd ed., p. 172)*

88. **(A)** The pulmonary trunk arises from the left ventricle continuing posteriorly to form the right and left pulmonary arteries. On cross-sectional images, as the trunk divides into the right and left arteries, it can be seen as a T-shaped structure. This structure is an important landmark when performing PE examinations. On the localizer image, the pulmonary trunk is slightly lower than the bifurcation of the trachea in most patients. *(Madden, 3rd ed., p. 240)*

89. **(B)** Size-specific dose estimate (SSDE) is a newer CT dose descriptor that is determined by multiplying the CTDI$_{volume}$ by a conversion factor based on the patient's effective diameter. The effective diameter is defined as the square root of the product of the anterior–posterior and lateral patient diameters. This value at present is not available on the CT scanner but could be calculated automatically by the scanner using patient localizer images. *(Mayer-Smith, 2014)*

90. **(B)** The formula to calculate CT number is as follows:

$$CT\,number = ((\mu(tissue) - \mu(water)) / \mu(water) \times 1,000$$
$$= ((0.0004 - 0.206) / (0.206)) \times 1,000$$
$$CT\,number = -0.998 \times 1,000$$
$$= -998\,HU$$

This HU number represents air.
(Seeram, 3rd ed., p. 200)

91. **(D)** The equation to determine volume amount when knowing the duration time and the flow rate is as follows:

$$contrast\,volume = flow\,rate \times time$$
$$= \frac{3\,cc}{sec} \times 40\,sec$$
$$= 120\,cc\,of\,contrast\,media$$

(Prokop, pp. 97–98)

92. **(B)** The principle behind shaded surface rendering (SSD) is to realistically produce a three-dimensional (3D) scene of the surface of a structure of interest from the acquired data set. This process uses a segmentation technique that separates the object of interest from the background. Light illumination is the key element in this processing technique. It is most commonly used for preoperative skeletal surgery. *(Prokop, p. 60)*

93. **(B)** The cardinal or Mackenrodt ligament forms the base of the broad ligament while passing laterally from the cervix to the upper vaginal fascia. Due to its position, it may not always be defined in its entirety on CT images. *(Prokop, p. 702)*

94. **(B)** The goal of uniformity is to maintain a constant CT value for water, over the entire cross section of a homogeneous water phantom. This test is performed using a 20-cm or a 32-cm water phantom. A region of interest (ROI) with the area measurement of 2 to 3 cm^2 is placed in the center of the phantom—one at the 12 o'clock position, one at the 3 o'clock position, one at the 6 o'clock position, and one at the 9 o'clock position. It is important to place the peripheral ROIs approximately one ROI diameter away from the edge. The measurements of each ROI should not deviate more than 4 to 5 HU of each other. *(Seeram, 3rd ed., pp. 487–488)*

95. **(A)** The fornix is the arch-shaped structure that lies below the splenium of the corpus callosum and creates the inferior margin of the septum pellucidum. It serves to combine the hippocampus with other functional areas of the brain. *(Madden, 3rd ed., p. 15)*

96. **(B)** Computer architecture refers to the overall structure of a computer, which includes the elements of hardware and software. CT architectures were developed to accommodate fast image reconstruction and other image processing functions, such as image manipulations, networking data to other systems, and archiving image data. *(Seeram, 3rd ed., pp. 34–35)*

97. **(D)** A Venturi mask is a high-flow oxygen mask that provides the proper volume of oxygen the patient requires. The concentration of O$_2$ (24–60%) is more accurately controlled with this type of mask. This mask is generally prescribed for patients with chronic obstructive pulmonary disease (COPD). *(Ehrlich, 8th ed., p. 298)*

98. **(B)** The spinal cord resides within the vertebral foramen extending from the foramen magnum to approximately the L1 level, ending as it tapers into the conus medullaris. The cauda equina or horse's tail appears at the S2 level, which is a bundle of nerves exiting at the neural foramina. *(Kelley, 3rd ed., pp. 210–215)*

99. **(C)** The modulation transfer function (MTF) is a mathematical formula that measures the ratio of the accuracy of the image compared to the actual object scanned, indicating its image fidelity. The MTF generates information concerning the entire frequency range (smooth through ultra-high) in a

quantitative and objective manner. *(Kalendar, 3rd ed., pp. 118–119)*

100. **(A)** Ruptured bladders can be caused from a blow to the lower abdomen when the bladder is extended and/or by pelvic fractures. A blow sustained to the lower abdomen may cause a sudden increase in pressure, rupturing the bladder at the dome. A fragmented piece of bone may lacerate the bladder due to a fractured pelvis. *(Webb, p. 204)*

101. **(A)** This patient is experiencing a mild reaction which occurs in approximately 3% of patients. Usually, no intervention or medication is required for this type of reaction; however, these reactions may progress into a more severe category, and that is why observation for 20 to 30 minutes or as long as necessary to determine clinical stability is essential. If the patient's symptoms worsen, treatment with an antihistamine may be required, but in most cases it is not necessary. *(The American College of Radiology Manual, p. 91)*

102. **(A)** The voxel dimension can be calculated when the pixel area and the slice thickness are known. In the question, the detector aperture is 1 mm in the z-direction, constituting a slice thickness of 1 mm. The next step is to determine the pixel size.

$$pixel\,size = \frac{FOV}{matrix}$$
$$= \frac{100}{512}$$
$$= 0.19\,mm$$

The next step is to take the pixel size and incorporate it into the equation to find the voxel volume.

$$voxel\,volume = pixel\,area \times slice\,thickness$$

Therefore, for this problem, the voxel volume = 0.19 mm × 0.19 mm × 1.0 mm.

(Sprawls, Computed Tomography Image Formation, 2014)

103. **(A)** A common cause of a pulmonary embolism is immobility, for which this patient has been restricted from movement due to the close quarters on an airplane. The other symptom that leads the ER physician to a PE is the leg swelling. The physician will order blood work to include renal function test along with a D-dimer test, then a CTA will be ordered if the patient does not have any contraindications to the examination. *(Grey, 2nd ed., p. 186)*

104. **(B)** The Image Wisely and Image Gently campaigns aid radiologists, patients, and referring doctors to choose care that is evidence based, not duplicative of other tests, free of harm, and truly indicated when diagnosing pediatric patients and adults alike. *(Mayer-Smith, 2014)*

105. **(D)** Due to the configuration of the third-generation scanner, there was a potential for small differences of the sensitivities between the detector channels for the fan beam systems with the rotating detectors causing a ring artifact. This artifact would also occur when a detector channel went out of alignment. *(Kalendar, 3rd ed., p. 365)*

106. **(C)** The technology utilized to improve sampling includes the quarter-shift detector system, which was employed in older CT models and shifted the detector rays by a quarter detector and the central ray a quarter of the sampling distance, thereby producing two measurements in the opposite direction. Newer CT models closely pack the detectors allowing for more detectors that are available for data acquisition. This ensures more samples per view and increases the total number of measurements taken. The most recent innovation is the z-Sharp Technology designed by Siemens Medical Solutions. This process employs a magnetic field that shapes and controls the beam within the tube. This field allows focus positions to switch, both in the fan direction and in the z-direction, to provide overlapping sampling. *(Seeram, 3rd ed., pp. 130–131; Kalendar, 3rd ed., p. 50)*

107. **(A)** Iodixanol a contrast agent, sold under the trade name Visipaque, is the only isosmolar contrast media available for intravascular use. It is also the only contrast media formulated with sodium and calcium in a ratio equivalent to blood serum. The toxicity of contrast agents decreases as osmolality approaches that of serum. This has been accomplished by developing nonionizing compounds and then combining two monomers to form a dimer. The ratio of iodine atoms to active particles is 6:1. *(Adler, 5th ed., p. 296)*

108.   **(B)** The transverse foramen is located within the transvers processes of the cervical vertebra. This circular area is the passage way for arteries and veins descending from the head. *(Kelley, 3rd ed., p. 179)*

109.   **(C)** The odontoid process is part of the second cervical vertebra (axis) projecting superiorly from the surface of the body. It projects into the anterior ring of the atlas to act as a pivot for the rotational movement of the atlas. *(Kelley, 3rd ed., p. 180)*

110.   **(D)** The first cervical vertebra is termed the atlas because it supports the head. Its structure is different from other vertebrae because it has no body. It consists of an anterior and posterior arch and two lateral masses. The posterior arch forms approximately two-fifths of the circumference of the ring. This arch does not have a true spinous process, but instead has a minute smaller posterior tubercle. *(Madden, 3rd ed., p. 173)*

111.   **(D)** Reconstruction algorithms possess a dramatic effect on contrast resolution. Low-pass algorithms (standard or smooth) are used for image smoothing. They enhance the perceptibility of low-contrast lesions, such as metastatic disease and brain and abdomen imaging, all of which demonstrates subtle differences in subject contrast. These algorithms suppress the high frequencies thus smoothening the image, reducing noise, and improving contrast resolution. *(Seeram, 3rd ed., p. 145)*

112.   **(A)** The mandibular condyle is the rounded process superior to the mandibular rami. The condyle articulates with the temporal bone to form the temporomandibular joint. *(Madden, 3rd ed., p. 10)*

113.   **(D)** The clivus is a bony structure located in the posterior cranial fossa between the dorsum sellae and the foramen magnum. The superior section of the clivus is formed by the body of the sphenoid bone, while the inferior part extends to the foramen magnum and is formed by the basilar part of the occipital bone. *(Madden, 3rd ed., p. 12)*

114.   **(B)** The middle ear, also known as the tympanic cavity, is an air-filled structure that communicates with the mastoid atrium and the nasopharynx. Air travels through the tympanic cavity via the eustachian tube. *(Kelley, 3rd ed., p. 37)*

115.   **(D)** The left gonadal vein drains into the left renal vein, which in turn drains into the inferior vena cava. The left phrenic vein also drains into the left renal vein. *(Kelley, 3rd ed., p. 487)*

116.   **(D)** A multidetector computed tomography scanner with 16 or greater detector rows produces a cone beam instead of a flat angle beam geometry. The resulting beam geometry images a wider volume of data with each revolution of the gantry, causing problems where the beam diverges along the z-axis. *(Seeram, 3rd ed., p. 148)*

117.   **(C)** Image data are the result of raw data being convoluted and processed by the computer. The computer uses the mathematical process of back projection to create a visible image that can be displayed on the computer monitor. *(Seeram, 3rd ed., p. 145)*

118.   **(D)** Distance is a major dose-reduction strategy, as dose is inversely proportional to the square of the distance. This radiation-protection action is achieved by positioning the patient isocentered in the gantry for precise anatomical imaging. Incorrect centering by only 2.2 cm degrades image quality and increases the dose to the patient by 23%, especially when using automated tube current modulation. If a patient is centered too close to the x-ray tube, there can be inappropriate magnification of the localizer image, resulting in higher CT outputs and increased dose. *(Mayer-Smith, 2014)*

119.   **(D)** The SFOV determines the fan beam angle to include the precise number of detectors in the x-direction. As radiation did not hit the detectors outside the prescribed SFOV, no intensity information was detected; therefore, the image cannot be reconstructed to be larger than 300 mm. DFOV is a subset of all the scan data available; therefore, the DFOV cannot be larger than the SFOV. *(Prokop, p. 5)*

120.   **(A)** The scalene muscle group is located on the anterolateral portion of the neck. This group divides into the anterior, middle, and posterior scalene muscle. They originate from the transverse process of the cervical vertebra and insert on the first and second ribs. The purpose of this muscle group is to elevate the upper two ribs and flex the neck. *(Kelley, 3rd ed., p. 297)*

121.   **(A)** When all technical factors remain constant, if one doubles the pitch, the patient exposure will

decrease by halve. As you can see, tube current and pitch have a directly proportional relationship. *(Mayer-Smith, 2014)*

122. **(D)** Sarcoidosis is a systemic disease primarily affecting the lungs. High-resolution CT imaging is the best modality for differentiating this disease, as it is interpreted as hilar and mediastinal lymphadenopathy and multiple round mass-like consolidations. *(Grey, 2nd ed., p. 192)*

123. **(B)** An isotropic digital image is one in which all sides are equal. Since the voxel volume is 0.125 mm³, the cube root of 0.125 mm³ is 0.5 mm representing the pixel size. The pixel area is the product of the pixel size in the x and y dimensions; therefore, the pixel area for this problem is equal to 0.25 mm². *(Sprawls, Computed Tomography Image Formation, 2014)*

124. **(D)** The vagina is situated below the uterus and can be described as a muscular tube lined with a mucous membrane that connects the uterine cavity with the exterior. It is located between the bladder and the rectum. *(Madden, 3rd ed., p. 397)*

125. **(B)** Patient education is an essential part of any CT examination. Patient unique identifiers are critical elements prior to performing a CT examination on a patient. Most institutions use the patient's date of birth and another formed question that matches the patient to the system. Obtaining a proper medical history provides the radiologist with information about the patient that may be excluded from the physician's orders. Finally, providing the patient with the proper instructions of the procedure lessens anxiety, reassures the patient they are receiving quality patient care, and enables them to cooperate more freely. *(Ehrlich, 8th ed., pp. 208–211)*

126. **(B)** The data acquisition system is a group of detector electronics positioned between the detector array and the computer. Its main functions are to measure the transmitted radiation beam, encodes these measurements into binary data, and, finally, to transmit the binary data to the computer. Each detector photodiode measures the transmitted beam from the patient and converts them into electrical energy. *(Seeram, 3rd ed., pp. 128–129)*

127. **(D)** Fresh hemorrhage is normally related with clot formation, in turn increasing the hematocrit of the collection corresponding with an increase of CT number. As the hemorrhage ages, it becomes less attenuated, as there is a breakdown of blood causing the CT number to decrease. An acute hemorrhage initially appears iso- or hyperdense with age and, with the breakdown of the plasma, it becomes hypodense. *(Prokop, p. 196)*

128. **(D)** Number of photons detected per pixel is referred to as signal-to-noise ratio (SNR). SNR compares the level of desired signal to the level of the background noise, as denoted in the following equation:

$$SNR = \frac{mean\,ROI}{background\,ROI}$$

(Kalendar, 3rd ed., p. 129)

129. **(C)** A tibial plateau fracture involves the proximal end of the tibia that carries the weight of the body across it. CT imaging employing 3D volume rendered or sagittal and coronal multiplanar reformations is a useful tool to evaluate the bony fragments and degree of displacement. *(Grey, 2nd ed., p. 414)*

130. **(D)** The lungs are considered a high-contrast examination, with large contrasts in attenuation properties between air and tissue, thus allowing the tube currents to be lowered, resulting in a reduction of radiation dose. *(Hale, 2013)*

131. **(A)** As its name indicates, raw data in the true sense are unprocessed computer data. Once measurement data has been preprocessed to correct for possible errors, it is sent to the ADC to convert the analog signal to discrete digital numbers where it becomes raw data. Raw data are archived in their digital form and can be retrieved to generate series of images with different convolution kernels. *(Seeram, 3rd ed., p. 144)*

132. **(B)** The superior mesenteric artery branches 1 cm below the celiac trunk at approximately the level of the first lumbar vertebra and extends downward. It supplies the head of the pancreas and the majority of the small and large intestines. Compared to the perpendicular origin of the celiac trunk, its oblique course can be a noticeable characteristic on sectional

images, especially reformatted sagittal images. The SMA appears as a hook descending downward over the horizontal portion of the duodenum. Fat planes that surround the artery are preferential sites for the spread of pancreatic cancer. *(Madden, 3rd ed., p. 327)*

133. **(A)** The large intestines lie inferior to the stomach and liver and almost completely frame the small intestine. The longitudinal muscle of the large intestine forms three thickened bands called the taenia coli, which gather the cecum and colon into pouch-like folds known as haustra. On the outer surface of the colon, the epiploic appendages, which are fat-filled sacs of omentum, attach the intestine to the abdominal wall. The ascending colon ascends the right lateral wall of the abdomen, curving sharply to form the hepatic flexure. This flexure marks the beginning of the transverse colon. *(Kelley, 3rd ed., pp. 462–463)*

134. **(C)** The renal pelvis is the enlarged upper end of the ureter. The pelvis is shaped somewhat like a funnel that is curved to one side, and is almost completely surrounded in the deep indentation on the concave side of the kidney. The large end of the pelvis has roughly cuplike extensions, called calyces, within the kidney. The calyces are cavities in which urine collects before it flows on into the urinary bladder. *(Madden, 3rd ed., p. 326)*

135. **(C)** Atelectasis is a collapse of a portion of lung tissue most commonly due to bronchial obstruction, pleural effusion, or other pleural processes. Types of atelectasis are distinguished according to their etiology. *(Webb, p. 124)*

136. **(C)** Out-of-field artifacts are caused by anatomy or objects that are outside of the selected SFOV. The extra tissues block the detectors and attenuate photons, resulting in a (hyperdense) bright rim at the edge of the field of reconstruction. *(Kalendar, 3rd ed., p. 132)*

137. **(C)** CT enteroclysis involves combining the techniques of conventional small bowel enteroclysis with those of CT enterography. Oral contrast agents are administered through an enteric tube whose tip is positioned in the proximal jejunum. This technique promotes more rapid and uniform small bowel distention than is seen during CT enterography. Although CT enteroclysis has shown great reliability for defining sites of partial small bowel

obstruction due to adhesions, neoplasms, or other causes, like conventional enteroclysis, this study has not been widely accepted due to its invasive nature. *(The American College of Radiology Manual, p. 63)*

138. **(A)** Parallel processing requires a type of computer that contains two or more processors running simultaneously. This process differs from other types of processors in that, as one processing task is completed, it will take on another no matter what the task involves. *(Seeram, 3rd ed., p. 35)*

139. **(B)** The spleen is located in the regional divisions of the left hypochondrium and partly in the epigastrium. It is located posterior to the stomach in the posterior aspect of abdomen between the fundus of the stomach and the diaphragm. It is a highly vascular organ with a spongy parenchyma. The spleen produces white blood cells, filters abnormal blood cells, stores iron from red blood cells, and initiates the immune response. *(Kelley, 3rd ed., p. 441)*

140. **(D)** The bronchus intermedius is a major branch of the right main bronchus which supplies air to the middle lobe and lower lobes of the chest. *(Madden, 3rd ed., p. 236)*

141. **(A)** When one wants to decrease the dimensions of a voxel, the most straightforward way is to decrease the slice width. Slice width is the direct indicator of volume of tissue in the area of interest in the z-axis direction. The voxel volume has a significant effect on image quality. As slice thickness decreases, spatial resolution increases; partial volume averaging decreases. *(Seeram, 3rd ed., p. 294)*

142. **(D)** The uterus is divided into three parts: the body, fundus, and the cervix. The cervix is the most inferior constricting region that opens into the vagina. *(Madden, 3rd ed., p. 397)*

143. **(B)** As a beam of radiation passes through an object, the long wavelengths will be absorbed in the object and the resulting beam's energy increases. *(Seeram, 3rd ed., pp. 89–91)*

144. **(B)** Urticaria is a skin eruption, manifested by an allergic reaction. They are seen on the skin as wheals of various sizes and shapes with well-defined erythematous margins and pale centers. They are also known as hives. *(Ehrlich, 8th ed., p. 481)*

145. **(B)** Islet cell tumors arise from endocrine cells located in the pancreas. Approximately 90% of these tumors are benign, with 75% being hormonally active. CT has a role in the preoperative localization of functioning tumors as well as staging of nonfunctional tumors. Contrast enhancement and proper scanning techniques are critical for their diagnosis. *(Prokop, p. 527)*

146. **(B)** Multi-planar reformation (MPR) software reformats two-dimensional images at arbitrary planes defined by the operator, using the pixel data from a stack of transaxial images. Each pixel in the 512^2 matrix, when used in conjunction with the slice thickness, forms a voxel or volume of data representing the digital values of the scanned object. The MPR software extracts only those voxels from the data volume positioned one above the other within the coronal or sagittal plane. An oblique or curved reformat is constructed in a similar way, but the image data need to be interpolated among adjacent voxels. *(Kalendar, 3rd ed., p. 232)*

147. **(A)** The thyroid gland is an endocrine gland located at the level of the cricoid cartilage, containing two lobes connected by a narrowed area known as the isthmus on the anterior trachea. On CT cross-sectional images, they are seen as high attenuation structures due to their iodine content. *(Madden, 3rd ed., p. 176)*

148. **(C)** Osteoarthritis, also termed as degenerative joint disease or degenerative arthritis, is usually caused by mechanical or biological events leading to the deterioration of the articular cartilage. It is the most common cause of work-related disabilities affecting the hand, wrist, shoulder, hip, knee, foot, and spine. Nonsteroidal drugs are used for pain, with various surgical interventions available. Patients are advised to take nutritional supplements (glucosamine sulfate and chondroitin sulfate). *(Grey, p. 396)*

149. **(C)** The formula for calculating beam collimation is as follows:

$$beam\ collimation = detector\ aperture\ size$$
$$\times number\ of\ detectors$$
$$= 0.3\ mm \times 64$$
$$= 19.2\ mm$$

(Seeram, 3rd ed., p. 274)

150. **(C)** The only effective treatment for pancreatic carcinoma is surgical intervention; therefore, staging is imperative. CT imaging when performed with optimal technical parameter and contrast enhancement aids the radiologist in defining the size and location of these tumors. Tumor staging includes: T1—limited to pancreas ≤2 cm; T2—limited to the pancreas and >2 cm in size; T3—invasion of duodenum, common bile duct, or peripancreatic fat; and T4—infiltration of the stomach, spleen, colon, and/or large vessels. *(Prokop, p. 524)*

151. **(C)** The intercostal muscles act to keep the intercostal spaces slightly rigid during respiration. These muscles also aid in forcing inspiration by elevating the ribs. *(Kelley, 3rd ed., p. 389)*

152. **(B)** Hypervascular lesions, after the appropriate contrast injection delivery and delay time, appear hyperdense on CT images. These lesions can be benign or malignant, with malignant tumors having a marked heterogeneous enhancement. Imaging performed in the arterial phase not only detects tumor diagnosis, but also can be used for preoperative evaluation of arterial variants in the upper abdomen. *(Prokop, p. 422)*

153. **(D)** Metal artifacts occur when the object(s) being imaged exceed the maximum attenuation value that a CT system can image. They appear as streaks on the reconstructed image, which can severely degrade the quality of the image. Metal artifacts are particularly pronounced with high atomic number metals, such as iron or platinum, and less pronounced with low atomic number metals, such as titanium. *(Boas, 2012)*

154. **(B)** The function of the bicuspid or mitral valve is to prevent a backflow of blood from the left ventricle up to the left atrium. *(Kelley, 3rd ed., p. 346)*

155. **(C)** A metropolitan area network (MAN) is a computer network larger than a local area network (LAN), covering an area of a few city blocks to the area of an entire city; hence, metropolitan, possibly including the surrounding areas. MAN links between local area networks with wireless links using either microwave, radio, or infrared laser transmission. *(Seeram, 3rd ed., pp. 37–38)*

156. (D) The left ventricle forms the apex, left border, and most of the inferior surface of the heart. It receives oxygenated blood from the left atrium and pumps it into the aorta for distribution throughout the systemic system. *(Kelley, 3rd ed., pp. 336–337)*

157. (C) Window width controls the contrast of the image by selecting a specific range of shades of gray from the Hounsfield scale displayed on the CT monitor. The window width is chosen according to the attenuation values inherited in the anatomy of interest. It is important to understand the effects window width has on image contrast. As the number of shades of gray decreases, image contrast increases, thus giving the reconstructed image a black and white appearance. On the contrary, image contrast decreases as the width increases because more shades of gray are available. *(Seeram, 3rd ed., pp. 170–177)*

158. (C) The cardinal ligament extends from the lateral wall of the cervix and vagina and then inserts in the wall of the lesser pelvis. Its main function is to suspend the uterus above the bladder and prevent its downward displacement. *(Kelley, 3rd ed., p. 528)*

159. (C) The formula for calculating detector rows is as follows:

$$number\ of\ detector\ rows = \frac{beam\ collimation}{aperture\ size}$$

$$= \frac{12\ mm}{0.5\ mm}$$

$$= 24$$

(Seeram, 3rd ed., p. 274)

160. (A) The large intestines lie inferior to the stomach and liver and almost completely frame the small intestine. The longitudinal muscle of the large intestine forms three thickened bands called the taenia coli, which gathers the cecum and colon into pouch-like folds known as haustra. On the outer surface of the colon are the epiploic appendages, which are fat-filled sacs of omentum attaching the intestine to the abdominal wall. The splenic flexure is located directly inferior to the spleen, marking the beginning of the descending colon. *(Kelley, 3rd ed., pp. 462–463)*

161. (C) The ileum is the longest portion of the small intestines situated in the right lower abdomen. The terminal end unites with the cecum at the ileocecal valve. During colonoscopy, the ileocecal valve is used, along with the appendiceal orifice, to identify the cecum. This is important as it indicates that a complete colonoscopy has been performed. *(Kelley, 3rd ed., p. 458)*

162. (D) Figure Q4.13 is considered the BE view, as it looks similar to anteroposterior view in conventional radiology. This 3D real-time visualization tool provides a guide for the user to explore in and around the colon. The 3D image demonstrates the anatomy of the colon from the rectum through the distal ileum separating the colon in search of polyps. *(Seeram, 3rd ed., p. 369)*

163. (B) In order to retrospectively reconstruct images, raw data are necessary. These data are archived in their digital form and can be retrieved to perform additional reconstructions as long as the data are still available. *(Seeram, 3rd ed., p. 144)*

164. (A) Avascular necrosis occurs as an interruption of the blood flow within the bone resulting in death of the cells within the bone. It occurs in patients between the ages of 30 and 70. In 50% of the cases, bilateral involvement may occur. The hip is the most common site for the development of avascular necrosis. *(Grey, p. 378)*

165. (A) The hybrid array detector system is similar to the matrix array detectors with the exception that the innermost rows are thinner than the outermost rows. The system described below is based on a 32-row detector array. The innermost rows can be 0.5 mm, while the outer rows increase to 1 mm in width. Here are a few possible combinations:

(1) 4×0.5 mm, beam collimation of 2 mm

(2) 4×1 mm, beam collimation of 4 mm

(3) 4×2 mm, beam collimation of 8 mm

(4) 4×4 mm, beam collimation of 16 mm

(5) 4×8 mm, beam collimation of 32 mm

(Prokop, p. 22)

Subspecialty List

43. Physics and Instrumentation — CT System Principles, Operations, and Components — Collimation/Beam Width
44. Imaging Procedures — Pathology — Kidney
45. Imaging Procedures — Imaging Processing — Reconstruction
46. Patient Care and Safety — Patient Assessment and Preparation — Laboratory Values
47. Imaging Procedures — Anatomy — Brain
48. Patient Care and Safety — Radiation Safety and Dosimetry — Dose Measurement
49. Imaging Procedures — Pathology — Soft Tissue
50. Patient Care and Safety — Contrast Administration — Administration Route and Dose Calculations
51. Physics and Instrumentation — Image Display — Matrix
52. Imaging Procedures — Anatomy — Heart
53. Imaging Procedures — Anatomy — Vascular
54. Physics and Instrumentation — CT System Principles, Operations, and Components — Detector Configuration
55. Patient Care and Safety — Patient Assessment and Preparation — Medications and Dosage
56. Imaging Procedures — Pathology — Chest
57. Physics and Instrumentation — Image Quality — Contrast Resolution
58. Imaging Procedures — Anatomy — Brain
59. Patient Care and Safety — Contrast Administration — Venipuncture — Aseptic and Sterile Technique
60. Physics and Instrumentation — Image Processing — Reconstruction
61. Imaging Procedures — Pathology — Abdomen
62. Imaging Procedures — Pathology — Brain
63. Patient Care and Safety — Radiation Safety and Dosimetry — Dose Measurement: $CTDI_{volume}$
64. Patient Care and Safety — Patient Assessment and Preparation — Management of Accessory Medical Devices
65. Imaging Procedures — Pathology — Spine
66. Physics and Instrumentation — Artifacts Recognition and Reduction — Metal Artifact
67. Imaging Procedures — Anatomy — Vascular
68. Physics and Instrumentation — Radiation Physics — Physical Principles (attenuation)
69. Physics and Instrumentation — Image Display — Field of View
70. Patient Care and Safety — Contrast Administration — Adverse Reaction
71. Physics and Instrumentation — CT System Principles, Operations, and Components — Collimation/Beam Width
72. Imaging Procedures — Pathology — Lower Extremity
73. Physics and Instrumentation — Image Quality — Temporal Resolution
74. Imaging Procedures — Pathology — Kidney
75. Patient Care and Safety — Contrast Administration — Contrast Media: Ionic, Nonionic
76. Physics and Instrumentation — Image Processing — Reconstruction
77. Imaging Procedures — Pathology — Chest
78. Patient Care and Safety — Radiation Safety and Dosimetry — Patient Dose Reduction and Optimization
79. Imaging Procedures — Anatomy — Pancreas
80. Patient Care and Safety — Contrast Administration — Injection Techniques
81. Physics and Instrumentation — Informatics — Networking
82. Imaging Procedures — Pathology — Soft Tissue
83. Physics and Instrumentation — CT System Principles, Operations, and Components — Detector Configuration
84. Imaging Procedures — Pathology — Brain
85. Patient Care and Safety — Patient Assessment and Preparation — Management of Accessory Medical Devices
86. Imaging Procedures — Pathology — Kidney
87. Physics and Instrumentation — Image Display — Windowing
88. Imaging Procedures — Anatomy — Vascular
89. Patient Care and Safety — Radiation Safety and Dosimetry — Dose Measurement
90. Physics and Instrumentation — Image Quality — CT number
91. Patient Care and Safety — Contrast Administration — Injection Techniques
92. Physics and Instrumentation — Postprocessing — 3D Reformation
93. Imaging Procedures — Anatomy — Reproductive Organs
94. Physics and Instrumentation — Image Quality — Uniformity
95. Imaging Procedures — Anatomy — Brain
96. Physics and Instrumentation — CT System Principles, Operations, and Components — Computer and Array Processor
97. Patient Care and Safety — Patient Assessment and Preparation — Management of Accessory Medical Devices
98. Imaging Procedures — Anatomy — Spine
99. Physics and Instrumentation — Image Quality — Spatial Resolution
100. Imaging Procedures — Pathology — Bladder

101. Patient Care and Safety — Contrast Administration — Adverse Reactions
102. Physics and Instrumentation — Image Display — Voxel
103. Imaging Procedures — Pathology — Vascular
104. Patient Care and Safety — Radiation Safety and Dosimetry — Patient Dose Reduction and Optimization
105. Physics and Instrumentation — Radiation Physics — Acquisition (Geometry)
106. Physics and Instrumentation — CT System Principles, Operations, and Components — Detector Configuration
107. Patient Care and Safety — Contrast Administration — Contrast Media
108. Imaging Procedures — Anatomy — Spine
109. Imaging Procedures — Anatomy — Spine
110. Imaging Procedures — Anatomy — Spine
111. Physics and Instrumentation — Image Quality Contrast Resolution
112. Imaging Procedures — Anatomy — Temporomandibular Joint
113. Imaging Procedures — Anatomy — Cranium
114. Imaging Procedures — Anatomy — Internal Auditory Canal
115. Imaging Procedures — Anatomy — Vascular
116. Physics and Instrumentation — Artifacts Recognition and Reduction — Cone Beam Artifact
117. Physics and Instrumentation — Image Processing — Reconstruction
118. Patient Care and Safety — Radiation Safety and Dosimetry — Patient Dose Reduction and Optimization
119. Physics and Instrumentation — Image Display — Field of View
120. Imaging Procedures — Anatomy — Soft Tissue
121. Patient Care and Safety — Radiation Safety and Dosimetry — Technical Factors Affecting Patient Dose
122. Imaging Procedures — Pathology — Chest
123. Physics and Instrumentation — Image Display — Voxel
124. Imaging Procedures — Anatomy — Reproductive Organs
125. Patient Care and Safety — Patient Assessment and Preparation — Education
126. Physics and Instrumentation — CT System Principles, Operations, and Components — Detector Configuration
127. Imaging Procedures — Pathology — Abdomen
128. Physics and Instrumentation — Image Quality — Contrast Resolution
129. Imaging Procedures — Pathology — Lower Extremity
130. Patient Care and Safety — Radiation Safety and Dosimetry — Patient Dose Reduction and Optimization
131. Physics and Instrumentation — Image Processing — Reconstruction
132. Imaging Procedures — Anatomy — Vascular
133. Imaging Procedures — Anatomy — GI Track
134. Imaging Procedures — Anatomy — Kidney/Ureters
135. Imaging Procedures — Pathology — Chest
136. Physics and Instrumentation — Artifact Recognition and Reduction — Out-of-Field Artifact
137. Imaging Procedures — Abdominal Procedures
138. Physics and Instrumentation — CT System Principles, Operations, and Components — Computer and Array Processor
139. Imaging Procedures — Anatomy — GI Tract
140. Imaging Procedures — Anatomy — Lungs
141. Physics and Instrumentation — Image Display — Voxel
142. Imaging Procedures — Anatomy — Reproductive Organs
143. Physics and Instrumentation — Radiation Physics — Physical Principles (Attenuation)
144. Patient Care and Safety — Contrast Administration — Adverse Reactions — Recognition and Assessment
145. Imaging Procedures — Pathology — Pancreas
146. Physics and Instrumentation — Postprocessing — 3D Reformation
147. Imaging Procedures — Anatomy — Neck Soft Tissues
148. Imaging Procedures — Pathology — Lower Extremity
149. Physics and Instrumentation — CT System Principles, Operations, and Components — Detector Configuration
150. Imaging Procedures — Pathology — Pancreas
151. Imaging Procedures — Anatomy — Chest Muscles
152. Imaging Procedures — Pathology — Liver
153. Physics and Instrumentation — Artifacts Recognition and Reduction — Metal Artifact
154. Imaging Procedures — Anatomy — Heart
155. Physics and Instrumentation — Informatics — Networking
156. Imaging Procedures — Anatomy — Heart
157. Physics and Instrumentation — Image Display — Windowing
158. Imaging Procedures — Anatomy — Reproductive Organs
159. Physics and Instrumentation — CT System Principles, Operations, and Components — Detector Configuration
160. Imaging Procedures — Anatomy — GI Track
161. Imaging Procedures — Anatomy — GI Track
162. Imaging Procedures — Procedures — GI Track
163. Physics and Instrumentation — Image Processing — Reconstruction
164. Imaging Procedures — Pathology — Lower Extremity
165. Physics and Instrumentation — CT System Principles, Operations, and Components — Detector Configuration

CHAPTER 5

Practice Test 2
Questions

1. What mater is located in the innermost layer of the meninges?

    (A) dura mater
    (B) pia mater
    (C) arachnoid mater
    (D) falx cerebri

2. Which of the following essential questions is not included in the patient history taking?

    (A) are you currently taking any medications
    (B) have you ever had a reaction to contrast media
    (C) have you ever received radiation treatments
    (D) how many children do you have

3. What type of radiation interaction with matter occurs when an incident x-ray photon is totally absorbed during the ionization of an inner shell electron?

    (A) Compton scatter
    (B) bremsstrahlung interaction
    (C) photoelectric interaction
    (D) stochastic effects

4. What tubular-shaped organ is found in males is located inferior to the bladder extending through the prostate, urogenital diaphragm, and penis?

    (A) urethra
    (B) ureter
    (C) corpus cavernosum
    (D) corpus spongiosum

5. Which of the following x-ray tube anodes is most likely used in spiral/helical computed tomography scanners?

    (A) tungsten target fixed anode tube
    (B) tungsten target rotating anode tube
    (C) molybdenum target rotating anode tube
    (D) rotating anode tube with a rhenium tungsten disk

6. Which of the following salivary ducts are responsible for the flow of saliva within the mouth?

    (A) Stensen's duct
    (B) Rivinus's duct
    (C) Wharton's duct
    (D) Treitz's duct

7. What reconstruction technique was used by Hounsfield in the first EMI brain scanner?

    (A) filtered back projection reconstruction
    (B) multiplanar reconstruction
    (C) iterative reconstruction
    (D) algebraic reconstruction

8. Which of the following radiation dose quantities is determined by multiplying $CTDI_{volume}$ by a conversion factor based on the patient's effective diameter?

    (A) absorbed dose
    (B) size-specific dose estimation
    (C) effective dose
    (D) $CTDI_{volume}$

9. Which of the following combinations will produce an image with the best spatial resolution?

   (A) large pixels and thin slice width
   (B) large pixels and thick slice width
   (C) small pixels and thick slice width
   (D) small pixels and thin slice width

10. What is the name of the ligament that extends between the patella and the tibial tuberosity?

    (A) medial collateral ligament
    (B) lateral collateral ligament
    (C) patellar ligament
    (D) ligamentum flava

11. Patient history taking in children usually does not typically include which of the following?

    (A) history of contrast reaction
    (B) Blood urea nitrogen (BUN) level
    (C) patient anxiety level
    (D) history asthma

12. Compared with conventional computed tomography scanners, slip-ring scanners offer a number of advantages. Which of the following is **not** an advantage of slip ring technology?

    (A) removal of cable wraparound
    (B) elimination of start–stop action
    (C) continuous rotation of x-ray tube with minimal interscan delays
    (D) inability to perform CT angiography

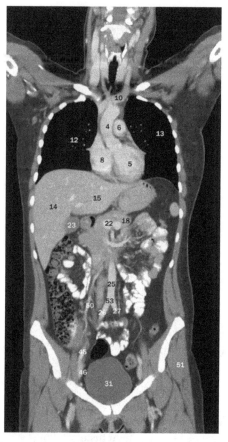

Figure Q5.1 Reproduced, with permission, from Weir J, Abrahams PH, Spratt JD, et al. *Imaging Atlas of Human Anatomy.* 4th ed. St MO: Mosby Elsevier; 2011.

Refer to Figure Q5.1 to answer Questions 13–16.

13. Which of the following is illustrated by label #22 in Figure Q5.1?

    (A) celiac trunk
    (B) splenic artery
    (C) portal vein
    (D) aorta

14. In Figure Q5.1 above, which of the following illustrates the right lobe of the liver?

    (A) 15
    (B) 14
    (C) 23
    (D) 18

15. What number in Figure Q5.1 illustrates the right external iliac artery?

    (A) 46
    (B) 45
    (C) 50
    (D) 26

16. Which of the following is illustrated by label #18 in figure Q5.1?

    (A) portal vein
    (B) splenic vein
    (C) stomach
    (D) pancreas

17. Which of the following is the term utilized for a defined set of instructions for solving a problem?

    (A) algorithm
    (B) Fourier transform
    (C) interpolation
    (D) convolution

18. What is the term used for the amount of friction generated by the molecules of a contrast media?

    (A) osmolality
    (B) viscosity
    (C) orinase
    (D) nasoenteric

19. What is the tale speed if the pitch is 1.5, the gantry rotation is 1 second, and the detector configuration is 16 × 1.2?

    (A) 19.2 mm/s
    (B) 28.8 mm/s
    (C) 13 mm/s
    (D) 16 mm/s

20. What meningeal space is filled with cerebrospinal fluid?

    (A) epidural
    (B) subdural
    (C) subarachnoid
    (D) subpial

21. A trauma patient enters the ER after sustaining a 20 foot fall from a building. Which of the following convolution kernels would be applied for both the prospective and retrospection reconstructions of the patient's trauma survey examination?

    (A) ultrasmooth and smooth
    (B) ultrasmooth and standard
    (C) standard and bone
    (D) bone and ultrasmooth

22. What is the term used to address the dose an individual receives annually or accumulates over a working lifetime?

    (A) stochastic effects
    (B) deterministic effects
    (C) dose justification
    (D) dose limitations

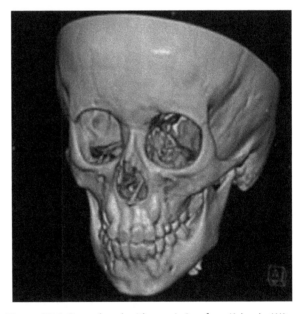

Figure Q5.2 Reproduced, with permission, from Kalendar WA. *Computed Tomography: Fundamentals System Technology, Image Quality, and Applications.* 3rd ed. Erlangen, Germany: Publicis; 2011.

23. Figure Q5.2 above specifically demonstrates which 3D-rendering technique?

    (A) volume rendered technique
    (B) multiplanar reformations
    (C) shaded surface display
    (D) maximum intensity projection

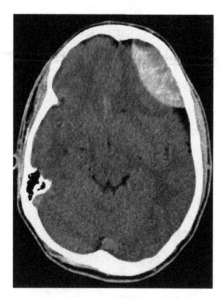

Figure Q5.3 Reproduced, with permission, from Grey ML, Ailinani JM. *CT and MRI Pathology: A Pocket Atlas.* 2nd ed. New York, NY: McGraw-Hill; 2012.

24. What pathological condition is demonstrated in Figure Q5.3?

    (A) epidural hematoma
    (B) subdural hematoma
    (C) subarachnoid hematoma
    (D) glomus tumor

25. Low contrast detectability can be defined by which of the following statements?

    (A) the ability to distinguish region whose attenuation coefficient are very close to each other
    (B) the ability to measure the smallest size structure that can be seen
    (C) the ability to freeze motion
    (D) the relationship between the linear attenuation coefficient and the HU

26. Which of the following laboratory values is a breakdown product of skeletal muscle?

    (A) creatinine
    (B) GFR
    (C) PT
    (D) INR

27. What area within the neck are common areas for foreign bodies to become lodged?

    (A) piriformis sinus
    (B) aryepiglottic folds
    (C) valleculae
    (D) rima glottis

28. Name an advantage of gas ionization detectors:

    (A) lower quantum detector efficiency
    (B) produce afterglow
    (C) utilize hydrogen in the ionization chamber
    (D) sensitivity of the individual chambers are uniform

29. What is the term used to describe the instrumentation and method used to measure patient dose from a CT scanner?

    (A) CT dosimetry
    (B) CT absorptiometry
    (C) radiation intensity
    (D) dose distribution

30. What is described as any discrepancy between the reconstructed CT numbers in the image and the true attenuation coefficients of the object?

    (A) artifact
    (B) noise
    (C) spatial resolution
    (D) low-contrast detectability

31. Which of the following medication has the potential risk of producing lactic acidosis?

    (A) Heparin
    (B) Advil
    (C) Lasix
    (D) Metformin

32. What is deemed an overlapping reconstruction interval?

    (A) slice thickness 5 mm, slice interval 5 mm
    (B) slice thickness 3 mm, slice interval 7 mm
    (C) slice thickness 1 mm, slice interval 2 mm
    (D) slice thickness 1 mm, slice interval 0.5 mm

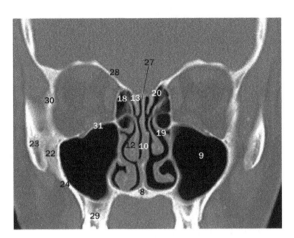

Figure Q5.4 Reproduced, with permission, from Weir J, Abrahams PH, Spratt JD, et al. *Imaging Atlas of Human Anatomy.* 4th ed. St. Louis, MO: Mosby Elsevier; 2011.

Refer to Figure Q5.4 to answer Questions 37–39.

33. What ligament extends across the ring of C1 to form a sling over the posterior surface of the odontoid process?

    (A) transverse ligament
    (B) anterior longitudinal ligament
    (C) posterior longitudinal ligament
    (D) supraspinous ligament

34. Which of the following CT examinations is temporal resolution of great importance?

    (A) HRCT chest
    (B) inner ear
    (C) cardiac angiography
    (D) bone mineral density

35. A particular CT examination requires the patient to receive 75 cc of nonionic contrast delivered over a 30-second duration time. What would the flow rate be for this study?

    (A) 1.5 cc/s
    (B) 2.0 cc/s
    (C) 2.5 cc/s
    (D) 3.0 cc/s

36. Name a characteristic of image data:

    (A) can be retrieved for later use
    (B) is subjected to preprocessing
    (C) can be sent to the CD burner
    (D) is a nonvisible digital image

37. In Figure Q5.4 label #31 represents which of the following structures?

    (A) orbital floor
    (B) inferior rectus muscle
    (C) middle rectus muscle
    (D) inferior oblique muscle

38. Which of the following is illustrated by label #9 in Figure Q5.4?

    (A) ethmoid sinus
    (B) maxillary sinus
    (C) sphenoid sinus
    (D) bony erosion of the orbital floor

39. Label #18 in Figure Q5.4 represents which of the following structures?

    (A) ethmoid sinus
    (B) maxillary sinus
    (C) sphenoid sinus
    (D) lacricmal duct

40. When speaking of radiation dose, a low pitch ratio >1 will produce what effect on dose?

    (A) decrease dose
    (B) increase dose
    (C) dose is not dependent on pitch
    (D) a pitch ratio >1 is never used in CT

41. What arteries join together to form the basilar artery?

    (A) internal carotid arteries
    (B) common carotid arteries
    (C) vertebral arteries
    (D) posterior cerebral arteries

42. A sudden change in mental activity may indicate that a patient is experiencing a serious condition; which of the following level of consciousness can be described as—only vigorous and repeated stimuli will arouse the individual?

    (A) stupor
    (B) lethargy
    (C) clouding
    (D) coma

43. Which of the following spine fractures is due to a severe compression of the vertebral body?

    (A) Jefferson's fracture
    (B) Hangman's fracture
    (C) burst fracture
    (D) vacuum phenomenon

44. Which CT scanner is based on a fan beam geometry and complete rotation of the x-ray tube and detectors?

    (A) first generation
    (B) second generation
    (C) third generation
    (D) fourth generation

45. Which of the following cranial nerves supplies motor fibers for the muscles of mastication?

    (A) olfactory
    (B) trochlear
    (C) abducens
    (D) trigeminal

46. In recent years, CT dose has been become a hot topic in the radiology community; therefore, many institutions have developed dose reduction team members to assess the radiation dose of each patient protocol. Which of the following is **not** a role of the CT dose reduction team?

    (A) identify examinations for dose reduction
    (B) review service logs
    (C) perform image quality review for each protocol
    (D) communicate changes with radiologists

47. What is the detector aperture size of a particular MDCT scanner with the beam collimation of 60 mm and 128 detector rows?

    (A) 1.2 mm
    (B) 0.46 mm
    (C) 0.3 mm
    (D) 1.5 mm

48. Which of the following structure reside in the retroperitoneal cavity?

    (A) spleen
    (B) liver
    (C) kidney
    (D) ileum

49. Which of the following forms of consent is used when a patient is unconscious in the emergency room?

    (A) simple consent
    (B) implied consent
    (C) formal consent
    (D) expressed

50. What pathological disorder presents with fluid in the posteribasal region forming a crescent-shaped collection that borders the chest wall?

    (A) pleural effusion
    (B) pulmonary embolism
    (C) pneumothorax
    (D) hemothorax

51. What pathological condition is characterized by submucosal edema with ulcerations involving a thickened segment of distal ileum?

    (A) small bowel obstruction
    (B) Crohn's disease
    (C) diverticulosis
    (D) pelvic inflammatory disease

52. Which of the following places a patient at greater risk for developing a chemotoxic adverse reaction to iodinated contrast media?

    (A) pregnancy
    (B) cirrhosis
    (C) pre-existing renal insufficiency
    (D) pre-existing renal calculi

53. What technique is used to ensure optimum evaluation of the urinary tract?

    (A) compression device
    (B) high mAs with low kVp
    (C) high mAs with high kVp
    (D) thick slice acquisition

54. The pituitary gland lies within what structure of the cranium?

    (A) pituitary stalk
    (B) sella turcica
    (C) cavernous sinus
    (D) sphenoid sinus

55. Documentation is imperative whenever IV contrast is administered. Which of the following is **not** a method used for medication reconciliation of IV contrast?

    (A) time the drug was administered
    (B) name and strength of the medication
    (C) scan delay time
    (D) patient's tolerance

56. What section of the large intestine is an *S*-shaped structure located at the terminal end of the descending colon originating at the lower left side of the abdominal cavity extending to midline?

    (A) ascending colon
    (B) rectum
    (C) splenic flexure
    (D) sigmoid

57. Which of the following networking topologies uses a common channel to connect all devices?

    (A) star networking
    (B) ring networking
    (C) redundant array of independent disks topology
    (D) bus networking

58. How long following the administration of an IV contrast media should a dialysis patient be dialyzed?

    (A) within 2 hours
    (B) within 6 hours
    (C) within 12 hours
    (D) when they are regularly scheduled

59. What type of detector array system contains detectors in which their width gradually increases in thickness as it moves away from the center of axis rotation?

    (A) hybrid array
    (B) adaptive array
    (C) matrix array
    (D) uniform array

60. Which of the following superficial muscles of the vertebral column are located on the posterior and lateral aspect of the cervical and upper thoracic spine?

    (A) splenius muscles
    (B) erector spinae muscle
    (C) transversospinal muscles
    (D) gluteal compartment

61. A dedicated CT examination of the liver was performed on a male patient with elevated LFTs. One image revealed a shading appearance on the right lobe of the liver and an erroneous HU measurement. The radiologist requested the technologist to perform thinner slices; what could be the reason for this request?

    (A) bean hardening artifact
    (B) cone beam artifact
    (C) partial volume averaging artifact
    (D) motion artifact

62. Immobilization devices prevent a patient from undesirable motion during the CT examination. Which of the following is categorized as a restraint and requires physician's orders?

    (A) tape
    (B) leather wrist guards
    (C) velcro straps
    (D) sponges

63. What is the principal advantage that 180-degree linear z-interpolation has over 360-degree linear *z*-interpolation?

    (A) better temporal resolution
    (B) better spatial resolution
    (C) fewer image artifacts
    (D) better *z*-axis resolution

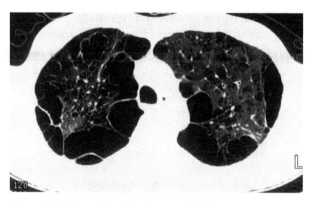

Figure Q5.5 Reproduced, with permission, from Grey ML, Ailinani JM. *CT and MRI Pathology: A Pocket Atlas.* 2nd ed. New York, NY: McGraw-Hill; 2012.

64. What pathological syndrome is depicted in Figure Q5.5?

    (A) pleural effusion
    (B) asbestosis
    (C) emphysema
    (D) pneumothorax

65. What new technique employed in multislice CT leads to a reduction of radiation dose?

    (A) slip rings
    (B) size of the detector aperture
    (C) automatic tube current modulation
    (D) subsecond scanning

66. Of the following, which organ is located in the right upper quadrant?

    (A) ileum
    (B) gall bladder
    (C) descending colon
    (D) fungus of the stomach

67. The left subclavian artery is a branch of which of the following artery?

    (A) arch of the aorta
    (B) descending aorta
    (C) ascending aorta
    (D) brachiocephalic trunk

68. The liver is surrounded by a strong connective tissue, which gives shape and stability to the soft hepatic tissue. What is this tissue called?

    (A) Gibson's compartment
    (B) Gerota's fascia
    (C) Morrison's pouch
    (D) Glisson's capsule

69. Which of the following statements is **true** concerning sequential access storage?

    (A) files are faster to read and write if you always access records in the same order
    (B) uses a disk drive to access files at any point on the disk without passing through all intervening points
    (C) gives the operator the ability to read and write data in a random order
    (D) makes use of magnetic or floppy disk for storage

70. Following the injection of 100 cc of iodinated contrast media a patient exhibits a severe vagal reaction that includes bradycardia. Which of the following drugs would be used for the initial treatment of this condition?

    (A) atropine
    (B) epinephrine
    (C) ranitidine hydrochloride (Zantac)
    (D) albuterol sulfate (Proventil)

71. Which of the following primary cancer usually does not metastasize to the lungs?

    (A) kidney
    (B) bone
    (C) breast
    (D) colon

72. What pathological condition occurs due to a sufficiently reduced spinal canal resulting in nerve root impingement from causes such as: osteophyte formation, disc herniation, and ligamentum flava hypertrophy?

    (A) spinal bifida
    (B) spondylolysis
    (C) disc herniation
    (D) spinal stenosis

73. Which of the following reconstruction algorithms is used as a means of reducing patient dose?

    (A) filtered back projection
    (B) algebraic reconstruction
    (C) iterative reconstruction
    (D) convolution reconstruction algorithms

74. What structure separates the lateral ventricles?

    (A) choroid plexus
    (B) septum pellucidum
    (C) falx cerebri
    (D) corpus callosum

75. What bone of the lower leg is situated most lateral in the anatomical position?

    (A) fibula
    (B) tibia
    (C) cuboid
    (D) navicular

76. Which of the following CT examination is performed with the use of an intrathecal injection?

    (A) CT angiography
    (B) virtual colonoscopy
    (C) CT enteroclysis
    (D) CT myelography

77. Which detector characteristic refers to the reliability of producing a useful signal?

    (A) response time
    (B) dynamic range
    (C) efficiency
    (D) stability

78. What is the first midline branch of the abdominal aorta?

    (A) inferior mesenteric artery
    (B) superior mesenteric artery
    (C) renal artery
    (D) celiac artery

79. With a window width of 1800 and a window level of –650, which of the following CT numbers would appear white in the image?

    (A) CT numbers above 250
    (B) CT numbers below –1,550
    (C) CT numbers between 250 and –1,550
    (D) CT number above –1,550

80. The pulse or heart rate is defined as the rate at which the heart beats in 1 minute. A pulse can be palpable where an artery is near the surface of the body. Where can the dorsalis pedis pulse be found?

    (A) lateral aspect of the wrist
    (B) behind the knee
    (C) apex of the heart
    (D) over the instep of the foot

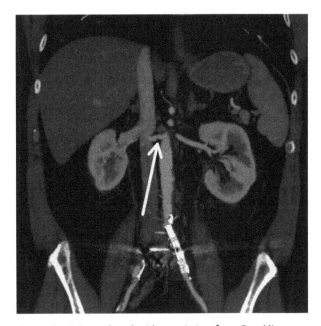

Figure Q5.6 Reproduced, with permission, from Grey ML, Ailinani JM. *CT and MRI Pathology: A Pocket Atlas.* 2nd ed. New York, NY: McGraw-Hill; 2012.

81. In Figure Q5.6, what pathological disorder is depicted in the coronal MPR image?

    (A) double renal artery
    (B) hydronephrosis
    (C) Nutcracker syndrome
    (D) renal artery stenosis

82. What is the main goal of computed tomography?

    (A) calculate the linear attenuation coefficients for image reconstruction
    (B) increase superimposition
    (C) decrease image contrast
    (D) utilize thick sections to increase spatial resolution

83. Special considerations are taken with patients at risk for developing an adverse event following the administration of IV contrast media. Which of the following conditions would not put the patient at risk for an allergic reaction?

    (A) patients with shellfish allergies
    (B) patients who had a prior reaction to contrast media
    (C) asthmatic patients
    (D) patients with low cardiac output

84. Which of the following chest muscles lies on the anterior surface of the third to fifth ribs?

    (A) pectoralis major muscle
    (B) pectoralis minor muscle
    (C) subclavius muscle
    (D) serratus anterior muscle

85. What reconstruction algorithm was developed to eliminate the star pattern typically seen in back projection?

    (A) filtered back projection reconstruction
    (B) adaptive statistical iterative reconstruction
    (C) modeled-based iterative reconstruction
    (D) algebraic reconstruction

86. What is the purpose of the taenia coli?

    (A) gathers the cecum and colon into pouch-like folds
    (B) attaches the intestine to the abdominal wall
    (C) sphincter muscle to control the flow of material from the ileum into the cecum
    (D) extracts water and salt from solid wastes before they are eliminated from the body

87. What is the general iodine concentration of water-soluble contrast media for gastrointestinal opacification during routine abdominopelvic CT examinations?

    (A) 5 to 10 mg I/mL
    (B) 13 to 15 mg I/mL
    (C) 20 to 30 mg I/mL
    (D) 50 mg I/mL

88. The same $CTDI_{volume}$ was used on two different patients, one with a small habitus and the other patient was extremely large. What would the absorbed dose be to the smaller patient as compared with the larger patient?

    (A) lower
    (B) stay the same
    (C) higher
    (D) half of the larger patient's dose

89. What benign pathological condition that occurs in women is seen on CT images as a well-defined mass with fluid density usually in the range of $+/- 15$ HU?

    (A) pelvic inflammatory disease
    (B) ovarian cancer
    (C) ovarian cyst
    (D) uterine cancer

90. What is the reconstructed DFOV, when the pixel area is 0.49 mm^2 with a 512^2 matrix?

    (A) 250 mm
    (B) 731 mm
    (C) 358 mm
    (D) 1,044 mm

91. Which artery may compress the left renal vein against the aorta causing venous stasis or Nutcracker syndrome?

    (A) iliac artery
    (B) inferior mesenteric artery
    (C) superior mesenteric artery
    (D) right renal artery

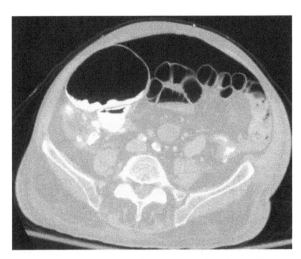

Figure Q5.7 Reproduced, with permission, from Grey ML, Ailinani JM. *CT and MRI Pathology: A Pocket Atlas*. 2nd ed. New York, NY: McGraw-Hill; 2012.

92. What types of artifacts can arise from insufficient projection sampling or from insufficient view sampling?

(A) aliasing
(B) motion
(C) beam hardening
(D) interpolation

93. Optimal IV access for CT procedures is achieved with what size angiocatheter when utilizing a power injector?

(A) 1 inch, 24 gauge
(B) 1 inch, 20 gauge
(C) .75 inch, 24 gauge
(D) .75 inch, 22 gauge

94. Which of the following characteristics contributes to heat dissipation in a CT x-ray tube?

(A) high-frequency generator
(B) increased beam filtration
(C) large diameter disk
(D) precise beam collimation

95. What ligament is longest and strongest tendon in the lower leg?

(A) anterior cruciate
(B) Achilles
(C) posterior cruciate
(D) medial meniscus

96. What pathological condition is demonstrated in Figure Q5.7?

(A) intraperitoneal free air
(B) small bowel obstruction
(C) peritoneal metastases
(D) colitis

97. What is the region called that is on the medial side near the center of both the right and left lungs, and is the where the bronchi, veins, and arteries enter and exit the lungs next to the heart?

(A) pulmonary trunk
(B) hilum
(C) left atrium
(D) carina

98. Which of the following image display techniques has become the principal mode of image evaluation with the onset of MDCT?

(A) region of interest
(B) multiplanar reformation (MPR)
(C) pixel analysis
(D) cine mode

99. Bolus or power injection of IV contrast material is superior to drip infusion for enhancing normal and abnormal structures during body CT examinations. Which of the following is **not** considered the proper technique to avoid the potentially serious complications of contrast media extravasation and/or air embolism?

(A) the patient's full cooperation should be obtained whenever possible
(B) use of a clean syringe
(C) once the syringe has been purged of air, keep the syringe in the upright position
(D) catheter tip should be checked for venous backflow

100. CT manufacturers and professional associations are all working towards a better method of tracking and documenting patient doses. What organization is responsible for setting the reference levels for tracking patient dose?

(A) NEMA and ACR

(B) OSHA

(C) HIPPA

(D) ACR

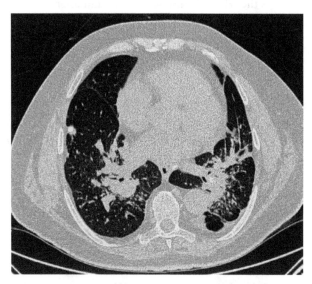

Figure Q5.8 Reproduced, with permission, from Grey ML, Ailinani JM. *CT and MRI Pathology: A Pocket Atlas.* 2nd ed. New York, NY: McGraw-Hill; 2012.

101. The HRCT of the chest in Figure Q5.8 demonstrates increased opacification in the mid lung and atelectasis in the middle lobe and lingual. Which of the following window widths was most likely used to display the image?

(A) 2,000

(B) −800

(C) 450

(D) 80

102. The endocrine system is a collection of glands that produce hormones that regulate your body's growth, metabolism, and sexual development and function. Which of the following organs accelerates metabolism and energy and are responsible for the body's "fight or flight" response?

(A) thymus gland

(B) thyroid gland

(C) adrenal gland

(D) pituitary gland

103. Which of the following ligaments join the laminae of adjacent vertebral arches to preserve the normal curvature of the spine?

(A) ligamentum flava

(B) supraspinous ligament

(C) anterior longitudinal ligament

(D) transverse ligament

104. Surgical aseptic techniques should be employed during which of the following CT procedures?

(A) administration of rectal contrast

(B) unenhanced sequences

(C) administration of oral contrast

(D) interventional CT procedures

105. A dedicated CT examination of the kidneys was performed on a patient complaining of frequent urination, upon the radiologist review, a small lesion with the μ of .189 was discovered. What did the radiologist attribute this measurement to be in HU?

(A) water

(B) air

(C) fat

(D) calcium

106. A radiologist is viewing the images of an abdomen and pelvis CT examination on the PACS workstation using a WW of 450 and a WL of 50, and notices there is a dense area on the patient's iliac crest. Which of the following adjustments can be made to make the image appear darker so that bony structures can be evaluated?

(A) increase the window level

(B) decrease the window level

(C) increase the window width

(D) decrease the window width

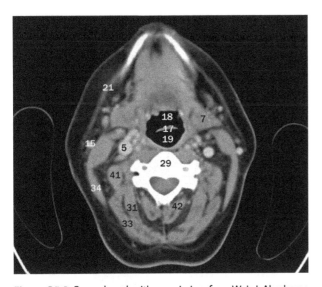

Figure Q5.9 Reproduced, with permission, from Weir J, Abrahams PH, Spratt JD et al. *Imaging Atlas of Human Anatomy*. 4th ed. ST. Louis, MO: Mosby Elsevier; 2011.

Refer to Figure Q5.9 to answer Questions 107–109.

107. Label #5 in Figure Q5.9 represents which of the following structures?

(A) common carotid artery

(B) internal jugular vein

(C) internal carotid vein

(D) external carotid vein

108. Which of the following is illustrated by label #17 in figure Q5.9?

(A) hyoid bone

(B) vallecular

(C) epiglottis

(D) piriformis sinus

109. In Figure Q5.9, the semispinalis capitis muscle is illustrated by which of the following numbers?

(A) 41

(B) 33

(C) 31

(D) 42

110. The American College of Radiology (ACR) publishes guidelines on ways of reducing radiation levels for various types of scans. Which of the following is **not** a way of minimizing radiation dose to patients?

(A) safety checks

(B) dose customization

(C) increasing tube potential output

(D) duplicate examination prevention

111. What is the purpose of the analog-to-digital converter?

(A) convert digital data to analog form

(B) convert transmitted data into attenuation and thickness data

(C) encode the analog measurements into binary data

(D) send data to the optical receiver array

112. Which of the following CT examinations utilizes the injection of contrast media and air into a joint space?

(A) CT angiogram of the aorta

(B) CT cystogram

(C) CT portogram

(D) CT arthrogram

113. When the SFOV is reduced for a particular image it results in what structure change?

(A) spatial resolution increases

(B) display image appears smaller

(C) display image appears larger

(D) fan angle increases

114. When imaging the adrenal glands, the density of lipid-poor adenomas may resemble that of nonadenomas, since their kinetics are similar to lipid-rich adenomas. Which of the following equations would be used to determine the relative percentage washout?

(A) $\dfrac{enhanced\,CT(HU) - delayed\,CT(HU)}{enhanced\,CT(HU)} \times 100\%$

(B) $delayed\,CT(HU) - enhanced\,CT(HU)$
$\times unenhanced\,CT(HU)$

(C) $\dfrac{unenhanced\,CT(HU) \times enhanced\,CT(HU)}{delayed\,CY(HU)} \times 100\%$

(D) $\dfrac{unenhanced\,CT(HU) - enhanced\,CT(HU)}{delayed\,CT(HU)} \times 100\%$

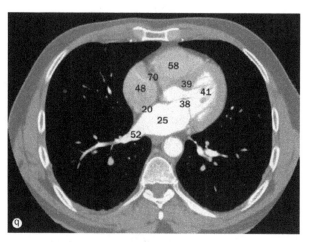

Figure Q5.10 Reproduced, with permission, from Weir J, Abrahams PH, Spratt JD et al, *Imaging Atlas of Human Anatomy*, 4th ed., ST. Louis, MO: Mosby Elsevier; 2011.

Refer to Figure Q5.10 to answer Questions 115–117.

115. In Figure Q5.10, label #38 represents what anatomical structure?

(A) tricuspid valve
(B) semilunar aortic valve
(C) semilunar pulmonary valve
(D) mitral valve

116. Which of the following is demonstrated by label #52 in Figure Q5.10?

(A) left atrium
(B) right inferior pulmonary vein
(C) left ventricle
(D) right inferior pulmonary artery

117. Label #70 in figure Q5.10 represents which of the following structures?

(A) tricuspid valve
(B) semilunar aortic valve
(C) semilunar pulmonary valve
(D) mitral valve

118. What classification of computer systems does a CT scanner utilize?

(A) supercomputer
(B) mainframe
(C) minicomputer
(D) microcomputer

119. What is considered the basic principle of estimating an unknown value of a function from two or more known values of the same function?

(A) filtered back projection
(B) z-interpolation
(C) algorithm
(D) convolution

120. What is the dose limit for radiation workers in the USA?

(A) 20 mSv/year
(B) 50 mSv/year
(C) 75 mSv/year
(D) 100 mSv/year

121. The purpose of contrast media is their ability to differentiate between radiographic densities and enable differences in anatomic tissues to be visualized. Which of the following contrast media agents is considered a negative agent?

(A) omnipaque
(B) carbon dioxide
(C) diatrizoate meglumine
(D) iohexol

122. What are the two muscles found on the anterior surface of the chest having their primary function to move of the upper limbs?

(A) trapezius muscles
(B) rhombus muscles
(C) pectoralis muscles
(D) scalene muscles

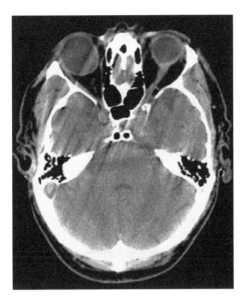

Figure Q5.11 Reproduced, with permission, from Seeram, Euclid. *Computed Tomography: Physical Principles, Clinical Applications, and Quality Control.* 3rd ed. St. Louis, MO: Saunders Elsevier; 2009.

123. Figure Q5.11 above represents which of the following CT artifacts?

(A) cone beam

(B) motion

(C) partial volume averaging

(D) metal

124. The kidneys are located in the retroperitioneum and are bound by a band of fibrous connective tissue; what is the name of this fibrocartilagenous tissue?

(A) Cooper's ligament

(B) Fascia of Camper

(C) linea alba

(D) Gerota's fascia

125. What is the voxel volume of a CT digital image having a 320 mm field of view (FOV), a 512^2 matrix, and a slice thickness of 3 mm?

(A) 0.625 mm^3

(B) 1.17 mm^3

(C) 0.39 mm^2

(D) 1.17 mm^2

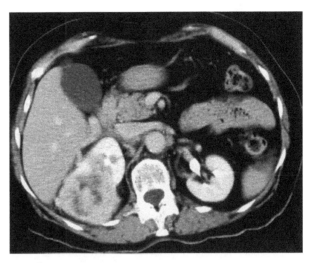

Figure Q5.12 Reproduced, with permission, from Grey ML, Ailinani JM. *CT and MRI Pathology: A Pocket Atlas.* 2nd ed. New York, NY: McGraw-Hill; 2012.

126. Figure Q5.12 demonstrates a large solid mass in the posterior aspect of the right kidney containing low-density area within the mass consistent with necrosis. What pathological condition does this image demonstrate?

(A) renal cell carcinoma

(B) polycystic kidney disease

(C) renal calculi

(D) horseshoe kidney

127. Image magnification is a basic visualization tool integrated into the CT system. Which of the following is an effect of image magnification?

(A) degrades the image display resolution

(B) changes the apparent noise in the image

(C) uses raw data to decrease the display FOV

(D) uses the segmentation process to give the illusion of depth

128. What is described as reduction of the intensity of a beam of radiation as it passes through an object?

(A) attenuation

(B) filtration

(C) collimation

(D) kerma

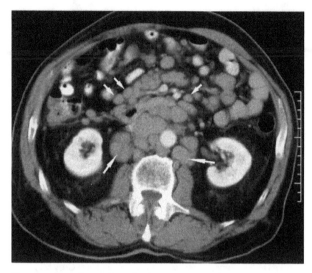

Figure Q5.13 Reproduced, with permission, from Grey ML, Ailinani JM. *CT and MRI Pathology: A Pocket Atlas.* 2nd ed. New York, NY: McGraw-Hill; 2012.

129. What pathological condition is demonstrated in Figure Q5.13?

(A) soft tissue sarcoma

(B) lymphoma

(C) peritonitis

(D) abdominal aortic aneurysm

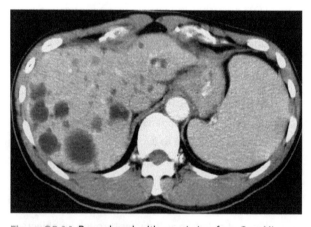

Figure Q5.14 Reproduced, with permission, from Grey ML, Ailinani JM. *CT and MRI Pathology: A Pocket Atlas.* 2nd ed. New York, NY: McGraw-Hill; 2012.

130. In Figure Q5.14 the radiologist interpreted the case as low-density lesions in the liver having a near water CT attenuation value and smooth margins. What is the diagnosis?

(A) hepatic abscesses

(B) hepatic cysts

(C) hepatocellular carcinoma

(D) metastatic lesions

131. Which of the following statements defines quality control?

(A) is any systematic process of checking the CT scanner's performance

(B) reviews the results of standard measurements and takes steps to correct any discrepancies

(C) ensures you are doing the right things, the right way

(D) concept that covers all policies and systematic activities implemented within a quality system

132. Which of the following pathological conditions can lead to mesothelioma?

(A) histoplasmosis

(B) emphysema

(C) asbestosis

(D) cystic fibrosis

133. What is the matrix size if the isotropic voxel volume equals 0.125 mm^3 with a 256 display field of view?

(A) 256

(B) 320

(C) 512

(D) 1024

134. Which of the following pathological conditions is caused by the compression of the flexor retinaculum?

(A) carpal tunnel syndrome

(B) Guyon's canal

(C) avascular necrosis

(D) Kienbock disease

135. Which of the following medication is delivered orally prior to a CT of the abdomen/pelvis examination?

  (A) barbiturate sedative medications before CT scanning
  (B) nonionic contrast media
  (C) suppository
  (D) diatrizoate meglumine

136. What type of data are also known as scan data?

  (A) raw data
  (B) measurement data
  (C) image data
  (D) convoluted data

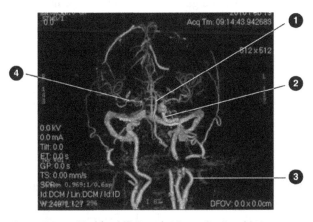

Figure Q5.15 Madden ME. *Introduction to Sectional Anatomy: Workbook and Board Review Guide.* 3rd ed. Philadelphia, PA: Wolters Kluwer; Lippincott Williams & Wilkins; 2013.

Refer to figure Q5.15 to answer Questions 137–139.

137. The structure labeled #4 in Figure Q5.15 is the:

  (A) posterior cerebral artery
  (B) vertebral artery
  (C) middle cerebral artery
  (D) common carotid artery

138. Which of the following is illustrated by label #3 in Figure Q5.15?

  (A) internal carotid artery
  (B) external carotid artery
  (C) middle cerebral artery
  (D) posterior communicating artery

139. What number in Figure Q5.15 illustrates the anterior cerebral artery?

  (A) 1
  (B) 2
  (C) 4
  (D) 5

140. A trauma patient received a chest/abdomen/pelvis study with a total beam collimation of 153.6 mm and the detector aperture size equaled 1.2 mm, what detector row scanned was this procedure on?

  (A) 32
  (B) 64
  (C) 128
  (D) 320

141. Which of the following flow rates is utilized for a CTA examination of the chest for pulmonary embolism?

  (A) 1 to 2 cc/s
  (B) 2 to 3 cc/s
  (C) 4 to 5 cc/s
  (D) 7 to 10 cc/s

142. Which of the following pathological conditions is characterized by inflammation of the bowel mucosa, bowel wall, and mesentery with marked submucosal edema?

  (A) appendix
  (B) angiomyolipoma
  (C) kidney stones
  (D) Cohn's disease

143. Which of the following pathological processes has an attenuation value of near water and accumulates in the greater peritoneal space?

  (A) cyst
  (B) abscess
  (C) ascites
  (D) hemorrhage

144. If a hepatic tumor is said to be hypervascular, it enhances during which phase of injection?

 (A) bolus

 (B) venous

 (C) nonequilibrium

 (D) delayed

145. Which of the following is **not** a characteristic of CT collimation?

 (A) ensure a constant beam width at the detectors

 (B) reduce patient dose

 (C) increase scatter radiation

 (D) improve image quality

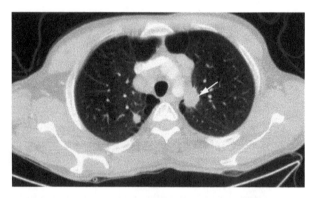

Figure Q5.16 Reproduced, with permission, from Grey ML, Ailinani JM. *CT and MRI Pathology: A Pocket Atlas.* 2nd ed. New York, NY: McGraw-Hill; 2012.

146. What is the pathological process demonstrated in Figure Q5.16?

 (A) cystic fibrosis

 (B) metastatic lung disease

 (C) lung abscess

 (D) bronchogenic carcinoma

147. A CT image of a homogeneous phantom is said to be uniform, what does this refer to?

 (A) constant CT numbers of an object

 (B) isotropic voxels

 (C) matrix detector array

 (D) accurate CT numbers

148. The heart is divided into four chambers, which chamber of the heart receives blood from the SVC, IVC, cardiac sinus, and cardiac veins?

 (A) right atrium

 (B) left atrium

 (C) right ventricle

 (D) left ventricle

149. Which of the following is a manufacture features that aids in the rectification of metal artifacts?

 (A) cardiac gating

 (B) use of low HU-value oral contrast

 (C) dual energy CT scanners

 (D) interpolation techniques to substitute the over range values in attenuation profile

150. What type of tumors show greater enhancement then the surrounding parenchyma during the arterial phase of injection?

 (A) hypervascular tumors

 (B) peripherally enhancing tumors

 (C) hypovascular tumors

 (D) complex cyst

151. Extravasated iodinated contrast media are toxic to the surrounding tissues, particularly to the skin, producing an acute local inflammatory response that sometimes peaks within how many hours post injection?

 (A) 1 to 5 hours

 (B) 10 to 12 hours

 (C) 24 to 48 hours

 (D) 60 to 72 hours

152. If one wants to improve spatial resolution, which of the following combinations of FOV and matrix size would be most effective?

 (A) FOV 10 cm, matrix 256^2

 (B) FOV 10 cm, matrix 512^2

 (C) FOV 15 cm, matrix 512^2

 (D) FOV 25 cm, matrix 256^2

153. What pulmonary disease may be caused by an elevation of pulmonary venous pressure?

    (A) pulmonary edema
    (B) pulmonary embolism
    (C) pulmonary fibrosis
    (D) cystic fibrosis

154. What measures the strength of a radiation field at some point in air?

    (A) exposure
    (B) absorbed dose
    (C) dose equivalent
    (D) dose rate

155. The ratio of the largest signal to the smallest signal measured by a CT detector is considered:

    (A) response time
    (B) dynamic range
    (C) efficiency
    (D) stability

156. Which of the following correctly describes the position of the seminal vesicles in the male pelvis?

    (A) posterior to the bladder and anterior to the rectum
    (B) superior to the rectum and inferior to the prostate
    (C) anterior to the bladder and superior to the prostate
    (D) inferior to the bladder and posterior to the rectum

157. Contrast resolution can be improved by which of the following?

    (A) imaging faster
    (B) reducing image noise
    (C) using a bone reconstruction filter
    (D) using low kVp

158. The wall of the uterus is composed of glandular and muscular linings, which lining of the uterus is highly vascular and responsible for the main contraction force during childbirth?

    (A) endometrium
    (B) epimetrium
    (C) myometrium
    (D) perimetrium

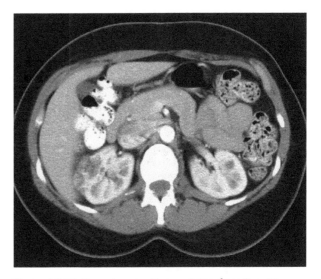

Figure Q5.17 Reproduced, with permission, from Grey ML, Ailinani JM. *CT and MRI Pathology: A Pocket Atlas.* 2nd ed. New York, NY: McGraw-Hill; 2012.

159. What pathological condition is demonstrated in Figure Q5.17?

    (A) soft tissue sarcoma
    (B) lymphoma
    (C) peritonitis
    (D) angiomyolipoma

160. Which of the following is **not** a function of the DAS?

    (A) measures the detected signal
    (B) converts the detected signal to analog form
    (C) transmits the detected signal to the computer
    (D) post processes the detected signal

161. What is the usual contrast delay when scanning the pancreas for hypervascular lesions or carcinomas using a flow rate of 4 to 5 cc/s?

(A) 15 to 20 seconds

(B) 30 to 40 seconds

(C) 70 to 80 seconds

(D) 120 to 180 seconds

162. What emotional state can lead to a severe adverse reaction to contrast media?

(A) confusion

(B) anxiety

(C) exaltation

(D) consciousness

163. The size of a pixel can be calculated by which of the following mathematical calculations?

(A) *pixel size = matrix × voxel size*

(B) *pixel size = FOV × matrix size*

(C) $pixel\ size = \dfrac{FOV}{the\ entire\ volume\ of\ tissue\ scanned}$

(D) $pixel\ size = \dfrac{FOV}{matrix}$

164. What is the largest and first carpal bone in the proximal row of the wrist?

(A) lunate

(B) capitate

(C) scaphoid

(D) hamate

165. Which of the following can occur if **not** enough samples are collected during data acquisition?

(A) beam hardening

(B) aliasing artifact

(C) image reconstruction is not possible

(D) blurry image

Answers and Explanations

1. **(B)** The pia mater is the innermost layer of the meninges surrounding the brain and the spinal cord. *(Madden, 3rd ed., p. 18)*

2. **(D)** A focused evaluation is necessary to assess the patient's degree of risk for adverse events during the computed tomography (CT) procedure and confirm the proper procedure that is being performed for the patient's specific signs and symptoms. Most institutions provide a written health assessment questionnaire for the patient to complete. The only question that is not necessary to ask the female patient if she has any children. *(The American College of Radiology Manual, pp. 5–6)*

3. **(C)** Photoelectric interaction occurs when an incident x-ray photon is totally absorbed during the ionization of an inner shell electron (usually the K or L shell). The incident x-ray photon's energy must be greater than the binding energy of the inner shell electron. This interaction is predominant with low-energy x-rays and material with high atomic numbers (bone, iodinated contrast media). *(Sprawls, Radiation Interaction with Matter, online)*

4. **(A)** The urethra is tubular organ approximately 20 cm in length that passes through the prostate gland, the urogenital diaphragm, and the penis in males. The function of the male urethra is to drain the bladder of urine and also transmit sperm to the exterior during ejaculation. *(Madden, 3rd ed., p. 397)*

5. **(D)** Modern CT scanner employs a rotating anode tube with a rhenium tungsten disk. The base of the disk is composed of graphite to increase the heat storage capacity. These large lightweight disks have a large heat storage capacity and a fast cooling rate to accompany the high demands of spiral/helical scanning. *(Seeram, 3rd ed., pp. 116–117)*

6. **(B)** Rivinus's duct located within the sublingual gland is responsible for the flow of salvia within the mouth. *(Kelley, 3rd ed., p. 270)*

7. **(D)** The simplest form of reconstruction was the algebraic method of reconstruction performed by Hounsfield. This method used a linear system of equations to solve a problem. The mathematical steps were sequential since the first image matrices were 80×80, only 6,400 calculations were needed to be performed. Granted it took hours to perform these calculations, but an image was produced revolutionizing the world of radiology. As technology increased in the computer world, new reconstruction methods were tried and improved. *(Seeram, 3rd ed., p. 5)*.

8. **(B)** Size-specific dose estimate (SSDE) is determined by multiplying CT dose index (CTDI) volume by a conversion factor based on the patient's effective diameter. The effective diameter is defined as the square root of the product of the anterior–posterior and the lateral patient diameter while not currently displayed with other CT parameters such as the $CTDI_{volume}$ or the dose length product (DLP) on the DICOM header of an individual patient's studies, SSDE could be calculated automatically by the scanner using the patient localizer images. *(Mayer-Smith, 2014)*

9. **(D)** The combination of small pixels and thin slice widths produces images with the least amount of volume averaging yielding a sharper image; hence, better spatial resolution. When a region of interest is placed on an image with such a combination, the Hounsfield units (HU) will most likely represent the true extent of the object. (*Seeram, 3rd ed., pp. 189–196*)

10. **(C)** The patellar ligament is the largest ligament of the knee. Its extension is from the patella and the tibial tuberosity, and is an extension of the quadriceps femoris tendon below the level of the patella. (*Madden, 3rd ed., p. 566*)

11. **(B)** Measurement of blood urea nitrogen (BUN) concentration is a poor indicator of renal function in children. BUN concentration depends on numerous variables in addition to renal function, including daily dietary protein intake, hepatic function, and patient hydration. A popular manner by which to express renal function in children is estimated glomerular filtration rate (GFR). Glomerular filtration rate calculations in children require knowledge of patient serum creatinine concentration and height. Currently, the best equation for estimating GFR from serum creatinine in children is the Bedside Schwartz equation. This formula is for use with creatinine methods and calibration traceable to isotope dilution mass spectrometry. (*The American College of Radiology Manual, p. 50*)

12. **(D)** Slip ring technology facilitates continuous rotation of the x-ray tube in order to produce volume data that is so important with CT angiography protocols. (*Seeram, 3rd ed., pp. 112–113*)

13. **(C)** The portal vein carries nutrient-rich blood to the middle of the visceral surface of the liver and lies adjacent to the hepatic bile ducts and the hepatic artery. Lying adjacent to the hepatic bile duct and the hepatic artery proper, it forms part of the porta hepatis. This vein is found in the retroperitoneum by a joining of the splenic vein and the superior mesenteric. Porta hepatis is a transverse fissure on the visceral surface of the liver, where the portal vein and the hepatic artery enter and the hepatic ducts leave. (*Madden, 3rd ed., p. 332*)

14. **(B)** The right lobe of the liver is the largest lobe separated from the left lobe by the interlobar fissure. This lobe is divided in anterior and posterior segments by the right hepatic vein and transversely by the right and the left portal veins. (*Kelley, 3rd ed., p. 416*)

15. **(B)** The external iliac artery becomes the femoral artery as it enters the anterior section of the thigh behind the inguinal ligament. The artery is rather superficial and easily palpable supplying all the compartments of the thigh and the skin of the anterior abdominal wall, inguinal region, and external genitalia. As it descends the thigh through the abductor muscles, it becomes the popliteal artery. (*Madden, 3rd ed., p. 392*)

16. **(D)** In this coronal image, the label represents the body of the pancreas. The body is the largest divisional section of the pancreas lying transversely to the left. As demonstrated in this image, it is anterior to the aorta and the superior mesenteric artery. (*Kelley, 3rd ed., p. 437*)

17. **(A)** In CT, an algorithm is a process or set of step-by-step rules to be followed in calculations or other problem-solving operations by the computer. (*Seeram, 3rd ed., p. 135*)

18. **(B)** Viscosity is the amount of friction generated by the concentration and the size of the contrast molecules. The higher the viscosity, the thicker the agent, and the more difficult to inject. Rapid injection with a higher viscosity agent can trigger the body's pressure sensors causing vessels to constrict and making injection painful. Heating the agent to body temperature reduces the viscosity of the agent. It is important to remember nonionic media are more viscous than ionic media at similar iodine concentrations. (*Adler, 5th ed., p. 296*)

19. **(B)**

$$pitch = \frac{table\ speed\left(\dfrac{mm}{sec}\right) \times gantry\ rotation\,(sec)}{total\ beam\ collimation}$$

$$1.5 = \frac{X\ table\ speed\left(\dfrac{mm}{sec}\right) \times 1\ sec}{16 \times 1.2}$$

$$1.5 = \frac{x}{19.2}$$

$$table\ speed = \frac{28.8\ mm}{sec}$$

(*Kalendar, 3rd ed., p. 89*)

20. **(C)** The subarachnoid space is the interval between the arachnoid membrane and the pia mater containing cerebrospinal fluid and vessels. *(Kelley 3rd ed., p. 100)*

21. **(C)** When a patient sustains a fall from that far of a distance the physician's major concerns are for internal abdominal bleeding and bone fractures. To enhance the abdominal cavity, a standard convolution is applied in order to demonstrate soft tissue structures and detailed peripheral borders. The bone or high-pass kernel is used to enhance bony details where fine hair-lined fractures could be seen. *(Seeram, 3rd ed., pp. 75–76)*

22. **(D)** The concept of dose limitations is a major integral component of regulatory guidance on radiation protection. This concept addresses the dose an individual receives annually or accumulates over a working lifetime. *(Seeram, 3rd ed., p. 243)*

23. **(C)** The principle behind the shaded surface rendering is to realistically produce a 3D scene of the surface of a structure of interest from the acquired data set. This process uses a segmentation technique that separates the object of interest from the background. The simplest way of generating these images is to define the object (skull, mandible, or an abdominal organ) and defining the range of CT numbers, whose voxel attenuation threshold values do not exceed the threshold value of the volume of interest. Light illumination is the key element in this processing technique. *(Seeram, 3rd ed., pp. 347–348)*

24. **(A)** An epidural hematoma appears as a classic biconvex (lentiform or football), shaped lesion with the dura bulging inward. Blood collects between the dura matter and the skull that is mainly caused as a consequence of a blunt force trauma. In CT imaging during the acute stage, the hemorrhage appears hyperdense, but as it proceeds into the subacute and chronic stage, the hemorrhage becomes isodense to hypodense. Skull fractures are usually present with an epidural hematoma. *(Grey, 2nd ed., pp. 82–83)*

25. **(A)** Contrast resolution can be described as the ability to distinguish one soft tissue from another with similar densities as their background. The term low-contrast detectability (LCD) is used to describe contrast resolution in CT. CT has the capability to image tissues that vary only slightly in density and atomic number, thus detecting density difference from 0.25% to 0.5%. When the difference between the object and the background is small, LCD improves. *(Seeram, 3rd ed., pp. 196–198)*

26. **(A)** Creatinine is a breakdown product of skeletal muscle, and its rate of production is proportional to muscle mass. Muscle mass depends on a variety of factors, including patient age, gender, and level of physical activity. Creatinine clearance testing is a test that utilizes creatinine assays from both serum and urine to detect very early loss of kidney function before abnormal increases in serum levels of BUN or creatinine arise. *(Ehrlich, 8th ed., pp. 223–224)*

27. **(C)** The valleculae are spaces on either side of the glossoepiglottic fold. On cross-sectional images it can be seen posterior to the tongue and the epiglottis. It is a common site for foreign bodies to lodge. *(Madden, 3rd ed., p. 176)*

28. **(D)** Xenon gas chambers offer several advantages. First their construction is relatively simple in principle and the sensitivity of the individual chambers is exactly the same, since constant pressure exists for the complete set of detector pressure channels. *(Kalendar, 3rd ed., p. 54)*

29. **(A)** CT dosimetry is the term used to describe the instrumentation and methods of computing radiation exposure and the effects it has on technologist and the population. It is also a method to compare their institutions doses with that of the national average, and can be utilized to educate hospital personal on the dose a patient received from a CT examination. *(Mayer-Smith; Seeram, 3rd ed., pp. 223–224)*

30. **(A)** Artifacts occur when part of the contents of a CT image does not represent the physical object being imaged. They can appear as false structures or corruption of the CT number. *(Kalendar, 3rd ed., p. 130)*

31. **(D)** Metformin is excreted without any decomposition of the medication by the kidneys; therefore, the renal route eliminates approximately 90% of the absorbed drug within the first 24 hours. Metformin seems to cause increased lactic acid production by the intestines. Any factors that decrease

metformin excretion or increase blood lactate levels are important risk factors for lactic acidosis. Renal insufficiency, then, is a major consideration with this drug and should be taken into consideration with patients undergoing contrast enhanced CT examinations. *(The American College of Radiology Manual, p. 43)*

32. **(D)** An overlapping reconstruction interval is one in which the interval is half the thickness of the slice thickness. Overlapping intervals improve image quality and decrease partial volume averaging. *(Seeram, 3rd ed., pp. 260–262)*

33. **(A)** The transverse ligament contains longitudinal fibers that attach to the anterior margin of the foramen magnum and insert on the body of the axis. This ligament extends across the ring of C1 to form a sling over the posterior surface of the odontoid process. The function of this ligament is to hold the odontoid process against the anterior arch of C1. It is also known as the cruciform ligament due to its cross-like appearance. *(Kelley, 3rd ed., p. 193)*

34. **(C)** With the introduction of CT cardiac imaging, temporal resolution has become a hot topic. Even though modern multidetector computed tomography (MDCT) scanners have the capability of producing scan speeds as low as 33 milliseconds, it is not sufficient enough to completely freeze the motion of the beating heart; therefore, manufactures developed specific cardiac reconstruction algorithms. The 180-degree multi-cardio delta algorithm uses a half-scan along with the fan angle for the reconstruction process, which improves temporal resolution by 40%. Another algorithm termed the 180-degree multi-cardio interpolation utilizes the patient's EKG to reconstruct the data only during the selected heart phase. This technique allows for a significant reduction in the effective scan time (<100 ms). *(Kalendar, 3rd ed., p. 100)*

35. **(C)** The equation to determine flow rate when knowing the amount of contrast and the duration time is as follows:

$$flow\ rate = \frac{volume}{duration\ time}$$

$$flow\ rate = \frac{75\,cc}{30\,sec}$$

$$flow\ rate = \frac{2.5\,cc}{sec}$$

(Prokop, pp. 97–98)

36. **(C)** Image data are the result of raw data being convoluted and processed by the computer. Once this process is completed a visible digital image appears on the scanner console. The only operation that can be performed on this data is reformation in the form of multiplanar or 3D manipulations. Image data can be copied to a CD and reviewed by means of a DICOM viewer or it can be sent to a laser printer for hard copy viewing. *(Seeram, 3rd ed., p. 145)*

37. **(A)** The orbital floor, also known as the roof of the maxillary sinus is made up of the following bones: the maxilla, the zygoma, and the palatine bone. *(Kelley, 3rd ed., p. 83)*

38. **(B)** The maxillary sinuses are located well within the body of the maxilla, beneath the orbit, and lateral to the nose. These sets of sinuses are the largest of the paranasal sinuses. They contain pockets of air that empties in the nasal cavity through the middle meatus. *(Madden, 3rd ed., p. 10)*

39. **(A)** The ethmoid sinuses are located within the labyrinths of the ethmoid bone (between the nose and the eye). The primary function of the ethmoid sinus (like all the sinus cavities in the skull) is to provide lubrication (mucus) to the inner nose. *(Madden, 3rd ed., p. 9)*

40. **(B)** Pitch can be described as the ratio of the distance the table travels per one revolution of the x-ray tube to the total collimated beam width. If the mAs is kept constant as the table moves, the radiation dose is proportionally decreased as pitch is increased. When increasing the pitch by a factor of two and all other factors remaining the same the dose is decreased by one-half. When moving in the opposite direction, if the pitch ratio is decreased, the dose will increase; therefore, pitch is inversely proportional to dose. *(Mayer-Smith, 2014)*

41. **(C)** The arterial system of the brain commences with the basilar artery. It is found at the midline on the anterior surface of the pons. It originates from the junction of the right and left vertebral arteries. *(Madden, 3rd ed., p. 21)*

42. (A) A stupor is the lack of critical cognitive function and a level of consciousness in which an individual is almost entirely unresponsive and only responds to base stimuli. This change in a patient's ability to respond, react, and cooperate normally usually results from illness, injury, medication, alcohol, or drugs. It is important as a technologist to remember, a patient in a stupor may not respond to simple instructions and are not responsible for their actions or answers. *(Ehrlich, 8th ed., p. 117)*

43. (C) A burst fracture occurs when there is hyperflexion and axial loading on the spine. It most commonly occurs in the thoracic and lumber spine. It involves the posterior body and the posterior longitudinal ligament with the compressed disc herniating into the vertebral body. *(Prokop, p. 954)*

44. (C) The third-generation CT scanners employed the rotate–rotate scanning geometry principle with the fan beam geometry. This principle allowed the x-ray tube and detectors to make a complete 360-degree rotation around the patient in order to collect a large set of data samples for the reconstruction process. *(Prokop, p. 3; Seeram, 3rd ed., p. 104)*

45. (D) The trigeminal is a motor and sensory nerve of the face consisting of three major divisions ophthalmic (V1), maxillary (V2), and mandibular (V3). It supplies motor fibers for the muscles of mastication. *(Madden, 3rd ed., p. 14)*

46. (B) The major roles of the team are to identify examinations for dose reduction, perform image quality review of each examination, and communicate the changes made with radiologists. Each member of the team has their own responsibility, but the primary goal with dose reduction endeavors is to uphold the diagnostic performance of CT, which in turn is influenced by the image quality. *(Mayer-Smith, 2014)*

47. (B)

$$Detector\ aperture\ size = \frac{beam\ collimation}{detector\ rows}$$

$$Detector\ aperture\ size = \frac{60\,mm}{128}$$

$$Detector\ aperture\ size = 0.46\,mm$$

(Seeram, 3rd ed., p. 274)

48. (C) Retroperitoneum consists of structures posterior to the peritoneum. The retroperitoneal space is located between the diaphragm and the pelvic brim and is divided into the anterior pararenal, perirenal, and posterior pararenal compartments by the anterior and posterior renal fascia. It houses organs such as: the kidneys, ureters, adrenal glands, and pancreas, most of the duodenum, ascending and descending colon, aorta, inferior vena cava (IVC), and uterus. *(Kelley, 3rd ed., p. 410)*

49. (B) Implied consent is utilized when a patient's decision-making capabilities are compromised due to their medical condition and consent cannot be taken from an appropriate designee in a timely manner. In these situations, a "reasonable person" can authorize consent and the required procedure may be performed without liability for failure to attain consent. A "reasonable person" is one who has full knowledge and understanding of the situation and would consent to the procedure under these circumstances. *(Gurley, 7th ed., pp. 145–147)*

50. (A) Pleural effusion is the abnormal collection of fluid between the pleural layers. Fluid within the pleural space will only be detected if the volume is 15 mL or greater. A thoracentesis is useful in defining the underlying cause of the fluid. *(Grey, 2nd ed., p. 184; Prokop, p. 398)*

51. (B) Crohn's disease is characterized by submucosal edema with ulcerations involving a thickened segment of distal ileum. The terminal ileum is affected in 80% of patient, while the colon is affected in 50%. *(Webb, p. 331)*

52. (C) Chemotoxic reactions result from the physicochemical properties of the contrast media that can result in contrast-induced nephropathy (CIN). The most important risk factor for CIN is pre-existing renal insufficiency. There are other known factors such as diabetes mellitus, dehydration, cardiovascular disease, diuretic use, advanced age, multiple myeloma, hypertension, hyperuricemia, and multiple iodinated contrast media doses in a short time interval (<24 hours) but these have not been rigorously confirmed as independent risk factors. *(The American College of Radiology Contrast Manuel, p. 33)*

53. **(A)** A compression device placed over the L5 region applies pressure to the ureters restricting the flow of contrast. A scan is performed, with the device inflated, from the kidneys to the iliac crest. Once the compression is released, the pelvic scan must be performed. This will demonstrate a urinary flow into the bladder. *(Prokop, p. 646)*

54. **(B)** The pituitary gland is an endocrine gland connected to the hypothalamus. It is nestled in the sella turcica at the base of the brain. It is known as the master gland, since it controls and regulates the functions of many other glands through the action of its six major types of hormones. *(Kelley, 3rd ed., p. 113)*

55. **(C)** Medication reconciliation is a formal process in which healthcare providers ensure accurate account of the contrast media given to each individual patient. The documentation should include the contrast media's name and strength, volume, route, date, and time of administration along with the patient's tolerance of the medication (whether an adverse event occurred). Medication reconciliation is a legal significance and should not be taken lightly by the technologist. *(Ehrlich, 8th ed., pp. 285–286)*

56. **(D)** The sigmoid colon can be found at the terminal end of the descending colon. It is the terminal portion of the descending colon and curves toward the midline to cross the sacrum where it turns downward to end in front of S3 at the rectum. *(Madden, 3rd ed., p. 392)*

57. **(D)** The bus network topology uses a common channel to connect all devices. A single cable (Ethernet cable) function as a shared communication medium that devices, such as, computers and printers, attach or tap into with an interface connector. This topology works best when there are a limited number of devices. *(Bradley, 2015)*

58. **(D)** According to the American College of Radiology (ACR) manual on contrast media, a dialysis patient undergoing an enhance CT examination does not need to be immediately dialyzed, since contrast agents are not protein-bound. They have relatively low molecular weights, and are readily cleared by dialysis. Unless an unusually large volume of contrast media is administered or there is substantial underlying cardiac dysfunction, there is no need for urgent dialysis after intravascular iodinated contrast media administration. *(The American College of Radiology Manual, p. 40)*

59. **(B)** Adaptive, variable, or nonuniform array detectors consist of detector rows that grow in width from the center of the section to the periphery. The aperture size of the center rows are usually 1 mm with the outer most row being 5 mm. Depending on the total beam collimation all or only a specific number of detectors will be exposed. For example:
    1) 2×0.5 mm, beam collimation 1 mm—in this case the DAS divided the signal of each 1-mm detector to reconstruct two images each 5 mm in width
    2) 4×1 mm, beam collimation of 4 mm
    3) 4×2.5 mm, beam collimation of 10 mm
    4) 4×5 mm, beam collimation of 20 mm
    5) 2×8 mm, beam collimation of 16 mm *(Prokop, p. 21; Seeram, 3rd ed., p. 287)*

60. **(A)** The splenius muscles are located on the posterior and lateral aspect of the cervical and upper thoracic spine. They are divided into a cranial segment, the splenius capitis, and the cervical segment, the splenius cervicis. The functions of these muscles are to extend the head and the neck. *(Kelley, 3rd ed., p. 201)*

61. **(C)** Partial volume averaging arises when tissues of widely different absorption are encompassed on the same CT voxel producing a beam attenuation proportional to the average value of these tissues. Using thinner slices will differentiate the different tissue types eliminating the shading artifact that appeared on the liver as in the above situation. *(Kalendar, 3rd ed., p. 132)*

62. **(B)** Restraints are devices utilized to restrict patient movement and to ensure their safety. Apparatuses such as leather wrist guards are used to prevent patients from injuring themselves and/or others or from disengaging therapeutic devices such as IV lines, suction catheters, or oxygen masks. *(Ehrlich, 8th ed., pp. 199–200)*

63. **(D)** The 180-degree linear *z*-interpolation technique substantially narrowed the slice sensitivity profile because the distance between corresponding projections in the real and virtual spirals are

less than between the corresponding projections in the real spiral alone. The data set generated by the virtual spiral is termed complementary data. The major advantages of 180-degree *z*-interpolation include: improved *z*-axis resolution, the generation of thinner slices, and scanning at higher pitches. *(Prokop, p. 11)*

64. **(C)** Emphysema is free air trapped with the lungs during the inhalation process with the inability to be exhaled. Cigarette smoking is the major culprit of this disease. *(Grey, 2nd ed., p. 180)*

65. **(C)** Tube current modulation (mA modulation) is an essential tool to ensure proper patient exposure with CT examinations. It allows the tube current to be actively modulated during the scan to more efficiently apply radiation to the patient. This potentially saves dose because instead of using a fixed tube current optimized for the thickest part of the patient, the scanner will produce fewer x-ray photons in regions of lower attenuation and modulate higher values of tube current in regions of higher attenuation. *(Mayer-Smith, 2014)*

66. **(B)** The midsagittal plane and transverse plane intersect at the umbilicus to divide the abdomen into four quadrants. The right upper quadrant consists of: right lobe of the liver, gallbladder, right kidney, portions of the stomach, small bowel, and large intestines. *(Kelley, 3rd ed., p. 7)*

67. **(A)** The left subclavian artery is the first branch of the aortic arch from left to right and is posterior to the left common carotid artery. This artery like it's counterpart the right subclavian artery, arches toward the axilla, and continues as the axillary artery. *(Kelley, 3rd ed., p. 363)*

68. **(D)** The liver is surrounded by a strong connective tissue referred to as Glisson's capsule that gives shape and stability to the soft hepatic tissue. *(Kelley, 3rd ed., p. 412)*

69. **(A)** Sequential access is referred to as reading or writing data records in sequential order, that is, one record after the other. Sequential-access files are faster to read and write if you always access records in the same order, but became very time consuming when a study in the middle of the tape needed retrieving. *(Seeram, 3rd ed., pp. 41–42)*

70. **(A)** Bradycardia refers to a decrease in heart rate for which the drug atropine is the initial treatment of choice. Atropine is an anticholinergic drug that acts as a vasoconstrictor, which increases the patient heart rate. *(Ehrlich, 8th ed., p. 319)*

71. **(B)** The lungs are the most common site of metastatic disease from primary cancers outside the lungs. Primary cancers such as colon, breast, kidney, pancreas, and uterus are most likely to metastasize to the lungs. The disease spreads through blood circulation and lymphatic system. *(Grey, 2nd ed., pp. 190–191)*

72. **(D)** Spinal stenosis is a condition where the spinal canal is sufficiently reduced in diameter size resulting in nerve root impingement from such causes as osteophyte formation and/or disc herniation. The acquired form is probably due to one of the following: degenerative disc disease, ligamentum flava hypertrophy, spondylolisthesis, and disc bulging and/or trauma. *(Grey, 2nd ed., p. 98)*

73. **(C)** The sophisticated iterative reconstruction algorithm starts with an initial guess of the object and iteratively improves on the initial estimate of the attenuation value by comparing the estimated noise projection with the acquired projection data and making an incremental model-based change to the previous guess. This mathematical noise guess allows for a decrease in tube output, thus reducing patient dose. *(Mayer-Smith, 2014)*

74. **(B)** The septum pellucidum is a thin partition in cerebral hemisphere located between the columns of the fornix and the corpus callosum separating the anterior horns of the lateral ventricles. *(Madden, 3rd ed., p. 15)*

75. **(A)** The fibula is located on the lateral aspect of the lower leg. The bone is rather thin with expanded proximal and distal ends. The proximal aspect of the bone articulated with the lateral condyle of the tibia creating the tibiofibular joint. The distal end of the bone articulates with the talus forming a section of the ankle joint. *(Madden, 3rd ed., p. 565)*

76. **(D)** A CT myelogram commences with an injection of contrast media in the patients intrathecal

space, which is located in the space around the spinal cord. The purpose of this procedure is to demonstrate the spinal cord, spinal canal, and nerve roots. (*Adler, 5th ed., p. 217*)

77. **(D)** Stability refers to the steadiness of the detectors' response. Instability causes a signal not to be useful. It is an important characteristic of detectors, since it will be free or almost free from change, variation, or fluctuation, and will produce a uniform signal. (*Seeram, 3rd ed., p. 123*)

78. **(D)** The celiac artery or trunk is the first unpaired branch of the abdominal aorta. It is a very short vessel that leaves the anterior wall of the aorta just after the aorta passes through the diaphragm at the level of T12–L1. (*Madden, 3rd ed., p. 327*)

79. **(A)** The range of CT numbers for this particular WW and WL is 250 at the upper level to −1550 at the lower level. Since the upper level is 250 all CT numbers above will appear white. To calculate the range of CT numbers use the following equation:

$$WL + \frac{WW}{2} \quad WL - \frac{WW}{2}$$

$$-650 + \frac{1,800}{2} \quad -650 - \frac{1,800}{2}$$

$$-650 + 900 \quad -650 - 900$$

$$250 \quad -1,550$$

The range of CT numbers for this window width and level calculated to 250 to −1,550. (*Seeram, 3rd ed., p. 172*)

80. **(D)** The dorsal most prominence of the navicular bone provides a bony landmark to readily locate the dorsalis pedis artery. This pulse is significant when there is a question of poor peripheral circulation. (*Ehrlich, 8th ed., pp. 217–218*)

81. **(D)** This coronal MPR demonstrates atherosmatous plaque along the aortic wall and small filling defect in the proximal right renal artery resulting in renal artery stenosis. (*Grey, 2nd ed., p. 296*)

82. **(A)** The main goal in CT is to calculate the linear attenuation value along each ray to the source detectors. This is accomplished through the Lambert Beer Law, but taking into account the attenuation from the photoelectric absorption and Compton scatter. (*Kalendar, 3rd ed., pp. 24–26*)

83. **(A)** Shellfish allergies were once considered contraindications to IV contrast, but the predictive value of shellfish and dairy allergies have proved to be unreliable. A significant number of healthcare providers continue to inquire specifically into a patient's history of a shellfish allergy, but there is no evidence to support the continuation of this practice. (*The American College of Radiology Manual, p. 5*)

84. **(B)** The pectoralis minor muscle lies directly behind the pectoralis major on the anterior surface of the third through fifth ribs. It acts to elevate and protract the scapula. (*Kelley, 3rd ed., p. 394*)

85. **(A)** Filtered back projection is a type of reconstruction method known as the convolution method and was developed in order to eliminate the star pattern typical of the back projection method. This analytic method uses the Fourier Transform to convert a signal in the spatial location domain to a signal in the spatial frequency domain. The first advantage of the data being in the frequency domain is that it can be manipulated by changing the amplitudes of the frequency components in determining the properties of the reconstructed image in terms of spatial resolution and image noise. The second advantage is the frequency information can be used to measure image quality. (*Seeram, 3rd ed., pp. 142–144*)

86. **(A)** The taenia coli is made up of three narrow but distinct longitudinal bands of smooth muscle running along the entire length the cecum and colon gathering them into pouch-like folds known as hastra. The taenia coli are not present on the rectum, anal canal, and vermiform appendix. (*Kelley, 3rd ed., p. 462*)

87. **(B)** Various iodine concentrations of water-soluble contrast media ranging from 4 to 48 mg I/mL, but in general, a solution containing 13–15 mg I/mL is recommended for oral and rectal administration in adults undergoing CT examinations. (*The American College of Radiology Manual, p. 61*)

88. **(C)** The absorbed dose to the smaller patient would be higher because the larger patient will have a more diluted deposition of absorbed dose, since the same dose is distributed over a larger mass than a smaller patient exposed to the same radiation. A fixed exposure setting (not using tube current modulation) results in an unnecessarily higher absorbed dose for the smaller and risks poor image quality in large patients. *(Mayer-Smith, 2014)*

89. **(C)** On CT imaging, ovarian cysts are homogeneous near water densities and have thin well-defined walls. *(Webb, p. 368)*

90. **(C)** The DFOV can be calculated by the produce of the pixel size and the matrix size. The equation is as follows:

$$DFOV = pixel\ size \times matrix\ size$$

Since the problem above gives the pixel area, the first step is to take the square root of the pixel area; therefore, the pixel size is calculated as 0.7 mm.

$$\sqrt{0.49} = 0.7$$
$$DFOV = 0.7 \times 512$$
$$DFOV = 358\ mm$$

(Seeram, 3rd ed., p, 193)

91. **(C)** The superior mesenteric artery extends from the aorta and branches into several arteries that supply blood to the majority of the small intestine and ascending and transverse colon. Due to the location of the left renal vein passing posterior to the superior mesenteric artery, the artery may compress against the left renal vein compromising the drainage of the vein into the IVC. *(Kelley, 3rd ed., p. 479)*

92. **(A)** Image quality depends on the number of projections to reconstruct an image. If not an adequate number of samples are collected, it results in misregistration by the computer of information relating to sharp edges and small objects. This artifact appears as evenly spaced lines that are easy to distinguish from anatomic structures and seldom render an image undiagnostic. *(Seeram, 3rd ed., p. 213)*

93. **(B)** CT injection procedures require the use of a power injector to administer contrast media with consistent flow rates and duration times. Due to the mechanism of the power injectors, a 20-gauge, 1-in angiocatheter is optimal, since they provide stability when the power injector releases pressure. *(Ehrlich, 8th ed., pp. 273–274)*

94. **(C)** The anode is the positive terminal and part of the tube where the target material is located. The spiral/helical scanners employ a 200 mm diameter rotating anode disk allowing for the use of higher tube currents in the range of 120 to 140 kVp. The heat storage capacity with these disks is increased with an improvement in heat dissipation. *(Seeram, 3rd ed., p. 115)*

95. **(B)** The Achilles tendon is the longest and strongest tendon of the foot and the ankle. An Achilles tendon injury usually occurs from trauma (sports injury or strenuous activity). These tears are classified as complete or partial with complete requiring surgical intervention and partial only needing immobilization and reduce weight bearing. *(Grey, 2nd ed., p. 420)*

96. **(A)** Intraperitoneal free air is a collection of air or gas in the peritoneal cavity, which can be caused by surgical perforation, ruptured intestine, or penetrating trauma. CT images viewed in the lung window demonstrate good subject contrast between oral contrast in the bowel and air within the cavity. In many cases, scanning in the decubitus position aids the radiologist in determining the exact location. *(Grey, 2nd ed., p. 231)*

97. **(B)** The hilum is a depression or pit where structures are attached. As in the chest, the hilum is part of the lungs where structures such as blood vessels and nerves enter. *(Madden, 3rd ed., p. 236)*

98. **(D)** The cine mode is an interactive display tool that gives the observer the ability to view large data sets in a comparatively short amount of time. Using this mode, the viewer has the capability of examining images in the axial, coronal, or sagittal planes alone or using a combination of planes. The user has full control of the cine loop with the use of a mouse or trackball. *(Prokop, p. 48)*

99. **(C)** The main steps in avoiding a potentially serious complication associated with the use of a power injector is to obtain complete cooperation

from the patient, if possible. Communication is a key with the patient before the examination and during the injection to reduce the risk of contrast media extravasation. To avoid unnecessary infections, a clean syringe (one in which the sterile packaging has not been tampered with) must be utilized. Standard procedures should be used to clear the syringe and pressure tubing of air, after which the syringe should be reoriented with the tubing directed downward. Before initiating the injection, the position of the catheter tip should be checked for venous backflow. Lastly, the power injector and tubing should be positioned to allow adequate table movement without tension on the intravenous line. (*The American College of Radiology Manual, p. 13*)

100. **(D)** The ACR in use with their CT Accreditation Program are working toward a better method of tracking and documenting patient doses in addition to ensuring that examinations are conducted with the least amount of radiation possible. The ACR has established reference levels for each specific patient protocol requiring an institution to investigate a protocol if it exceeds the reference levels and then determine if a lower radiation level can be utilized without a loss of image quality. (*Hale, 2013*)

101. **(A)** Window width controls the contrast of the image by selecting a specific range of shades of gray from the Hounsfield scale displayed on the CT monitor. The window width is chosen according to the attenuation values inherited in the anatomy of interest. Images of the lungs require a window width from 1,000 to 2,000 shades of gray to accentuate the air spaces and bronchioles as seen in Figure Q5.8. (*Kalendar, 3rd ed., p. 32*)

102. **(C)** The adrenal glands produce the hormones epinephrine and norepinephrine. These hormones secrete into the body's system to influence the body's metabolism, blood chemicals, and body characteristics, as well as influence the part of the nervous system that is involved in the response and defense against stress; hence, "fight or flight" response. (*Kelley, 3rd ed., pp. 442–443*)

103. **(A)** The ligamentum flava is located on either side of the spinous process consisting of strong yellow elastic tissue. Its purpose is to join the laminae of

adjacent vertebral arches to preserve the normal curvature of the spine. (*Kelley, 3rd ed., p. 201*)

104. **(D)** Surgical asepsis is the protection against infection before, during, and after a surgical procedure by utilizing sterile techniques. Interventional CT procedures require the use of a sterile techniques that include a sterile tray and sterile drapes. It is imperative to confirm the packages are clean and dry, have not been previously opened, or the expiration date has passed to be considered sterile. The other procedures that were mentioned in question 104, require aseptic techniques with the goal of preventing the spread of pathogens and/or harmful microorganisms. (*Adler, 5th ed., p. 217*)

105. **(C)**

$$CT\,number = \frac{\mu(tissue) - \mu(water)}{\mu(water)} \times 1,000$$

$$CT\,number = \frac{0.189 - 0.206}{0.206} \times 1,000$$

$$CT\,number = -0.802 \times 1,000$$

$$CT\,number = -82\,HU$$

On the HU scale −82 HU represents fat. (*Seeram, 3rd ed., p. 200*)

106. **(A)** Window level controls the brightness of an image on the computer monitor. Other names for window level are window center and window length. Within the range of CT numbers as in question 106, the window level is found in the center of the range of number and is placed on the Hounsfield scale closest to the attenuation value of the area of interest. By increasing the window level from 50 to 500, the image will have a darker appearance lending to a better analysis of the bony structures. (*Kalendar, 3rd ed., p. 32*)

107. **(B)** The jugular veins are the largest vascular structures of the neck. They drain blood from the face and the neck. The IJV commence at the jugular foramen and descend the lateral portion of the neck to unite with the subclavian vein to form the brachiocephalic vein. The enlargement of the jugular foramen is the jugular fossa. (*Kelley, 3rd ed., pp. 305–306*)

108. **(C)** The epiglottis differs from the other cartilages in that it is elastic and allows movement. During

swallowing it folds back over the larynx, preventing the entry of liquids and solid food from entering the respiratory passage. When swallowing solid or liquid material, the tongue shifts posteriorly bending the epiglottis over the opening of the larynx. *(Madden, 3rd ed., p. 175)*

109. **(C)** The splenius muscles are located on the posterior and lateral aspect of the cervical and upper thoracic spine. The splenius capitis is the cranial portion originating on the spinous processes of C7–T3 and inserting on the mastoid process of the temporal bone. *(Kelley, 3rd ed., p. 201)*

110. **(C)** Safety checks provide procedures for checking and double-checking patient information and the type of exam to be performed to prevent a patient from receiving an unnecessary examination. CT vendors have employed in their modern scanners new technology with the ability to intelligently customize the radiation dose according to the patient's weight, age, medical history, and the body part being scanned. Many Radiology Information Systems (RIS) have the ability to warn a physician when the patient had a similar exam recently or when a similar exam has already been scheduled. *(Mayer-Smith, 2014)*

111. **(C)** The purpose of the analog-digital-converter (ADC) is to divide the electrical signal into multiple parts, the more divisional parts, and the greater the accuracy. The parts are measured into bits, 1-bit divides the signal into two digital values. The ADC's dynamic range must be large to preserve the large dynamic range of the x-ray image. Converters with 16-bit resolution or greater are common in CT. These values determine the gray-scale resolution of the image. *(Seeram, 3rd ed., pp. 128–129)*

112. **(D)** A CT arthrogram study employees the use of a nonionic contrast media and air into a joint space. It is most commonly utilized in the shoulder for the evaluating the labrum and the joint capsule, when joint instability is suspected. *(Prokop, p. 958)*

113. **(A)** As the SFOV decreases, going from a 500 mm to a 250 mm view, the fan angle decreases resulting in a reduction of radiation hitting the object outside the field. A narrow fan angle results in increased sampling rate which in turn improves spatial resolution. *(Kalendar, 3rd ed., p. 121)*

114. **(A)** The relative washout to determine the morphology of an adrenal lesion is as follows:

$$\frac{enhanced\ CT\,(\mathrm{HU}) - delayed\ CT\,(\mathrm{HU})}{enhanced\ CT\,(\mathrm{HU})} \times 100\%$$

(Prokop, pp. 636–637)

115. **(D)** The mitral valve also known as the bicuspid valve is located at the entrance of the left ventricle. It functions to maintain a one-way directional blood flow from the left atrium into the left ventricle. *(Kelley, 3rd ed., p. 346)*

116. **(B)** The right inferior pulmonary artery is located in the right lower lobe of the lung crossing behind the right atrium to the left atrium. *(Kelley, 3rd ed., p. 350)*

117. **(A)** The tricuspid valve is located at the entrance of the right ventricle. It functions to maintain a one-way directional blood flow from the right atrium into the right ventricle. *(Kelley, 3rd ed., p. 346)*

118. **(C)** The midrange or minicomputer is the computer system used in CT. The midrange computer deals efficiently with the convoluted mathematical input and produces output data at subsecond time intervals. Its major characteristics are its large storage capacity and fast and efficient processing of various kinds of data. *(Seeram, 3rd ed., p. 33)*

119. **(B)** In mathematics, engineering, and science the basic idea of interpolation is to estimate an unknown value of a function from two or more known values of the same function. The two types of interpolation are known as 360-degree interpolation and 180-degree interpolation with 180-degree interpolation being the technique of choice especially with MDCT. *(Kalendar, 3rd ed., pp. 90–94)*

120. **(B)** Dose limitation is a major integral component of regulatory guidance on radiation protection. International organizations such as the ICRP and the National Council on Radiation Protection recommend that radiation workers do not exceed 50 mSv/year to reduce the probability of stochastic effects and to prevent detrimental deterministic effects. *(Seeram, 3rd ed., p. 220)*

121. **(B)** The body absorbs photons according to the various atomic numbers and the amount of

matter per volume of tissue, since carbon dioxide has an atomic number of 6, it is considered a negative agent. This agent is relatively lucent to x-rays; therefore, the areas filled by this agent appear dark on CT images due to increased density. Carbon dioxide gas is used in virtual colonoscopy to distend the colon and to aid in distinguishing polyps from residual stool. *(Adler, 5th ed., p. 291)*

122. **(C)** The pectoralis muscles are two muscles found on the anterior surface of the chest with their primary function being movement of the upper limbs. The pectoralis major muscle is most anterior and aids in the flexion, abduction, and rotation of the arms. Its other function is to expand the thoracic cavity during deep inspiration. The pectoralis minor muscle lies directly behind the pectoralis major on the anterior surface of the third through fifth ribs. It acts to elevate and protract the scapula. *(Kelley, 3rd ed., p. 394)*

123. **(B)** Motion artifacts appear as streaks that are tangential to high-contrast edges on the moving part. They result from the computer's inability to calculate the data possessing inconsistencies in their voxel attenuation arising from the edge of the moving part. *(Seeram, 3rd ed., pp. 206–207)*

124. **(D)** Gerota's fascia is perirenal fat that surrounds and protects the kidneys. *(Kelley, 3rd ed., p. 446)*

125. **(B)**

$$voxel\ volume = pixel\ area^2 \times slice\ thickness$$

$$pixel\ size = \frac{FOV}{matrix}$$

$$pixel\ size = \frac{320\,mm}{512}$$

$$pixel\ size = 0.625$$

$$pixel\ area^2 = 0.625 \times 0.625$$

$$pixel\ area^2 = 0.39\,mm^2$$

$$voxel\ volume = 0.39\ mm^2 \times 3\ mm$$

$$voxel\ volume = 1.17\ mm^3$$

(Sprawls, Computed Tomography Image Formation, 2014)

126. **(A)** The image in Figure Q5.12 demonstrates low-density areas within the mass consistent with necrosis.

It is not uncommon for the renal cell tumors to contain internal hemorrhage, cystic necrosis, and coarse and irregular calcifications. *(Grey, 2nd ed., p. 300)*

127. **(A)** Image magnification is a computer software program that changes the size of the pixels on the computer monitor. As the pixel resolution becomes larger, the image appears blurry on the display monitor. Image magnification should not be confused with targeting an area of interest. Magnification uses image data only for the purpose of enlarging the image on the screen, while targeting employs raw data to decrease the display field of view (FOV) in order to enhance a particular area of interest. *(Sprawls, Computed Tomography Image Formation, 2014)*

128. **(A)** The principle of attenuation is the reduction in the intensity of an x-ray beam when passing through matter. The extent of attenuation is a property of the material which is exposed to radiation and is quantitatively described by the linear attenuation coefficient. *(Kalendar, 3rd ed., p. 368)*

129. **(B)** On CT images affected lymph nodes have the same attenuation value as muscle tissue. Lymphomas tend to form conglomerate masses, which may encase the mesenteric vessels known as the "sandwich" sign. *(Webb, p. 189; Grey 2nd ed., p. 327)*

130. **(B)** Hepatic cysts appear as homogeneous, well-defined, round, or oval-shaped thin-walled lesions that have a near water attenuation value and should not enhance with IV contrast. *(Grey, 2nd ed., p. 270)*

131. **(B)** The terms "quality assurance" and "quality control" are often used interchangeably and should not be confused even though, both refer to ways of ensuring the quality of a CT scanner. Quality control on the other hand reviews the results of the quality assurance testing and makes corrections to improve the scanner's performance. *(Seeram, 3rd ed., pp. 478–482)*

132. **(C)** Asbestosis is the inhalation of asbestos fiber causing scarring of the lungs that can lead to lung CA (Mesothelioma). On CT images it may show ground-glass opacities and honeycomb patterns. *(Grey, 2nd ed., p. 176)*

133. **(C)** The first problem to solve is determining the pixel size. Since an isotropic voxel contains three equal sides, the cube root of 0.125 mm³ is equal to 0.5-mm pixel size. The following equation is utilized to find the matrix:

$$\sqrt[3]{125} = 0.5 \, mm$$

$$matrix = \frac{FOV}{pixel \, size}$$

$$matrix = \frac{256 \, mm}{0.5 \, mm}$$

$$matrix = 512^2$$

(Seeram, 3rd ed., p. 193)

134. **(A)** Carpal tunnel syndrome occurs when there is compression of the median nerve and is associated with repetitive activity, such as typing. Injections of hydrocortisone may be very beneficial to most patients, but surgery may be needed to release the flexor retinaculum. *(Grey, 2nd ed., p. 366)*

135. **(D)** Diatrizoate meglumine is intended to be therapeutically and biologically inert when ingested/injected into the body for use in organ or tissue enhancement. It is particularly suited for times when a more viscous agent such as barium sulfate (not water soluble) is not feasible or is potentially dangerous. *(The American College of Radiology Manual, pp. 56–57)*

136. **(B)** Measurement data, also known as scan data, are the transmitted intensities hitting the detectors. The measured attenuation profiles undergo a number of corrections to adjust for errors that may have occurred from beam hardening, variations of the sensitivity, and distance between detector channels, or scatter radiation. *(Seeram, 3rd ed., p. 144; Kalendar, 3rd ed., p. 364)*

137. **(C)** The image in Figure Q5.15 represents a CTA volume rendered technique of the arteries within the brain. The middle cerebral arteries branch from the internal carotid arteries transversing laterally through the Sylvain fissure. These arteries supply blood to the parietal and temporal lobes. *(Madden, 3rd ed., p. 22)*

138. **(B)** The external carotid arteries ascend the neck and pass through the parotid gland to the level of the temporalmandibular joint. The ECA bifurcates into terminal branches to supply blood to the face

and the neck. Their location in relationship to the internal carotid artery changes through its course. The ECA is lateral to the ICA at the level of C1, whereas it is medial to ICA at the vertebral levels of C3–C2. *(Kelly, 3rd ed., p. 300)*

139. **(A)** The anterior cerebral arteries are also branches of the internal carotid arteries running anterior into the interhemispheric fissure. These arteries are somewhat smaller in size than the middle cerebral arteries distributing blood to the frontal lobe and the medial part of the parietal lobe. *(Madden, 3rd ed., p. 22)*

140. **(C)**

$$number \, of \, detector \, rows = \frac{total \, beam \, collimation}{detector \, aperture \, size}$$

$$number \, of \, detector \, rows = \frac{153.6 \, mm}{1.2 \, mm}$$

$$number \, of \, detector \, rows = 128 \, rows$$

(Seeram, 3rd ed., pp. 272–274)

141. **(C)** A 4–5 cc/s is the protocol for PE studies. This fast injection rate with a short delay time will enable the contrast media to enhance the pulmonary arteries in order to depict a filling defect within the artery. *(Webb, p. 45)*

142. **(D)** The key characteristics of Cohn's disease include bowel wall thickening, submucosal edema with ulcerations involving a thickened segment of distal *ileum*. *(Grey, 2nd ed., p. 226; Webb, p. 331)*

143. **(C)** Ascites is the common term for the collection of serous fluid in the peritoneal cavity. Serous ascites has a CT attenuation value between −10 to a +15 HU and has the tendency to accumulate in the greater peritoneal space. Due to its isodensity, unenhanced CT studies will suffice. Ample bowel opacification aids in the detection of small amounts of fluid in the infracolic spaces. *(Webb, p. 176)*

144. **(A)** The arterial or bolus phase of injection is used to visualize hypervascular lesions such as hepatomas, carcinoid metastases, and focal nodular hyperplasia, mainly because these lesions are supplied by the hepatic artery. *(Webb, p. 211)*

145. **(C)** The purpose of collimation is to protect the patient by restricting the beam to the anatomy of interest. They are arranged to ensure a constant beam width at the detectors. Collimators affect patient dose and image quality by removing scatter radiation, which improves axial resolution. *(Seeram, 3rd ed., pp. 272–274)*

146. **(D)** Bronchogenic carcinoma will appear as an irregular shaped mass with speculated margins. CT is useful for radiation planning, radiotherapy, monitoring the response to chemotherapy, and the selection of patients for surgical resection. *(Prokop, p. 305)*

147. **(A)** The end result of the CT measurement is the CT number, calculated from the linear attenuation coefficient of the object, by scaling with the respective coefficient for pure water and given in HU. Using the scaling factor of water, it is safe to say, the accuracy of all CT numbers depends on the CT number for water in a homogeneous material; therefore, CT number is an important QA test. *(Kalendar, 3rd ed., p. 112)*

148. **(A)** The right atrium is the drainage point of the SVC and IVC, which pumps venous blood into the right ventricle via the tricuspid valve. The right atrium is located in the mediastinum slightly superior to the right ventricle. *(Madden, 3rd ed., p. 238)*

149. **(D)** The large gaps in detector measurements created by metal edges are amplified by the filter in filter back projection; therefore, interpolation techniques are used to substitute for the over range values in the attenuation profile. The metal objects are usually considered opaque and the data corresponding to the rays through the metal objects are defined as missing data. The inaccurate metal data are then replaced with forward projected values. *(Boas, 2012)*

150. **(A)** Hypervascular tumors have a good blood supply causing enhancement of the tumor as compared with the adjacent parenchyma and appear as a focus with transient hyperattenuation during the arterial or the bolus phase of injection. *(Prokop, p. 206)*

151. **(C)** Extravasation is the accidental administration of intravenous contrast media into the extravascular space/tissue around the infusion site by an indirect or direct leakage. Extravasation of contrast media produces an acute local inflammatory

response usually within 24 to 48 hours following the accident. A vast majority of patients in whom extravasations occur recover without any significant injury. Only rarely will a low-osmolality contrast media extravasation injury proceed to a severe adverse event, but special care should be taken to avoid such an event. *(The American College of Radiology Manual, p. 17)*

152. **(B)** The smaller the pixels the better the spatial resolution. Small pixels are produced with a combination of a small FOV and a large matrix with the assumption that the entire area of interest is covered. Pixel size is related to the matrix and the FOV by the following equation:

$$pixel\ size = \frac{FOV}{matrix}$$

When calculating the pixels size from each of the choices in question 152, the results are as follows:

$a = 0.39\ mm$, $b = 0.19\ mm$, $c = 0.29\ mm$, $d = 0.97\ mm$

Therefore; the FOV of 100 mm and the matrix size of 512^2 produced the smallest pixels, producing the best spatial resolution.

(Seeram, 3rd ed., p. 193)

153. **(A)** Pulmonary edema has two mechanical processes, an elevation of pulmonary venous pressure or an increased permeability of the alveolar capillary membrane. As the edema manifest, fluid leaks into the alveolar airspaces from the interstitium tissue. *(Prokop, pp. 341–343)*

154. **(A)** Exposure is a measure of the strength of a radiation field at some point in air. This is the measure made by a survey meter. The most commonly used unit of exposure is the roentgen (R). *(Seeram, 3rd ed., pp. 219–220)*

155. **(B)** The dynamic range is the ratio of the largest signal to be measured to the precision of the smallest signal to be discriminated. In other words, it can be described as the range of voltage or input signals that result in a digital output. The dynamic range for many modern CT scanners today is a million to one (1,000,000:1). *(Seeram, 3rd ed., p. 123)*

156. **(A)** The seminal vesicles are located superior to the prostate gland and bladder and anterior to the

rectum found on either side of the ductus deferens. *(Madden, 3rd ed., p. 396)*

157. **(B)** Contrast and noise have a direct relationship. Noise can be defined as the unwanted fluctuation of pixel values in an image of a homogeneous material. The LCD definition concludes that the visibility of an object depends not only on the size of the object, but on its contrast to the background; therefore, this visibility is highly dependent by the presence of noise. *(Seeram, 3rd ed., p. 197)*

158. **(B)** The myometrium is the middle muscular layer, highly vascular and the thickest lining of the uterus. Its muscular function is to contract during childbirth forcing the baby through the vaginal canal. *(Kelley, 3rd ed., p. 526)*

159. **(D)** Angiomyolipomas are common benign renal tumors composed of blood vessels, smooth muscle, and fat. The detection of fat within these renal masses confirms their diagnosis and distinguishes them from renal cell carcinoma. *(Grey, 2nd ed., pp. 286–287)*

160. **(D)** The data acquisition system's main functions are to measure the transmitted radiation beam, encode these measurements into binary data, and lastly to transmit the binary data to the computer. Each detectors photodiode measures the transmitted beam from the patient and converts them into electrical energy. The energy is proportional to the light striking the diode. At this point, the electrical energy is so weak that it must be amplified by the preamplifier before it can be analyzed further. The transmission measurement data must then be transformed into attenuation and thickness data through a process known as the logarithmic conversion. Following the conversion, the data are sent to the ADC. The purpose of the ADC is to divide the electrical signal into multiple parts, the more divisional parts, the greater the accuracy. The parts are measured into bits, 1-bit divides the signal into two digital values. The ADC's dynamic range must be large to preserve the large dynamic range of the x-ray image. Converters with 16-bit resolution or greater are common in CT. These values determine the gray-scale resolution of the image. The final stage of DAS is transmission of the data to the computer. The output of the ADC data are routed to an image signal processor over a high-speed optoelectronics by the use of lens and light diodes to facilitate data transmission for further signal processing and image reconstruction. *(Seeram, 3rd ed., pp. 128–129)*

161. **(B)** The blood supply to the pancreas is completely arterial in nature; therefore, the attenuation of the parenchyma rises faster than the liver, but lasts for a shorter time because of the absence of the portal phase. Peak enhancement occurs 5 seconds after the aortic plateau. *(Prokop, pp. 518–519)*

162. **(B)** There is subjective evidence that severe adverse reactions to contrast media or to procedures can be alleviated to some extent by reducing anxiety. It may be beneficial to determine whether a patient is particularly anxious and to reassure and calm that patient before contrast injection. *(The American College of Radiology Manual, p. 6)*

163. **(D)** The pixel size is determined by the following mathematical equation:

$$pixel\ size = \frac{FOV}{matrix}$$

Once the individual pixel size is determined in the x-axis, the pixel area can be calculated by squaring the determined size.

$$pixel\ area^2 = x\text{-}axis \times y\text{-}axis$$

164. **(C)** The scaphoid bone is the largest carpal bone in the wrist located in the proximal row. It is the only bone that articulates with the radius and is a frequent site for fracture due to a force from a fall. *(Madden, 3rd ed., p. 545)*

165. **(B)** The aliasing artifact can occur if the appropriate number of samples is not achieved during data acquisition. It appears in the final image as fine streaks and web-like patterns. *(Kalendar 3rd ed., 350)*

Subspecialty List

40. Patient Care and Safety — Radiation safety and Dosimetry — Pitch
41. Imaging Procedures — Anatomy — Brain Vascular
42. Patient Care and Safety — Patient Assessment and Preparation — Level of Consciousness
43. Imaging Procedures — Pathology — Spine
44. Physics and Instrumentation — Radiation Physics — Acquisition (Geometry)
45. Imaging Procedures — Anatomy — Cranial Nerves
46. Patient Care and Safety — Radiation safety and Dosimetry — Patient Dose Reductions
47. Physics and Instrumentation — CT System Principles, Operations, and Components — Detector Configuration
48. Imaging Procedures — Anatomy — Kidney/Ureters
49. Patient Care and Safety — Patient Assessment and Preparation — Consent
50. Imaging Procedures — Pathology — Chest
51. Imaging Procedures — Pathology — Colorectal
52. Patient Care and Safety — Contrast Administration — Adverse Reactions — Recognition and assessment
53. Imaging Procedures — Procedures — Kidney
54. Imaging Procedures — Anatomy — Pituitary Gland
55. Contrast Administration — Venipuncture — Documentation
56. Imaging Procedures — Anatomy—Colorectal
57. Physics and Instrumentation — Informatics Networking
58. Patient Care and Safety — Contrast Administration — Contrast Media—Dialysis
59. Physics and Instrumentation — CT System Principles, Operations, and Components — Detector Configuration
60. Imaging Procedures — Anatomy — Spine
61. Physics and Instrumentation — Artifacts Recognition and Reduction — Partial Volume Averaging
62. Patient Care and Safety — Patient Assessment and Preparation — Immobilization
63. Physics and Instrumentation — Image Reconstruction — Interpolation
64. Imaging Procedures — Pathology — Chest
65. Patient Care and Safety — Radiation safety and Dosimetry — Dose Modulation Techniques
66. Imaging Procedures — Anatomy — Biliary
67. Imaging Procedures — Anatomy — Chest Vascular
68. Imaging Procedures — Anatomy — Liver
69. Physics and Instrumentation — Informatics Archive
70. Patient Care and Safety — Contrast Administration — Adverse Reaction — Recognition and Assessment
71. Imaging Procedures — Pathology — Chest
72. Imaging Procedures — Pathology — Spine
73. Patient Care and Safety — Radiation Safety and Dosimetry — Iterative Reconstruction
74. Imaging Procedures — Anatomy — Brain
75. Imaging Procedures — Anatomy — Lower Extremity
76. Patient Care and Safety — Contrast Administration — Administration Routes and Dose Calculations — Intrathecal
77. Physics and Instrumentation — CT System Principles, Operations, and Components — Detector Configuration
78. Imaging Procedures — Anatomy — Abdomen Vascular
79. Physics and Instrumentation — Image Display — Windowing
80. Patient Care and Safety — Patient Assessment and Preparation — Vital Signs
81. Imaging Procedures — Pathology — Kidney Vascular
82. Physics and Instrumentation — Radiation Physics — Physical Principles (attenuation)
83. Patient Care and Safety — Contrast Administration — Special Contrast Considerations — Contraindications
84. Imaging Procedures — Anatomy: Chest Muscles
85. Physics and Instrumentation — Image Reconstruction — Iterative Reconstruction
86. Imaging Procedures — Anatomy — GI Tract
87. Patient Care and Safety — Contrast Administration — Contrast Media — Ionic Contrast
88. Patient Care and Safety — Radiation safety and Dosimetry — Dose Measurement
89. Imaging Procedures — Pathology — Reproductive Organs
90. Physics and Instrumentation — Image Display — Field of View
91. Imaging Procedures — Anatomy — Abdominal Vascular
92. Physics and Instrumentation — Artifacts Recognition and Reduction — Edge Gradient
93. Patient Care and Safety — Contrast Administration — Administration Route and Dose Calculations — IV
94. Physics and Instrumentation — CT System Principles, Operations, and Components — Tube

95. Imaging Procedures — Pathology — Lower Extremity
96. Imaging Procedures — Pathology — Abdomen
97. Imaging Procedures — Anatomy — Chest
98. Physics and Instrumentation — Image Display — Cine
99. Patient Care and Safety — Contrast Administration — Injection Techniques — Power Injector
100. Patient Care and Safety — Radiation safety and Dosimetry — Patient Dose Reduction and Optimization
101. Physics and Instrumentation — Image Display — Windowing
102. Imaging Procedures — Anatomy — Biliary
103. Imaging Procedures — Anatomy — Lower Extremity
104. Patient Care and Safety — Contrast Administration — Venipuncture—Aseptic and Sterile Technique
105. Physics and Instrumentation — Image Quality — CT number
106. Physics and Instrumentation — Image Display Windowing
107. Imaging Procedures — Anatomy — Neck Vascular
108. Imaging Procedures — Anatomy — Larynx
109. Imaging Procedures — Anatomy — Soft Tissue
110. Patient Care and Safety — Radiation safety and Dosimetry — Patient Dose Reduction and Optimization
111. Physics and Instrumentation — CT System Principles, Operations, and Components — Data Acquisition System
112. Imaging Procedures — Pathology — Lower Extremity
113. Physics and Instrumentation — Image Display — Field of View
114. Imaging Procedures — Pathology — Adrenal
115. Imaging Procedures — Anatomy — Heart
116. Imaging Procedures — Anatomy — Chest Vascular
117. Imaging Procedures — Anatomy — Heart
118. Physics and Instrumentation — CT System Principles, Operations, and Components — Computer and Array Processor
119. Physics and Instrumentation — Image Reconstruction — Interpolation
120. Patient Care and Safety — Radiation safety and Dosimetry — Dose Measurement
121. Patient Care and Safety — Contrast Administration — Contrast Media — Air
122. Imaging Procedures — Anatomy — Chest Muscles
123. Physics and Instrumentation — Artifacts Recognition and Reduction — Motion Artifact
124. Imaging Procedures — Anatomy — Kidney
125. Physics and Instrumentation — Image Display — Voxel
126. Imaging Procedures — Pathology — Kidney
127. Physics and Instrumentation — Image Display — Magnification
128. Physics and Instrumentation — Radiation Physics — Physical Principles (attenuation)
129. Imaging Procedures — Pathology — Abdomen
130. Imaging Procedures — Pathology — Liver
131. Physics and Instrumentation — Image Quality — QA
132. Imaging Procedures — Pathology — Chest
133. Physics and Instrumentation — Image Display — Matrix
134. Imaging Procedures — Pathology — Lower Extremity
135. Patient Care and Safety — Contrast Administration — Administration Routes and Dose Calculations — Oral
136. Physics and Instrumentation — Image Reconstruction — Raw data versus image data
137. Imaging Procedures — Anatomy — Brain Vascular
138. Imaging Procedures — Anatomy — Neck Vascular
139. Imaging Procedures — Anatomy — Brain Vascular
140. Physics and Instrumentation — CT System Principles, Operations, and Components — Collimation/Beam Width
141. Imaging Procedures — Procedures — Chest Vascular
142. Imaging Procedures — Pathology — Abdomen
143. Imaging Procedures — Pathology — Abdomen
144. Imaging Procedures — Pathology — Liver
145. Physics and Instrumentation — CT System Principles, Operations, and Components — Collimation/Beam Width
146. Imaging Procedures — Pathology — Chest
147. Physics and Instrumentation — Image Quality — Uniformity
148. Imaging Procedures — Anatomy — Heart
149. Physics and Instrumentation — Artifacts Recognition and Reduction — Metal Artifact
150. Imaging Procedures — Pathology — Abdomen

151. Patient Care and Safety — Contrast Administration — Adverse Reactions — Recognition and Assessment

152. Physics and Instrumentation — Image Quality Spatial Resolution

153. Imaging Procedures — Pathology — Chest

154. Patient Care and Safety — Radiation safety and Dosimetry — Dose Measurement

155. Physics and Instrumentation — CT System Principles, Operations, and Components — Detector Configuration

156. Imaging Procedures — Anatomy — Pelvis

157. Physics and Instrumentation — Image Quality — Contrast Resolution

158. Imaging Procedures — Anatomy — Pelvis

159. Imaging Procedures — Pathology — Kidney

160. Physics and Instrumentation — CT System Principles, Operations, and Components — Data Acquisition System

161. Imaging Procedures — Procedures — Pancreas

162. Patient Care and Safety — Contrast Administration — Adverse Reactions — Recognition and Assessment

163. Physics and Instrumentation — Image Display — Pixel

164. Imaging Procedures — Anatomy — Upper Extremity

165. Physics and Instrumentation — CT System Principles, Operations, and Components — Detector Configuration

Index

Note: Page numbers followed by f indicate figures.

To access your complimentary online practice exam, visit www.MHEAlliedHealth.com.

CPSIA information can be obtained
at www.ICGtesting.com
Printed in the USA
JSHW032021201122
33402JS00003B/115